BEYOND MEDICARE FOR ALL

Cracking the Code of the Healthcare Affordability Crisis

BY KEN TERRY

Foreword by David W. Johnson

AAPL

978-1-960762-61-0 print
978-1-960762-62-7 eBook

Published by **American Association for Physician Leadership, Inc.**
PO Box 96503 | BMB 97493 | Washington, DC 20090-6503

Website: www.physicianleaders.org

13 8 7 6 5 4 3 2 1

Copyedited, typeset, indexed, and printed in the United States of America

PUBLISHER
Nancy Collins

PRODUCTION MANAGER
Jennifer Weiss

DESIGN & LAYOUT
Carter Publishing Studio

COPYEDITOR
Hannah Irish

Dedication

To my children, Selene, Alycia, Adam and Justin, and my grandchildren. This book is about their future.

Acknowledgments

In this book — my third and final effort to chart a new course for U.S. healthcare — I stand on the shoulders of many people who educated and guided me through my journey over the past 30 years. The first of these guides was Steve Murata, the editor of *Medical Economics Magazine*, who threw the hardest stories at me and with whom I had long conversations about health policy. Healthcare consultant Jacques Sokolov taught me the fundamentals of managed care back in the 1990s. Another consultant, Mike LaPenna, has been a fount of hard-won practical knowledge about the business of medicine from A to Z.

I've learned much from a group of health policy experts in my interviews with them and in their writings. Paul Ginsburg, former chair of the Medicare Payment Advisory Commission and a professor at the University of Southern California, gave me a high-level view of the trends that shape U.S. health costs and government policy, and he wrote the foreword to my first book. Donald Berwick, MD, former president and CEO of the Healthcare Improvement Institute (IHI) and a former Administrator of the Centers for Medicare and Medicaid Services (CMS), has been a courageous and profoundly moral voice promoting patient safety, and he helped devise the Triple Aim that is the cornerstone of value-based care. IHI's idealized primary care practice model in the early 2000s showed me how the basic elements of practice could be improved. Robert Berenson, MD, another former CMS official and a senior fellow at the Urban Institute, has been an unfailing reality check on many of the health policy ideas circulating in the field, from value-based care to global hospital budgeting. David Eddy, MD, is a healthcare analyst and expert on clinical guidelines who influenced me with his thinking on medical necessity and what is required to control the diffusion of new medical technologies. And David B. Nash, MD, who wrote the foreword to my second book, has been a great source of knowledge on the disease management and population health management trends. Nash is the founding dean emeritus and a professor of health policy at the Jefferson College of

Population Health and the author of many books and hundreds of articles.

In the course of writing for *Medical Economics* and, later, for other healthcare publications, I also interviewed many physicians who imparted their perspectives on healthcare issues at the frontline level. Robert Kagan, MD, a Connecticut internist, has been especially helpful in this respect. I've cited his insights on everything from being a nursing home consultant to the pitfalls of certain medical devices to the reasons for selling his practice to a hospital. Similarly, I prize the conversations I've had with Kenneth Kubitschek, MD, another internist and the coleader of a medium-sized practice in Asheville, North Carolina. I've found his stories about some of his patients particularly revealing and insightful. Jeffrey Pearson, DO, of San Marcos, California, has been a superb source for what is going on in the home state of managed care. I especially appreciated his frank account of his unhappy odyssey as an employed physician and his decision to return to private practice.

This book's chapter on rural healthcare — a topic I had never researched before in depth — benefited from my interviews with rural physicians and experts in the field. I want to thank Jack Westfall, MD, who works for a critical access hospital in Yuma, Colorado; Michael Tuggy, a family physician in rural Washington; and Harold Miller, president and CEO of the Center for Healthcare Quality and Payment Reform.

My editor, Nancy Collins, has been a warm and supportive presence throughout the writing of this book and its predecessor. She deserves many thanks for believing in me and the importance of my message.

None of my books would have been possible without the support I've received from my wife Lisa from the very beginning. Lisa understood why I was writing about healthcare reform and what I hoped to achieve. Thank you, Lisa, from the bottom of my heart.

Table of Contents

About the Author

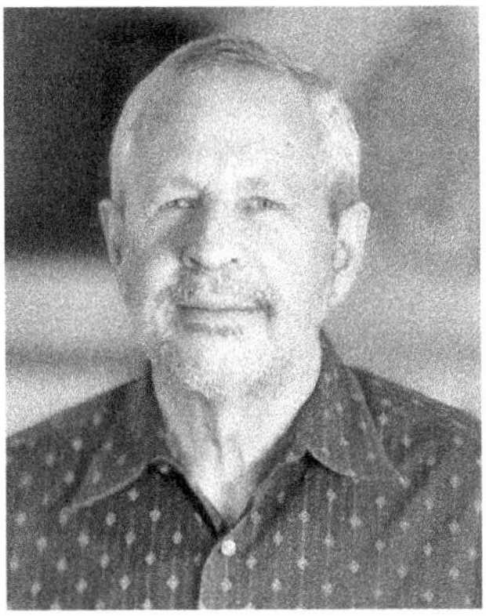

Ken Terry, the author of two previous books on healthcare reform, has been writing about the healthcare field for more than 30 years. As a senior editor at *Medical Economics* from 1993-2007, he covered many aspects of medical practice and the healthcare business, including managed care and information technology. In 2008, Terry began freelancing for such publications as Medscape Medical News, WebMD, cio.com, InformationWeek, and Fierce Healthcare.

Terry's first book, *Rx for Health Care Reform* (Vanderbilt University Press, 2007), won acclaim from several health policy experts and a favorable review in the *Journal of the American Medical Association.* Joseph E. Scherger, MD, then a professor at the University of California, San Diego, called the book "just the kind of bold analysis needed today to put reason and common sense back into health policy."

The American Association for Physician Leadership in 2020 published Terry's second book, *Physician-Led Healthcare Reform: A New Approach to Medicare For All.* Tom Bodenheimer, MD, MPH, founding director of the Center for Excellence in Primary Care, said this book "offers an encyclopedia of knowledge on the U.S. healthcare system, written in an engaging, popular style."

Terry also helped write Stephen K. Klasko's 2023 book, *Feelin' Alright: How the Message in The Music Can Make Healthcare Healthier*. In addition, he contributed to a 2016 book about population health management by several executives of IBM Watson Health.

Terry recalls how his baptism by fire at *Medical Economics* ignited his interest in fixing the healthcare system. When a friend got him hired at the magazine, the editor at the time, Steve Murata, was unconvinced he could do the job. So Murata threw at him the hardest, gnarliest assignments he could think of, including pieces on how preventive care and medical advances raise health costs. Terry survived and thrived, and this book presents everything he has learned about healthcare since then.

Foreword

American healthcare rarely changes quickly. For decades, the system has absorbed criticism, reform attempts, political battles, and economic shocks. Each time, the structure bends but does not break. Costs rise. Complexity deepens. Access remains uneven. Yet the underlying architecture stays largely intact.

Until it doesn't. Ernest Hemingway famously described bankruptcy as occurring "gradually and then suddenly." Healthcare transformations follow the same pattern. Systems weaken slowly. Pressures accumulate. Then the tipping point arrives. American healthcare is approaching this moment.

Ken Terry's book begins with a blunt assessment: The United States healthcare system is experiencing structural failure. Costs continue to outpace wages and economic growth. Employers struggle to provide coverage. Government programs strain under long-term fiscal pressure. Patients increasingly delay care because they cannot afford it.

Parts of the system in low-income urban and rural communities are already collapsing. Increasingly, middle-class Americans are struggling to cover their medical costs. Concurrently, the forces driving change are growing stronger.

In our recent book, *The Coming Healthcare Revolution: 10 Forces That Will Cure America's Health Crisis*, Paul Kusserow and I describe 10 macro and market forces that are pushing American healthcare toward inevitable transformation. Together, these forces are reshaping healthcare faster than many incumbents realize.

Ken Terry's work fits squarely within this emerging conversation. His analysis tackles a central question confronting healthcare reformers today: Who should control the incentives that drive healthcare? His answer is equally clear: physicians.

HEALTHCARE'S INCENTIVE PROBLEM

American healthcare does not lack expertise, technology, or clinical talent. It suffers from misaligned incentives as these bedrock features of U.S. healthcare illustrate:

- Hospitals make money when beds are full.
- Specialists are paid more than primary care physicians.
- Insurers earn profits by managing risk rather than improving health.
- Investors search for financial returns inside a $5 trillion healthcare economy independently of whether their investments create value.

Each of the above participants behaves rationally within healthcare's financial incentive structures. Unfortunately, the whole is less than the sum of its parts. The structure itself produces expensive and fragmented care.

The results of this dysfunctional incentive structure are visible for all to see. Healthcare spending approaches one-fifth of the U.S. economy. Yet Americans experience shorter life expectancy, higher rates of chronic illness, and greater barriers to care than people in other advanced nations. The system generates extraordinary medical innovation but struggles to deliver affordable, coordinated care.

The U.S. system excels at rescuing people when they're drowning but never teaches them to swim. This paradox defines American healthcare. Our nation possesses the world's most sophisticated medical capabilities and one of the least efficient healthcare delivery systems.

A Transformative Idea

Ken Terry proposes a different path. His argument is simple but disruptive: Physicians — particularly primary care physicians — should regain control over healthcare delivery and assume responsibility for managing the financial resources associated with patient care.

This proposal goes beyond traditional calls for physician leadership. Terry argues that physicians must assume greater financial accountability for the care they deliver. In effect, physicians would function as stewards of healthcare resources, responsible for managing both clinical decisions and cost outcomes.

For decades, physicians have operated primarily within fee-for-service reimbursement systems that reward volume rather than value. Hospitals and insurers have absorbed most financial risk. Physicians have focused on delivering individual services rather than managing population health.

Terry proposes reversing that dynamic. Under his model, physician-led organizations — especially those centered on primary care — would coordinate care, manage budgets, and accept financial responsibility for outcomes.

Terry's goal is straightforward: align incentives so that physicians succeed financially when patients become healthier, safer, and better served.

Physicians sit at the operational center of healthcare. They diagnose disease, order tests, prescribe treatments, and coordinate referrals. Their decisions trigger the majority of healthcare spending. No group understands clinical workflows better.

Primary care physicians, in particular, occupy a critical position. They see patients early in the course of illness. They manage chronic disease. They determine when specialty care is necessary and when preventive interventions can avoid more expensive treatment later.

Strong primary care systems consistently produce better outcomes at lower cost. Yet the American healthcare economy undervalues primary care. Only a small portion of healthcare spending flows to primary care services. The system's imbalance between pro-health expenditures and treatment-focused expenditures is breathtaking.

Terry's restructuring model attempts to correct that imbalance. By shifting responsibility and financial authority toward physician-led organizations, the system could reward prevention, care coordination, and population health management.

Done correctly, such a shift could reduce unnecessary utilization, improve patient outcomes, and stabilize healthcare spending. In theory, physician stewardship could create a more rational healthcare economy.

The Risks

Theory is not reality. Transferring financial risk to physicians carries substantial challenges.

Most physicians are trained as clinicians, not financial managers. Running risk-bearing healthcare organizations require expertise in actuarial analysis, capital management, and population health analytics. Many physicians understandably prefer to focus on patient care rather than corporate operations.

Scale also matters. Healthcare risk pools work best when they cover large populations. Small physician groups may struggle to absorb the financial volatility associated with expensive medical cases. Without adequate infrastructure and capital reserves, physician-led organizations could face financial instability.

There are ethical considerations as well. Physicians must always place patients' interests first. If physicians assume financial risk for the cost of care, conflicts could arise between financial stewardship and clinical decision-making. The perception of such conflicts could erode trust between physicians and patients.

Healthcare reform must tread carefully here. Aligning incentives is essential. Undermining clinical integrity would be disastrous. A refinement of Terry's proposal might be requiring all hospitals and health systems to divest or separate their primary care personnel from their organizations. Health and healthcare are not synonymous. As the system does a better job of health promotion, preventive care, and disease management (primary care's core elements), there will be less need for expansive acute care treatment.

A Necessary Conversation

Ken Terry's book does not offer easy solutions, but it nails the essential dilemmas confounding the policy debate for how best to reform America's broken healthcare system. As such, Terry challenges readers to reconsider fundamental assumptions about how healthcare should operate. His proposal to shift greater financial responsibility to physicians raises important questions about incentives, governance, and professional responsibility.

Some readers will find his ideas compelling. Others will view them as impractical or risky. Both reactions are valuable. Healthcare reform requires open debate about new models and alternative approaches. The stakes are too high for complacency.

The coming decade will determine whether the United States can build a healthcare system that delivers better outcomes at sustainable cost. The forces driving change are already in motion. Demographic pressures will intensify. Technology will accelerate care redesign. Consumers will demand greater transparency and value. Financial constraints will force difficult decisions.

Healthcare transformation is not optional. It is inevitable.

Ken Terry's contribution pushes the reform conversation forward. By exploring the possibility of physician-centered restructuring, he invites us to rethink the incentives that govern healthcare delivery.

Whether his model ultimately proves correct is less important than the dialogue it sparks. Healthcare's future belongs to organizations capable of aligning clinical excellence, financial discipline, and patient trust. Achieving that alignment is the central challenge of our time.

Ken Terry offers an intriguing path toward achieving that goal. The conversation he begins could not come at a more critical time.

David W. Johnson
CEO
4sight Health

Introduction

THE RUNAWAY TRAIN OF HEALTH COSTS

The longest federal government shutdown in history was mainly about healthcare. In fall 2025, Democratic Senators refused to fund the government until their Republican colleagues agreed to extend enhanced subsidies for Affordable Care Act (ACA) health plans that were due to expire at the end of the year. Large majorities of voters in both parties supported their demand. Yet the Republicans in the Senate refused to renew the tax credits that made insurance affordable for 22 million people on Obamacare plans.[1] In the end, the government reopened, and Republicans in both Houses of Congress continued to block the renewal of the subsidies. As a result, premium costs more than doubled for people on these plans, and about 4 million of them are expected to lose their health insurance.[2]

What this charade revealed, once again, is the failure of America's political class to come to terms with the reality of out-of-control health costs. The ACA, passed in 2010, was the most serious effort to tackle the problem since the passage of Medicare and Medicaid in the 1960s. Yet that legislation was a compromise that did not address the root causes of healthcare inflation. That's why its subsidies were insufficient to make Obamacare plans affordable even before the COVID-19 pandemic, and it's why enhanced subsidies are still necessary.

However, Republican attacks on Obamacare ring hollow, because the GOP has never had a real plan to bring down healthcare inflation. Republicans recently proposed a smorgasbord of strategies, including health savings accounts, association plans and high-risk pools. Over the years, all these ideas have proved to be dead ends.

The Trump Administration has also proposed to allow the sale on the ACA marketplace of "skinny" plans with out-of-pocket costs of up to $27,000 per year for family coverage and $15,600 a year for individual plans. Such insurance costs less than current ACA plans but provides no coverage below the catastrophic level.[3]

The proposals from the other side of the aisle have not been much better. The Democratic bills at the end of 2025 would have retained the enhanced subsidies for three more years with no changes in Obamacare. More broadly, the mainstream Democratic position has been to build on the ACA rather than replace it. On the far left, Medicare for All bills have been reintroduced every year for the past decade without any chance of passage.

So, at a time when healthcare is unaffordable for a growing number of Americans, the country's political parties are simply not addressing the core problem: Our profit-driven healthcare system is not designed to deliver affordable, high-quality care for all. To change that, we'd have to change the incentives of the major healthcare players.

Long History of Failure

Repeatedly over the past half century, American politicians have deplored the high level of healthcare costs and vowed to do something about it. This was the case when President Richard Nixon embraced HMOs in 1973 as an alternative to the Democrats' Medicare for All. At that time, healthcare spending comprised 7.7% of GDP. In 1993, when President Bill Clinton bowed the Clinton Health Care Plan, healthcare expenditures were 13.9% of GDP. And in 2009, when newly elected President Barack Obama warned that, unless we controlled healthcare spending, it would swallow the federal budget, the United States spent 17.6% of its GDP on healthcare.

In the decade after the Affordable Care Act (ACA) was implemented, the percentage of our national output devoted to healthcare remained at around that same level, except during the pandemic years of 2020-2021.[4] A number of explanations have been advanced for the flattening of health cost growth relative to GDP, including declining utilization, lower private hospital and physician prices, declining home health use, slower growth in insurers' administrative costs, and the law's promotion of value-based care.[5-6] But, in 2024, healthcare spending was projected to rise 8.2% to $5.26 trillion. While that still represented only 18% of GDP, the actuaries of the Centers for Medicare and Medicaid Services (CMS) predicted that national health expenditures would climb to $8.58 trillion, or 20.3% of national output, in 2033.[7]

Of course, this metric fails to show the unaffordability of healthcare for the average consumer. National health spending increased from $2.2 trillion in 2000 to nearly $4.9 trillion in 2023, after adjusting for inflation, and then soared to $5.3 trillion in 2024 — a huge jump in less than a quarter century.[8-9] Regardless of what percentage of the economy that is, it's a huge burden on consumers and taxpayers. Nevertheless, the relative stability of the healthcare spending-to-GDP ratio begs the question, how bad is the healthcare crisis?

The answer is that it's very bad and is careening toward catastrophe. Take employer-sponsored insurance (ESI), which covers roughly half of Americans. In 2025, according to a Kaiser Family Foundation report, the cost of family coverage under ESI leaped 6% to reach an average of $26,993 annually. While employers contributed an average of $20,143 for a family policy, employees paid $6,850, or $571 a month. For single coverage, employees paid $1,440 per year in insurance premiums.[10]

Over the past 25 years, the cost of employer-provided family health insurance has grown more than three times faster than workers' earnings[11] And, even as employees have paid much more for coverage, their out-of-pocket expenses in the form of deductibles, copayments and other forms of cost sharing have increased substantially.[12]

Unsurprisingly, about half of U.S. adults in a Kaiser survey said it was difficult to afford healthcare, and one in four said they or a family member had had problems paying for healthcare in the past 12 months. The high cost of care led one in four adults to skip or postpone needed care because of the cost, including 60% of uninsured people.[13] But bear in mind that most of the people who had trouble paying medical bills *were insured.*

About one in four adults reported that they had medical debts. And three in four people said they were worried about being able to afford unexpected medical bills or the cost of healthcare services. About half of the respondents said they'd be unable to pay an unexpected medical bill of $500 without going into debt.[14] The situation got so bad that, in January 2025, the Consumer Financial Protection Bureau (CFPB) promulgated a rule excluding medical debt from people's credit ratings. Unfortunately, a federal court later blocked that rule with the consent of the shrunken, Trump-controlled CFPB.[15]

Looking inside the latest ESI numbers, it's evident that some employers are paying a very high percentage of their payroll for health insurance. For example, if they pay a worker $60,000 a year, they're contributing about a third more than that for family coverage, on average. The go-to solution in the past was to increase cost sharing. For example, the portion of workers who had single coverage with a deductible of $2,000 or more jumped from 18% in 2014 to 34% in 2025.[16] But companies may be reaching the limit of how much they can pile on employees when half of their workers are having trouble affording care.

Most large employers are still offering health coverage. But smaller employers are rapidly shedding health insurance for their workers, according to the Employee Benefit Research Institute (EBRI). Less than half of small firms now offer insurance, a Commonwealth Fund report notes. Workers at small firms pay a higher percentage of premiums and have higher deductibles than those in big companies.[17-18]

Also, let's not forget the millions of people who don't get their health insurance through their employers. Many of them are on Medicaid, and many more have subsidized plans purchased on the ACA marketplaces. As a result of Obamacare, which prompted the Medicaid expansion that now encompasses most states, the uninsured rate in the United States sank from 16% in 2010, when the ACA was passed, to 8.2%, or about 27 million people, in the first quarter of 2024.[19]

Because of Trump Administration policies, however, the uninsured rate is expected to soar again. Under the One Big Beautiful Bill Act (OBBBA), which the Republican-controlled Congress passed in 2025, about 10 million people are expected to lose their Medicaid coverage, starting in 2027. Moreover, because Congress failed to address the expiration of ACA subsidies, as noted above, several million people will no longer be able to afford health insurance.[20]

Primary Care Shortage

Even people who can afford healthcare don't necessarily get what they pay for in this country. Healthcare spending per capita is much higher here than in other advanced countries, yet U.S. health outcomes are far worse than in those peer nations. Compared to them, our country has the lowest life expectancy at birth, the highest death rates for avoidable or treatable conditions, the highest maternal and infant mortality, and among the highest suicide rates. We also have the highest rate of people with multiple chronic conditions, and our obesity rate is nearly twice that in peer countries.[21]

Americans see physicians less often than do people in other advanced nations, and we have among the lowest rates of practicing physicians and hospital beds per 1,000 residents.[22] This is not the only reason for our poor outcomes, although the paucity of doctors and hospitals has certainly hurt healthcare in rural and inner-city areas. But the shortage of primary care physicians (PCPs) in the United States explains much of what's wrong with our system.

Just six years ago, when my book *Physician-Led Healthcare Reform: A New Approach to Medicare For All* was published, around a third of practicing U.S. physicians were in primary care. Now, in the wake of post-COVID retirements and with a dwindling share of medical students going into the field, only about a quarter of American doctors are delivering primary care.[23] Many studies have shown that primary care is fundamental to a sound healthcare system and that people have better health outcomes when more primary care doctors are available. The cratering of our primary care workforce is a clear and present danger to U.S. healthcare.

The number of nurse practitioners — many of whom work in primary care offices — has grown quickly in recent years. Just from 2022 to 2023, the number of NPs in the workforce increased by 8.5% to 385,000.[24] It is now common for PCPs to work with NPs or physician assistants. But, because the training of NPs is much shorter and less comprehensive than that of doctors, they can't do everything that a PCP can do. And, despite their growing numbers, it still takes a long time to get an appointment with a primary care provider.[25]

The Signs of an Impending Collapse

Looking at all the negative trends in U.S. healthcare, the idea of a systemic collapse occurring sometime in the next few years is not crazy. Sure, it didn't happen all the other times that people said the sky was falling; but the combination of steeply higher prices, the growing inability of average people to pay for care, and the alarming decline in primary care provides some reason to think that we're approaching a cliff.

I'm not the only one who thinks so. The Healthcare Financial Management Association (HFMA), which represents chief financial officers of hospital systems, convened an expert task force to consider the future of healthcare. When they met in 2024, most of these "high-level industry stakeholders," an HFMA spokesman told me, concluded that the current healthcare system is "not sustainable."[26]

A similar position is taken by the Purchaser Business Group on Health (PBGH), a West Coast-based coalition of 40 large private employers and public purchasers. "The current system does not work for employers, families or most health care providers, and the industry has demonstrated it will not reform itself to deliver high-quality care at lower costs," said Elizabeth Mitchell, president and CEO of PBGH, in a report to the new Congress in 2025. Her statement called on Congress and President Trump "to curb anticompetitive practices and enable accountability."[27]

A 2021 survey conducted by the PBGH and the Kaiser Family Foundation (KFF) found despairing attitudes about healthcare among representatives of 302 companies with 5,000 or more employees. Eighty-seven percent of the respondents agreed that the cost of providing health benefits would become unsustainable at some point in the next five to ten years; about the same portion of employers believed that the government would need to take a greater role in providing healthcare coverage.[28]

When and if the healthcare crunch comes, will private insurance become unaffordable? Not for everyone, but the number who can afford it, even with their employer's help, will be much smaller than it is today. An Ernest Hemingway character famously said that his bankruptcy happened "gradually and then suddenly." The same will occur with health insurance unless we figure out how to rein in cost growth. Who will pay hospitals and physicians their high prices when coverage disappears for a large part of the population? Not enough people to keep many of them in business, providing all the services we need. So, we're looking at sharply reduced access to lower-quality, more expensive healthcare.

This is the future we face unless we make drastic changes in our healthcare system.

Consolidation and Competition

How did we get here? At a 20,000-foot level, we reached this sorry state because the United States is a capitalist, free-enterprise society where everything is a product with a market price. Other countries that have much better healthcare systems are also capitalist, but not everything is subject to market forces. To start with, other advanced countries guarantee universal coverage of all necessary healthcare services. Also, the amount of cost sharing with patients is much lower in those nations than it is here. Although their systems vary from one country to another, all of them are based on a philosophy of social solidarity that is notably lacking in the U.S.

This is not only a problem in our private sector. Government healthcare agencies like Medicare and Medicaid, which finance nearly half of U.S. healthcare, are also buckling. As health costs rise and Congress addresses rival demands such as tax cuts for the rich, Medicaid and ACA health plans are under political assault. The 2025 tax legislation will cut funding for Medicaid, the Children's Health Insurance Program (CHIP), and ACA coverage by $803 billion over 10 years.[29]

Meanwhile, more than half of Medicare beneficiaries now belong to private Medicare Advantage plans, which in 2024 cost the government $88 billion more than traditional Medicare would have cost for the same people.[30] With the aid of this counterproductive privatization, Medicare's Hospital Trust Fund is projected to become insolvent in 2036.[31]

The market orthodoxy holds that competition will keep prices down. But this claim is inoperative in healthcare. The three major industry players — hospitals, insurers and drug manufacturers — are so consolidated that a handful of organizations dominate most of the markets that each of these players is in. Meanwhile, hospitals, insurers and other corporate entities now employ nearly 80% of physicians, eliminating most competition in that profession as well. While negotiations between big health systems and big insurers sometimes fail, the health systems tend to win, because health plans can't do without them in their networks. So, it's not surprising that the average prices that private insurers pay hospitals now exceed 240% of Medicare rates.[32]

The Profit-Making Imperative

The public tends to blame insurance and drug companies more than healthcare providers for the high cost of care.[33] In a Kaiser poll conducted in late 2024, two-thirds of consumers said insurers deserve "a lot of blame for high healthcare costs."[34] In a recent survey, 55% of respondents said they were dissatisfied with their plans.[35] Insurers are routinely attacked as greedy and callous.

Insurance companies do make a lot of money, and their consolidation has enabled them to raise prices in some markets.[36] But, since the turn of the century, their aggregate profits have not increased as fast as hospital margins have.[37] It is the provision of healthcare, not the financing of it, that is the biggest source of health spending growth.

In a recent *Health Affairs* article, Donald Berwick, president emeritus and senior fellow of the Institute for Healthcare Improvement, and several other health policy experts blamed the profit motive for the inexorable rise in health spending.

> Drug companies, health insurers, and hospitals have harvested steadily increasing profits, yet millions of Americans struggle to access needed care and pay health care bills. Market failures persist. At the heart of the problem lies a misalignment of incentives,

> in which profit seeking far too often takes precedence over the quest for patients' well-being...
>
> To reorient a system from focusing on acute illness to prioritizing preventive services and lifelong optimal health, policy makers will have to take on corporate health care interests heavily vested in the profits available in the status quo. Powerful interests make a lot of money in the failing US system. Financial incentives need to be realigned to focus on the goal of health for individual patients and populations.[38]

As Berwick *et al.* point out, policy makers have proposed and the government has implemented a number of patchwork solutions "to improve the public-private healthcare system without requiring too much government oversight. That has not worked; instead, it has stranded the system in a muddled middle ground, where neither solution is well executed."

The most extensive program of this kind, the Affordable Care Act, sharply reduced the number of uninsured, but it failed to make healthcare affordable or improve the quality of care. Medicare For All, which briefly looked like a politically feasible alternative in the runup to the 2020 election, was dead on arrival. The "public option," a public health plan that would have cost less than private plans, was dropped from the ACA. While it has been tried by a few states and is favored by the Berwick-led group of experts, there is no political appetite for it at present. Insurers oppose it because they believe it would lead to Medicare for All.

Criteria for a New System

What is abundantly clear is that, for any healthcare reform proposal to gain traction, it will have to give the dominant industry players a way to remain in business and be profitable, even if their enterprises are not as lucrative as they are today. At the same time, the industry must be largely restructured to have any chance of curbing costs. And the financial incentives for healthcare providers must be changed so that they earn money from health and reduced disability rather than from sickness.

It's also clear that physicians must run the system. Physicians are the only ones who know where the waste is in healthcare and how to eliminate it safely. And, unlike hospitals, insurers or drug companies, their first duty is to their patients. So, they should be the stewards of our scarce healthcare resources.

Primary care physicians, who are the furthest upstream from the expensive services provided by specialists, hospitals, and post-acute-care providers, should direct and take financial responsibility for most ambulatory care. Their worth is becoming more widely recognized as the value-based care movement gathers steam (see Chapter 3). But so far, that recognition has not been accompanied by a commensurate rise in their compensation. That needs to change so that more doctors will go into primary care and so that primary care physicians are adequately reimbursed for proactively managing the health of their patients.

How is it possible for primary care physicians to be in charge when most of them now work for health systems and corporate entities? That's a good question, and one that will be answered in due course. Suffice it to say here that PCPs must be liberated from practice owners that have agendas other than providing great healthcare.

This book is divided into three parts. The first part will consider where healthcare is now, starting with industry consolidation, primary care, and value-based care, along with several recent reform proposals. The second part will explain a new model of healthcare reform unlike any other that has been proposed. It has many features in common, however, with the system I proposed in my two earlier books; in addition, a key part of it is derived from a book I helped write for former Jefferson Health CEO Steve Klasko. In Part 3, I'll explain how this model would address or be affected by some other issues in healthcare, including information technology, rural healthcare, social determinants of health, and the spiraling costs of new drugs and medical devices. I'll also discuss the role of technology assessment in establishing and updating standardized insurance benefits.

To conclude, U.S. healthcare is in a crisis that is approaching the point of no return. While we shouldn't expect any beneficial reforms from the Trump Administration — which has already made the situation worse in numerous ways — the reform model described in this book could be politically feasible under a future government. Let's hope that that future arrives soon and that, when it does, our country will finally be ready to grapple with the challenge of giving all our people comprehensive, affordable healthcare.

PART 1.

Why Healthcare Is a Mess

CHAPTER 1.

The Corporate Grip Tightens

PRICES ARE ABOUT MARKET POWER

Four decades ago, Paul Starr noted in his landmark history of U.S. healthcare, *The Social Transformation of American Medicine*, that the industry had taken a decisive turn toward corporate ownership. "Medical care in America now appears to be in the early stages of a major transformation in its institutional structure," he wrote. "Corporations have begun to integrate a hitherto decentralized hospital system, enter a variety of other health care businesses, and consolidate ownership and control in what may eventually become an industry dominated by huge healthcare conglomerates."[1]

Starr's prediction has come true. Over two thirds of hospitals are now part of health systems, and some of those systems are multibillion-dollar, for-profit or not-for-profit corporations.[2] The majority of physicians work for hospitals or private companies, including insurers and other corporate entities.[3] Enormous retail chains like CVS, Walgreens and Walmart have displaced many community pharmacies and control nearly two-thirds of the pharmacy market.[4] Nursing home chains have taken over two-thirds of skilled nursing facilities.[5] Private equity firms own hundreds of hospitals and many physician practices.[6] The top 10 drug companies generated over a third of U.S. industry revenue in 2023.[7]

Health insurance companies have also consolidated across the country. Five insurers — United, Elevance, CVS/Aetna, Cigna, and Kaiser Permanente — together held 54% of the national market for private health insurance in 2022, and Blue Cross and Blue Shield plans owned most of the rest.[8] In 2023, according to the American Medical

Association, insurance was highly concentrated in 95% of markets, and at least one insurer held a commercial market share of 30% or greater in 89% of markets. In 47% of markets, a single insurer's market share exceeded 50%.[9] This consolidation has led to a rise in insurance costs in many areas.[10]

Where insurers have more market power than health systems do, they can negotiate better deals with the providers. Health plans argue that that reduces out-of-pocket costs for consumers, but the evidence doesn't support this contention. In fact, one study found that premiums increased in certain markets after insurance mergers. "This is likely because consolidated insurers face less pressure to keep premiums low, since their market power also puts them at lower risk of losing a significant number of customers to competitors," noted a report from the Center for American Progress.[11]

THE BIGNESS IMPERATIVE

As health insurers have grown bigger, health systems have done likewise, mainly to maintain or improve their negotiating positions. That has proved to be an effective strategy in many cases. Even dominant health plans cannot do without the largest health systems in their areas, especially when they employ many of the local physicians. Therefore, while the plans may push back against the providers' demands — and now and then even threaten to walk away — they eventually capitulate and pass on the higher costs to employers and individuals.

Hospitals usually give other reasons for their mergers. For example, they often claim that the consolidation will lead to greater efficiency because of economies of scale. But that rarely happens, notes healthcare consultant Michael La Penna. "Hospitals may consolidate laundry services and supply purchasing, but they won't close a department in one hospital and concentrate those services at another. They won't close down one of the ERs."

A PwC study of 5,600 healthcare facilities and 525 healthcare systems showed that large hospitals had a lower cost per patient encounter than small hospitals did. But PwC also found that in health systems with multiple facilities, there was no relationship between size and cost. Hospitals within merged health systems didn't centralize functions or stop competing on procedures. The real purpose of mergers, PwC concluded, was to gain negotiating leverage with insurers.[12]

Some hospitals have asserted that they need to build larger systems to meet the challenge of value-based care (see Chapter 3). But this is actually the opposite of most hospitals' business model. "It's hard to find systems that are really moving in this direction," La Penna says. "Value exists, but only a few health systems have really plunged in."

There is also an argument that larger, more organized systems are better equipped than smaller systems to improve the quality of care and engage in population health management. But David Blumenthal, former president of the Commonwealth Fund, hasn't seen that happen very often. "I think it does happen in some cases. I wish there were better evidence of real quality gains," he says. Other experts have observed poorer patient outcomes when hospitals face less competition.[13] One study found that hospital mergers did not reduce readmissions or mortality rates but were associated with a worse patient experience of care.[14]

In many mergers, large healthcare organizations acquire single hospitals or small hospital systems, La Penna observes. The smaller hospitals need capital and the large ones — which often include tertiary-care academic medical centers — are seeking patient referrals from the smaller institutions. He cites Northwell Health's acquisitions of hospitals on Long Island and in neighboring New York City as an example. Some academic medical centers have also picked up failing rural hospitals to protect their referral sources and keep lower-acuity patients out of their facilities.[15]

Some mergers are designed as defensive moves against other large healthcare systems. In March 2019, for instance, Boston, Massachusetts-based Beth Israel Deaconess Medical Center merged with Lahey Health to form a 10-hospital system with $6 billion in revenues. The systems maintained that they had to merge to counter Partners Healthcare, the largest healthcare organization in New England.[16]

Other mergers involve giants of similar size and scale. For example, Catholic Health Initiatives and Dignity Health completed their union in February 2019. The combined chains, which had roughly similar revenues, formed a new organization called CommonSpirit Health, which has 142 hospitals, 150,000 employees, and nearly $30 billion in revenues.[17]

Cross-state Mergers on the Rise

Cross-state mergers are also becoming more common. For example, in December 2022 Advocate Aurora Health, based in Chicago and Milwaukee, closed a merger with Atrium Health, based in Charlotte, North Carolina. The resultant Advocate Health is the country's fifth largest nonprofit health system, with 67 hospitals and $27 billion in revenue.[18]

Kaiser Permanente, the giant California-based health system, has followed a similar playbook, merging with Geisinger Health in Pennsylvania to form Risant Health in April 2023.[19] In December 2024, Risant acquired Cone Health, a medium sized system in Greensboro, North Carolina. Risant plans to acquire three or four more systems and aims to reach $35 billion in annual revenues in the next five years.[20]

Unlike most other entities that merge, Kaiser and Geisinger both include group-model HMOs. Although their care delivery systems have outside business, they have a vested interest in lowering costs and improving population health to maintain the profitability of their health plans. Their announced goal in forming Risant was to expand access to value-based care outside their organizations.[21] Risant also extended its value-based platform to Cone.

Extracting Higher Prices

A substantial body of research shows that health systems use their market power to raise prices. For example, a 2016 study found that hospital prices in California grew by an average of 76% per admission between 2004 and 2013. Prices at hospitals belonging to large, multi-hospital systems grew substantially more (113%) than prices paid to all other California hospitals (70%). By the end of the period, average prices per admission at hospitals in the largest systems exceeded prices at other hospitals by about $4,000, or 25%. After controlling for other factors, the authors concluded that the higher prices resulted from the greater market power of the biggest systems.[22]

A RAND study found that commercial insurers paid hospitals an average of 241% of Medicare rates in 2017. The private insurance payments to hospitals ranged from 150% to more than 400% of Medicare rates.[23] A 2022 analysis by the Congressional Budget Office (CBO) concluded that hospitals got an average of 240% of Medicare rates from private insurers for outpatient services and 182% for inpatient services. Commercial plans paid health systems a mean of 129% of Medicare rates for physician services, the CBO found.[24]

In discussing their results, the RAND researchers noted that some analysts interpret the high prices that hospitals demand from private payers as evidence that they need the money to cover the shortfalls from Medicare underpayments. "The other interpretation is that hospitals, especially 'must-have' hospitals, have used their negotiating leverage to extract unreasonable price concessions from health plans," the authors noted.

David Muhlestein, a healthcare expert at the Duke Margolis Institute for Health Policy, offers a franker assessment: "A dominant provider in the market can extract almost any price they want," he says.

Many hospitals have paper-thin margins, and others are losing money or are on the verge of bankruptcy.[25] But overall, hospitals are doing quite well. In 2024, hospital operating margins averaged 4.9%. Looking at the results by hospital size, there was a direct correlation between the number of beds in a hospital and the increase in its 2024 operating margin from that in the previous year. The average profit growth was 6.6% in hospitals with 25 or fewer beds, versus 13.8% for hospitals with 300-499 beds.[26]

Profit margins can increase because of higher utilization, higher prices or a combination of the two. Observers say that in the case of U.S. hospitals, prices are what's driving up costs. A recent paper in *Health Affairs* shows how consolidation has affected these prices. From 2012 to 2021, average per-case prices of system-affiliated hospitals grew 45% from $14,282 to $20,732. Prices among independent hospitals, in contrast, grew 35% from $13,460 to $18,197.[27]

Is There Hospital Competition?

If you've ever seen highway billboards claiming that one hospital has the best cardiac care or orthopedic care in the area — or is high up on the *U.S. News and World Report* rankings — you might have thought that that hospital was competing with other local facilities for patients. But those billboards are more likely public relations exercises than real signs of competition. Even where there is competition between hospitals, it rarely results in lower prices.

"Driven by a lack of competition, ever higher prices are being paid to hospitals, doctors and insurers without leading to better outcomes," declared health policy experts Martin Gaynor, Farzad Mostashari, and Paul Ginsburg in a 2017 *Forbes* article.[28]

Blumenthal agrees. "The evidence so far is that prices go up with more consolidation," he says. "The lack of competition increases the ability to charge high prices. But I don't think competition reduces prices in health care."

Traditionally, the Federal Trade Commission (FTC) has policed corporate mergers to deter those that reduce competition. But in 2014, a post on the FTC blog noted that the agency had challenged only two of 752 mergers, joint ventures, or other collaborations among healthcare providers on antitrust grounds. The following year, the FTC blocked a merger between Advocate Health Care and NorthShore University HealthSystem in Chicago and two smaller mergers.[29] But this flurry of activity was the exception, not the rule, for the FTC.

Over the past 20 years, there have been approximately 1,000 hospital or system mergers, and the FTC took enforcement action against only 13 of them. Researchers have estimated that, from 2002 to 2020, about a fifth of hospital mergers could have been flagged by the FTC.[30]

In summary, the healthcare industry is going through the same transition to a high concentration of ownership that other industries have made. This process has allowed the merged healthcare systems to extract more and more money from employers and consumers. The fire of consolidation, however, hasn't just devoured hospitals and other healthcare facilities; it is now roaring through the ranks of independent physician practices.

PHYSICIAN EMPLOYMENT

Physicians have been steadily moving away from private practice into employment by hospitals, large physician groups, and other entities for decades. But in the past several years, there has been a stunning increase in this activity. Just from 2019-2021, for example, over 100,000 formerly independent physicians became employed.[31] In 2023, Optum, a unit of UnitedHealth Group, signed up 20,000 physicians to reach a total of 90,000 employed and affiliated doctors.[32] From 2019-2023, hospitals and corporate entities hired 127,700 physicians, propelling their cumulative total to 503,000 doctors.[33]

According to a report by the Government Accountability Office (GAO), 47% of physicians worked for hospitals in 2024, up from 30% in 2012. Corporate entities, including insurers and private equity firms, employed 23% of doctors in 2024, versus 15% in 2019.[34] Overall, nearly 80% of doctors are now employed, including non-owners of group practices. Of all employed doctors, 55.1% work for health systems, 22.5% for corporate entities, and 22.4% for group practices.[35]

Many of the physicians employed by hospitals and health systems were formerly in private practice. They sold their practices to hospitals because of increasing overhead, dwindling reimbursement, and the rising administrative burdens of ownership, according to Jackson Healthcare, a physician recruiting firm. The Affordable Care Act also played a role in their decisions. Sixty-five percent of the doctors surveyed by Jackson had sold their practices since the ACA's passage in 2010, and many felt they didn't have the resources to comply with the ACA. Other formerly independent physicians went to work for hospitals or larger groups because they couldn't afford to buy electronic health record (EHR) systems.[36] The stresses of the COVID-19 pandemic, which hurt physician practices, also undoubtedly played a role.

The many negative factors affecting primary care (see Chapter 2) have also impelled a growing number of primary care physicians to seek employment. In 2018, 47% of general internists, 57% of family physicians and 56% of pediatricians were employed,[37] and at least 60% of PCPs work for another entity today.[38] There is evidence that this trend may be exacerbating the primary care shortage because employed doctors see fewer patients per day, on average, than do those in private practice.[39]

An increasing percentage of hospital-employed physicians are young doctors fresh out of residency training. A 2019 survey by Merritt Hawkins, another recruiting firm, found that 91% of final-year medical residents wanted to be employed and that only 1% wanted to start a private practice. Forty-five percent of the residents said they'd consider a job offer from a hospital — the highest percentage ever in Merritt Hawkins' ongoing survey.[40]

Why Hospitals Hire Docs

Hospitals say they acquire practices and build their physician groups to improve care coordination and lower costs, but some observers say it's mainly about patient referrals. According to a Stanford University study, a hospital's ownership of practices increases the odds that doctors will admit patients there instead of at another hospital. Because the hospitals that employ the referring physicians are not necessarily the best, hospital employment of doctors also boosts the chances that patients will go to higher-cost, lower-quality facilities.[41]

Hospitals and health systems benefit from employing doctors in other ways. Physicians in hospital groups order their tests from hospital labs and radiology centers. In addition, hospitals can bill Medicare for the ambulatory care provided by their doctors at a much higher rate than what Medicare pays to private practices for the same services. The hospitals have been allowed to do this because their employed practices are part of hospital outpatient departments (HOPDs). HOPDs, which also include emergency departments and same-day surgery units, charge not only professional fees, but also facility fees.[42]

Pursuant to a regulation authorized by the Bipartisan Budget Act of 2015, the Centers for Medicare and Medicaid Services (CMS) began paying new HOPDs and private practices the same for identical services in January 2019. In September of that year, however, a federal district court ruled that CMS had overstepped its statutory bounds by implementing these "site-neutral" payments.[43] CMS lost its appeal of this decision. In December 2023, the House of Representatives passed legislation to apply site-neutral payments to drugs administered in an outpatient setting. However, that bill died in the Senate.[44]

If the government had been able to enforce site-neutral payments, despite the opposition of health systems, it would have reduced hospitals' incentive to acquire practices, observers say. But, with most practices already owned by hospitals or corporate entities, that's now less important than it was.

Hospitals still have incentives to employ independent physicians. Their most important motive, La Penna says, is to lock up physicians so that other hospitals can't control them. Even if there's little overlap between two hospitals' service areas, he says, they want to make sure that the other hospital doesn't employ some of their referring doctors.

"When I ask a hospital board, 'Would you be buying practices if St. John's wasn't buying practices,' they say 'No,'" he points out. "They're buying their own distribution chain, which they already have for free."

Higher Insurance Payments

Getting higher Medicare rates for services provided by their physicians is not the only way that hospitals have driven up costs by buying practices and recruiting doctors out of residency. When health systems employ physicians, they can use their market power to negotiate higher commercial payment rates for those doctors. A study of claims data from commercial insurers found substantial differences between the prices negotiated by employed groups and private practices across the country.[45] In two-thirds of the areas included in the study, physician prices increased as the result of practice purchases by hospitals.[46] Another study found that physician prices rise nearly 14% when a hospital acquires a physician group.[47]

The higher private insurance payments to many hospital-employed groups — like the higher Medicare payments to HOPDs — put additional pressure on independent practices. The physicians who own those practices must meet payroll and cover other costs, yet they're getting paid less than the much bigger hospital groups with which they're competing. Besides the other reasons enumerated above, this factor has undoubtedly induced some private practice doctors to throw in the towel and go to work for a hospital.

Practice owners are also having an increasingly difficult time recruiting physicians to their groups. Because hospitals negotiate higher rates from commercial insurers, they can pay high starting salaries that private practices can't match.

Before retiring, family physician David Boles, DO, of Clarksville, Tennessee, told me that when he interviewed recent residency graduates, they wanted to start out at a salary "that's impossible to sustain under a production formula. If you start a family doc at $240,000 right out of residency — because that's the only way you can get one — the odds are that if that's a one-year contract, they're going to have to take a pay cut in the next year."

OTHER EMPLOYMENT ALTERNATIVES

While hospitals and health systems still employ the largest number of physicians, other types of organizations have acquired or formed a rapidly growing number of practices. These include insurance companies, private equity firms, retailers, and "advanced" primary care firms.

As noted earlier, Optum Health, a unit of insurance giant UnitedHealth Group, employs or contracts with more than 90,000 physicians, or about 10% of the national workforce. One reason why Optum employs so many doctors, according to some observers, is that United Healthcare can use them to get around an ACA provision that requires insurers to spend at least 80-85% of their premium revenue on patient care.[48] Optum pays its physicians 17% more than it pays comparable non-Optum physicians, and 60% of its revenue comes from United health plans. These inter-company transfers allow the insurance company to claim it is spending the required amount on patient care, shielding it from having to pay rebates to consumers and employers.[49]

Optum's largest purchase was of the Davita Medical Group, whose 17,000 doctors shifted to Optum in 2019.[50] Since then, Optum has continued to acquire large groups such as Crystal Run Healthcare, Kelsey-Seybold and Atrius Health.[51] In addition, Optum operates a chain of MedExpress urgent care centers and a national network of ambulatory surgical centers and surgical hospitals.[52] And it owns LHC, one of the nation's largest providers of home care.[53]

Humana is the other major employer of physicians among insurance firms. Unlike Optum, which has focused on acquiring large groups, Humana has established hundreds of CenterWell primary care clinics. These clinics provide value-based, senior-centered care in keeping with Humana's concentration on the lucrative Medicare Advantage market. As of June 2023, CenterWell had 250 clinics in 12 states, mostly in the South and Midwest. Many of them are located in rural communities where there was previously a lack of primary care.[54]

Elevance Health (formerly named Anthem) has also entered this territory, but to a much more limited extent. In 2024, Elevance announced that it had partnered with a private equity firm to provide digital "whole health" services to its 30 Carelon clinics and to a primary care-centric "platform" named MPG that serves 900 providers.[55]

Venture Capital Strategies

Always on the prowl for investment opportunities, private equity has rediscovered healthcare in the past 15 years. Worldwide, venture capital healthcare deals surged to a total value of $115 billion in 2024, their second highest level ever. Healthcare PE deals in North America accounted for 65% of global deal value. Biopharmaceutical investments in North America totaled $34 billion; "providers and related services" also received $34 billion in PE funding; medical technology (including IT) got $15 billion, and healthcare payers, $16 billion.[56] Over the past decade, PE has invested a staggering $750 billion in acquiring U.S. healthcare providers.[57]

In many of these deals, PE firms have acquired physician practices or companies that employ doctors. In 2018, for example, PE firm KKR spent $9.9 billion to acquire physician staffing company Envision Healthcare. Summit Partners and Optum acquired a controlling stake in Sound Inpatient Physicians for $2.2 billion.[58]

In 2021, PE firms made 484 United States practice deals, up from 75 in 2012. These practices tended to be in high-volume specialties such as dermatology, ophthalmology, gastroenterology, urology, and allergy. The doctors in these practices may have been attracted by the large upfront payments they were offered. They also may have wanted to sell to relieve financial pressures and gain negotiating clout with health plans.[59]

Many PE firms have pursued a strategy of rolling up practices in particular specialties to gain competitive advantages in individual markets. The number of PE-acquired physician practices sites increased from 816 in 2012 to 5,779 in 2021. Single PE firms had market share exceeding 30% in 108 markets and exceeding 50% in 50 of these markets.[60]

How much have these tactics driven up prices? According to one study of gastroenterology practices, after PE acquisition, their prices increased by an average of $92 per claim, or 28.4%, driven by a 78% increase in professional fees. At the same time, utilization of services such as colonoscopies increased.[61] Another paper on PE-acquired practices in three specialties found they raised healthcare spending by 32% compared to independent practices, partly through increases in patient visits and service use.[62]

Private equity buyouts may have some unfortunate consequences for both the quality and the cost of care, suggest the coauthors of another study:

> Evidence comparing the quality of private equity firm-owned practices with physician-owned practices is limited… However, the need for private-equity firms to achieve high returns on investment (often at least 2.5×) on a fast time horizon (approximately 6 years on average) may conflict with the need for investments in quality and safety. Additionally, the need for generating

> returns may create pressure to increase utilization, direct referrals internally to capture revenue from additional services, and rely on care delivered by unsupervised allied clinicians.[63]

The time to sale may even be shorter than these authors indicate. According to a recent Bain & Co. report on private equity deals in healthcare, only a small portion of buyout funds had a time horizon of six years or more. The largest number sold acquired companies within 3 years, followed by those selling within 4-6 years.[64]

This data is worth pausing over for a moment. In the larger corporate world, the buying and selling of assets is how investors earn profits, and they prefer to hold onto investments for as short a time as possible so they can deploy the money elsewhere. But in healthcare, where patients' lives and health are at stake, such a cold, calculating approach should have no place.

Retail Initiatives

Pharmacy chains have been involved in care delivery for a couple of decades. CVS operates about 900 MinuteClinics that provide minor acute care, usually delivered by nurse practitioners or physician assistants.[65] CVS also owns Aetna, a leading insurer, and it recently began expanding MinuteClinic services to include more primary care in certain markets, but only for Aetna members. Physicians will be involved only in a supervisory capacity.[66]

Other retail initiatives have been scaled back or shut down. Walgreens, which used to operate retail clinics similar to MinuteClinics, paid $5.2 billion to acquire a controlling interest in primary care network VillageMD in 2021.[67] Walgreens planned to expand VillageMD with hundreds of primary care clinics in its stores, and it opened 200 such clinics. But recently, it announced it would shut down more than 160 VillageMD clinics after losing $6 billion on the operation. CVS has also shuttered some MinuteClinics, and in 2024, Walmart closed all 51 of its standalone primary care clinics in five states because they had lost money.[68]

The thrust into retail primary care has not paid off for several reasons. First, primary care reimbursement is low. Unless a company can profit from referrals to more profitable specialists and hospitals, as health systems do, there's not much money in it. When pharmacy chains focused on minor acute care as a loss leader, it was a sensible business proposition. But as soon as they invested in full-service primary care, the business case went south.[69]

'Advanced' Primary Care Clinics

Another area of care delivery where CVS is forging ahead is known as "advanced" primary care. This rubric covers a cluster of approaches to reducing the cost and increasing the quality of care by emphasizing better preventive and chronic care and improving care coordination. In 2023, CVS bought Oak Street Health, a senior-focused primary care company, for $10.5 billion. Oak Street now has about 230 locations, with plans to increase that to 300 by 2026.[70]

The sweet spot for companies like Oak Street, ChenMed, and Iora (part of One Medical) is the Medicare Advantage business. CMS pays MA plans a fixed sum, based on traditional Medicare rates, to cover all care for beneficiaries. These plans lay off some of the financial risk to advanced primary care companies. Both the insurers and the primary care companies benefit when providers trained in value-based-care techniques deliver care for less than their budgets.

One Medical is an interesting hybrid of this approach with concierge care — a primary care model in which patients pay a monthly fee to get extra medical attention, sometimes including telehealth visits. Acquired by Amazon in 2023 for $4 billion,[71] One Medical now offers memberships to Amazon Prime members for $99 per year.[72] While accepting regular medical insurance, One Medical provides longer appointments quicker than do traditional primary care offices, as well as 24/7 online care. It has recently formed partnerships with Cleveland Clinic and Hackensack Meridian Health to open new locations.[73]

The "value-based care" trend that these advanced primary care firms embody will be discussed at greater length in Chapter 3. The important point here is that big corporations view this change in care delivery as a profit opportunity. In that regard, they are ahead of most healthcare systems, which still see value-based care as a threat to their business model.

Independent Groups Dwindling Fast

At one time, many doctors seeking employment signed up or merged with large independent groups. But far fewer of them are still looking in that direction, because there aren't many of those groups left. Most have been snapped up by health systems, Optum, or PE firms.

One indication of this switch is a 2023 article in *Becker's Hospital Review*, which listed "the 15 largest independent physician groups." All but one of those groups was an independent practice association (IPA). IPAs are networks of small independent practices that band together for economies of scale and, in some cases, to negotiate contracts with payers.[74] This finding suggests that most of the bigger integrated groups have been acquired.

The American Medical Group Association (AMGA), the trade association for big groups, still claims to have more than 400 members, roughly the same number as five years ago. But the focus of efforts to maintain independent practice has shifted to IPAs and clinically integrated networks (CINs). A recent paper in the *New England Journal of Medicine* notes:

> Physicians in smaller, independent practices — those that are owned by one or more physicians — have sought alternative forms of practice affiliation to leverage the advantages of being part of a larger organization while honoring the ability of physicians to practice as they see fit. These physician-led structures include independent physician associations (IPAs) and physician-owned clinically integrated networks (CINs). Yet recent legal and regulatory uncertainty has led to concerns about the long-term viability and efficacy of these organizational structures as an alternative to corporate control.[75]

The main problem is that federal antitrust statutes still prohibit IPAs from negotiating prices unless they use the ineffective "messenger model." CINs, which are more integrated and have a more explicit focus on clinical or financial integration, can enter into group contracts and share risk. Government regulations, the article concludes, are out of step with the current wave of corporatization — which, as we've seen, is hardly constrained by antitrust considerations.

CONSOLIDATION AND SUSTAINABILITY

The corporate grip on healthcare has tightened considerably since 2020, when my last book on healthcare reform was published. Just a few data points show how far this has gone: The largest health systems now have, on average, a combined 43.1% of the market share for inpatient care in each state. The top three large-group insurers hold an average of 82.2% of the market share in each state.[76] And over three-quarters of physicians, as stated earlier, are now employed by health systems or corporate entities.

This consolidation has raised prices without improving quality — and, in some cases, has degraded the quality of care delivered. Horizontal hospital mergers increase hospital prices from 20% to 40%. Vertical hospital-physician consolidation raises the cost of professional services from 14% to 33.5%.[77] And acquisitions of physician practices by PE firms, as noted above, pump up prices by nearly a third, on average.

The reasons for the intense interest in healthcare mergers and acquisitions vary from one sector to another. For example, health systems want to increase their negotiating power and control their physicians, while PE firms want to make a quick buck.

Corporations increasingly see a pot of gold in value-based care (VBC), which aims to cut health costs, reduce the amount of waste, and improve population health. The long-term monetary value of this opportunity has been estimated at up to $1 trillion.[78] Whoever can grab some of that money stands to make a bundle.

CMS's stated intention of having all Medicare beneficiaries in VBC arrangements by 2030 has heightened interest in the providers who can make this happen — particularly primary care physicians. According to McKinsey & Co., private capital inflows to VBC companies — which include advanced primary care companies, management services organizations, and infrastructure vendors — increased fourfold just from 2019 to 2021.[79]

Consolidation Is a Prime Suspect

Yet, primary care continues to decline, and value-based payment is still considered a weak alternative to the dominant fee-for-service payment structure. Meanwhile, the health of Americans continues to lag behind that of citizens in other advanced countries. "Among 10 [of those] nations, Americans die the youngest and live the sickest lives, despite the United States spending the most on health care," states the latest international survey of the Commonwealth Fund.[80]

The report also finds that, among the countries compared, Americans face the most barriers to getting and affording health coverage. Despite the gains produced by the Affordable Care Act, 25 million Americans remain uninsured, and nearly a quarter of us cannot afford healthcare when we need it.

In a commentary on the report, David Blumenthal, Evan Gumas and Arnav Shah note that the U.S. health system has profound problems that result in huge inefficiencies and excessive costs. Besides the worsening shortage of primary care, they point to the high prices charged by U.S. healthcare facilities and professionals. For that, they blame the consolidation of healthcare organizations and the expansion of private equity in healthcare.[81]

In an article on the healthcare affordability issue, Michael McWilliams and Stacie B. Dusetzina also cite industry consolidation as a key concern. "In the commercially insured market, affordability is most compromised by excessively high prices charged by health care provider organizations with market power amassed over decades of local consolidation," they write.

Government intervention is needed where the market has failed, these experts note. But antitrust action is not the solution. "Given the market power already attained by provider organizations, attempting to rein in commercial prices by challenging a greater number of new mergers and acquisitions is probably too little, too late."

The other avenue the federal government could take to lower prices is to regulate them, they point out, but "insurance regulation is traditionally the states' responsibility." Thus, "while pressure for reform will continue to mount, it's challenging to predict the origin and extent of movement on this front."[82]

The previously cited *Health Affairs* article by Donald Berwick, *et al.*, about the failing U.S. healthcare system focuses on systemic factors other than consolidation. But the commentary cites the excessive profits that have been enabled by consolidation as the primary barrier to affordability. It also says PE firms should be prohibited from acquiring or controlling healthcare organizations.

"Profiteering in its many forms must be made unacceptable and, indeed, illegal," Berwick and his colleagues declare.[83]

Meanwhile, Americans are losing their patience with a system that seems to prioritize profits over people's heath. In a March 2025 article, David W. Johnson and Paul Kusserow noted that the 2024 murder of United Healthcare CEO Brian Thompson ignited a powder keg of simmering anger against U.S. healthcare. "Upon his death, Thompson became a symbol of the harm the nation's dysfunctional health system inflicts on everyday Americans," they stated.[84]

United is the poster child for healthcare consolidation, as described earlier. The huge power of this company to determine healthcare prices and coverage, along with its consistently high profits, represent everything that people see as wrong with the system. But it's unreasonable to expect this company, or any other profit-making entity, to act differently. United's actions are a natural outgrowth of the barely restrained capitalism that has been allowed to make a public good into just another profit-making activity.

Healthcare is often described as the most regulated industry in the United States. Yet, because of its enormous lobbying power, as well as widespread political support for doctors and hospitals, the industry manages to work around or defeat most regulations designed to limit its autonomy. That's why antitrust regulation of the industry has mostly failed. It's why CMS has been unable to enforce its site-neutral regulations to hold down outpatient prices. And it's why government lawsuits against several large insurers for illegally pumping up Medicare Advantage payments have disappeared without a trace.

No matter how you slice it, the tightening grip of corporate America has not been good for healthcare. It is one of the chief reasons why our system is heading for collapse. And nowhere is the mechanism paving the way for that collapse more evident than in the mass takeover of physician practices and the way that assimilation has affected physician morale and the doctor-patient relationship. That, and the precipitous decline of primary care, are among the topics discussed in the next chapter.

CHAPTER 2.

A Clinical Workforce in Distress

THE DOWNSIDES OF VERTICAL INTEGRATION

Considering what a mess hospital systems and corporate players have made of running U.S. healthcare, perhaps it's time for a reboot. Maybe physicians, the ones who actually diagnose and treat patients, should be in charge. Because of their hands-on understanding of healthcare, physicians are the only ones who know how to improve it and how to reduce the systemic waste in patient care.

However, placing physicians in charge of healthcare is much harder than it sounds. It would require a complete restructuring of the healthcare system. The argument of this book is that such a reorganization is necessary and feasible.

In this chapter, I discuss the employment-related factors that might make many doctors receptive to such sweeping changes. In addition, I explain the reasons for the catastrophic decline of primary care and how it can be reversed. Without an adequate primary care workforce, it will be impossible to rescue our healthcare system from its impending collapse.

WHY EMPLOYED DOCS ARE UNHAPPY

As explained in Chapter 1, many physicians sold their practices to health systems or corporate entities because of a confluence of factors. Among their motivations were increasing overhead, dwindling reimbursement, growing administrative burdens, and the cost of electronic health records (EHRs). Moreover, the high prices being paid for practices in some specialties were an inducement to many physicians. Most young physicians coming out of residency opt to work for a hospital or a corporation because they've been told how challenging it is to start their own practice in the current market conditions.

This doesn't mean, however, that employed physicians are necessarily happy with their choice. For starters, physicians who work for health systems or private equity firms usually have to see a certain number of patients per day or per week, and a large part of their compensation is tied to their productivity. Coupled with the need to document every encounter in the EHR, that often means not spending enough time with patients or failing to attend to all their health needs.

Particularly in primary care, physicians are like hamsters running on a wheel, never getting ahead. According to a recent report, physician productivity continues to climb, even as reimbursement lags behind. Clinicians' productivity has risen 7% since 2023, the report found, but their compensation has risen only 6%.[1]

In addition, employed doctors' clinical autonomy is more limited than it would be in private practice. Not only are hospital-employed doctors expected to order tests from their hospital's lab or imaging center, but they also are incentivized to admit patients to a system hospital and refer patients to specialists within the system.[2] The same can be true for physicians working for insurers or PE firms, who may be forced to refer to certain hospitals or specialists to curb costs.

Government regulations prohibit health systems from making an employed physician's compensation contingent on the volume or value of his or her hospital referrals.[3] But a health system can decline to renew the contract of a doctor who frequently refers to hospitals or specialists outside the system.

Unsurprisingly, doctors tend to refer within their health system. For example, one study found that when a patient's primary care doctor entered hospital employment, there was a 7.3% increase in the probability of a patient with cancer being referred for post-discharge follow-up to an oncologist in that health system.[4]

Quality Down, Burnout Up

In a 2023 survey, nearly 60% of physicians employed by health systems, insurers, staffing agencies and private equity firms said that the employment trend has hurt patient care quality, mainly because of a lack of clinical autonomy and an increased focus on cost savings. About half of the respondents said that practice guidelines or incentives had induced them to change a patient's treatment options to reduce costs.[5]

The switchover to physician employment has also contributed to burnout. According to a Physicians Foundation survey, six in 10 physicians and residents reported burnout in 2024. Before the pandemic, it was four in 10 physicians. Besides the added stress of caring for patients with COVID, the marked increase in physician employment during that period seems to have played a role in this shift.[6]

"Respondents said changes in the healthcare environment fueled by acquisitions, mergers, and private equity are contributing to the burnout crisis," the report said. "Among those who have experienced mergers or acquisitions, many said that it negatively impacted their job satisfaction (50%), the quality of patient care (36%), patient healthcare costs (30%), as well as independent medical judgement (35%). Plus, most respondents…said that consolidation is having a negative impact on patient access to high-quality and cost-efficient care."

According to a 2025 Medscape survey, about half of employed physicians liked having jobs because of the stable income and not having to run a business. But here's what they disliked about their jobs: less autonomy (48%), less income potential (33%), more workplace rules (31%), company management (30%), and mandatory performance targets (27%).[7]

Debra Glasser, MD, a retired internist in Portland, Oregon, was in private practice for many years and later worked in the VA system. She says that the corporatization of healthcare has played a major role in physician burnout.

"Back in the day when we were in private practice, our patients came to us by choice, and we were committed to them and stood by them as primary care doctors. There was a lot of relationship building and reward from that relationship and that commitment. Now that's all gone. Doctors are all employed, and, while the relationship with the patient is important, the doctor is not rewarded for that. And something about that loss of connection leads to burnout."[8]

The biggest downside to physician employment, Yul D. Ejnes, MD, of Cranston, Rhode Island, recently wrote in *Health Affairs*, is the "deprofessionalization" that results from doctors' lack of independence in clinical decision making.

> In many large organizations, what is 'special' about physicians is stripped away, perhaps unintentionally yet with potentially devastating consequences. Not only do physicians face external threats to their professionalism from those who pay for care and the commodification of medicine; there are internal ones as well, from the organizations that employ them.[9]

Concierge Care in Employed Groups

These conditions have made some employed physicians consider moving back to private practice. A Bain & Co. survey found that nearly 25% of physicians in health system-led organizations were considering a change in employers; of those doctors, 37% wanted to move to independent physician groups. But not many doctors have made the switch.[10]

Instead, some physicians offer "concierge care" — private healthcare in return for out-of-pocket payments by patients — while continuing to work for hospitals.[11] Some hospitals, including top academic medical centers such as Johns Hopkins and Mass General Brigham, even offer their own concierge arrangements. In their telling, this is being done to promote more personalized, patient-centered care.[12]

But there may be other reasons, as well, says Travis Singleton, president of Green Staff Medical, a nurse staffing agency, and a former physician recruiter. Health systems, he argues, "have to give their patient base — especially the affluent part of it — an outlet. It's partly for marketing to all patients, but it's also to ensure the hospital keeps the profitable parts of its base and makes sure they don't go elsewhere."

Physician Unions on the Rise

Another outcome of the mass migration of physicians to employment has been the rise of physician unions. Although the majority of their members are doctors in training, some board-certified physicians are also participating.

For example, several hundred primary care physicians at Mass General Brigham (MGB) in Boston notified the National Labor Relations Board (NLRB) in 2024 that they wanted to unionize. A spokesman for the unionizing doctors told *MedPage Today* that he and his colleagues needed better access to MGB leadership to resolve workplace issues. These included being required to work longer hours than doctors in other specialties, staff turnover issues that impeded care, inadequate call coverage, and overwhelming workloads related to patient emails.[13]

Across the country, the number of union petitions to the NLRB with physicians in the bargaining unit has spiked in recent years. From 2000-2022, there were 44 such petitions. In contrast, 33 were filed just in 2023-2024. Of the 66 union petitions to which the NRLB has responded, 41 were certified. Most of the union campaigns were motivated by working conditions (85%), lack of a voice in management (81%), and patient care concerns (54%). Only one campaign cited financial compensation.[14]

Private Equity Makes It Worse

As mentioned in Chapter 1, private equity firms have targeted several physician specialties. While many physicians have gladly taken their money, PE acquisitions have increased physician turnover. In ophthalmology practices, one study found, the share of physicians leaving PE-acquired practices increased by 265% after acquisition, relative to non-PE-acquired practices.[15]

"PE acquisitions may increase physician turnover if acquisitions are accompanied by changes to practice management and operations that affect clinicians' autonomy, practice conditions, and job satisfaction," the researchers noted.

Peter Ubell, MD, a behavioral scientist at Duke University, noted in a *JAMA* article that PE firms can offer valuable administrative support to practices. But their practice purchases often have ethically troubling consequences. For example, they may pressure clinicians to see more patients, perform more procedures on those patients, and/or upsell patients on products not covered by insurance, such as acne creams in dermatologists' offices. After PE acquisitions, Ubell said, practices may also raise their prices, reducing access for less well-off patients.[16]

One study of prices in primary care offices found that, relative to independent practices, negotiated prices for office visits were 11% higher in hospital-affiliated and 8% higher in PE-affiliated practices.[17] While relatively few PE-owned practices deliver primary care, another study found that gastroenterologists also raised their fees after PE firms bought their groups.[18]

There are indications that PE ownership is associated with lower quality of care. For example, after PE acquisition of hospitals, one study found, Medicare beneficiaries admitted to those hospitals had a 25% increase in hospital-acquired conditions compared with those at control hospitals. These included central line-associated bloodstream infections and surgical site infections.[19]

THE CLINICAL WORKFORCE

In order to revamp our healthcare system, we first must get a handle on our clinical workforce, which includes physicians, nurse practitioners (NPs) and physician assistants (PAs), among other healthcare professionals.

As anyone who has tried to get a physician appointment recently knows, it takes longer than ever to see a doctor. In 2022, the average length of time to obtain a new patient appointment in 15 metropolitan areas was 26 days, an 8% increase from 2017 and a 24% jump from 2004.[20]

The researchers who did this survey looked at five specialties, including obstetrics/gynecology, cardiology, orthopedic surgery, dermatology, and family medicine. The waiting time for medical and surgical specialties increased sharply; ob/gyn patients had the longest wait at 31.4 days. Family medicine's average waiting time, in contrast, dropped 30% to 20.6 days from 29.3 days in 2017. This was attributed mainly to more people accessing primary care through urgent care centers, retail clinics and telemedicine — venues that are typically staffed by nurse practitioners.

Overall, these waiting times suggest that there is an undersupply of physicians in the United States. The U.S. average of 2.7 doctors per 1,000 people is below the median of 3.5 per 1,000 for all advanced countries.[21]

The American Association of Medical Colleges (AAMC) now projects the United States is going to be short about 86,000 physicians by 2036, if current utilization patterns continue and the distribution of physicians remains about the same.[22] The second caveat reveals a key truth: the U.S. physician population is severely maldistributed, with more doctors per capita on the coasts and in major urban centers than in the center of the country and in rural areas. If underserved areas were properly served, the AAMC estimates, we'd need 200,000 more doctors by 2036 than we had in 2021, the beginning of their prediction period.

In addition, the AAMC estimate doesn't sufficiently consider the serious shortage of primary care doctors across the country. The National Center for Healthcare Workforce Analysis predicts that, by 2036, the United States will have shortages of more than 68,000 primary care physicians, 62,400 psychologists, 42,100 psychiatrists, 6,600 obstetrician/gynecologists, and 33,100 family medicine physicians, besides deficits in other specialties.[23]

How Many Doctors Do We Need?

Jonathan Weiner, PhD, professor of health policy and management at the Johns Hopkins Bloomberg School of Public Health, agrees that many Americans lack adequate access to physicians. But he doesn't know whether we need tens of thousands of new doctors. "It would probably be a good thing to have 86,000 new doctors. But there never will be enough, because the market is imperfect, and we don't have a way to get services to all of the people who need them. We currently have one physician, NP or PA in active practice for every 220 Americans. We could do better than that."

The other key factor in the AAMC projection is the assumption that Medicare will continue to fund graduate medical education (GME) positions for resident physicians at their current rate. In 1997,

Congress placed a cap on the number of GME positions. It added funding for an extra 1200 positions under bills passed in 2021 and 2023.[24]

Weiner is skeptical about AAMC's claim that the physician shortage will grow if GME funding isn't maintained or augmented. Aside from the obvious self-interest in this argument, he doesn't think we need more specialists. "If we're going to add more doctors, I'd prefer them to be in primary care," he says.

Weiner notes that about 30,000 U.S.-born physicians graduate from residency programs each year, along with around 8,000 international medical graduates (IMGs). If any Medicare-funded slots are lost, he says, that might mean fewer positions for IMGs, who now form about a fifth of the physician workforce.

The Trump Administration has thrown up obstacles to the training of IMGs. In spring 2025, it delayed appointments for J-1 visas needed to enter the United States. Since then, the government has barred citizens of 39 countries from coming in or restricted their ability to do so.[25] These actions have made it impossible for thousands of foreign doctors accepted into U.S. residency programs to start their postgraduate training.[26]

The government has also erected a high barrier to hiring highly skilled, foreign-born workers such as doctors by demanding that they or their employers pay a $100,000 fee for an H-1B visa. This new requirement has created turmoil in rural healthcare, where IMGs are in great demand. Rural hospitals and practices can't afford to pay the fee, so many of the doctors they have recruited from abroad have been left hanging.[27]

Some states are moving in the opposite direction. Since 2023, nine states have eased training requirements for IMGs, and a dozen others are in the process of doing the same to expand their physician workforces. About 10 of these bills or laws stipulate that the IMGs must practice in rural areas for several years.[28] If the Trump Administration persists in its foolhardy policies on legal immigration, however, these efforts will come to naught.

Another consequence of these anti-immigration policies is that they harm primary care, where IMGs are well represented, especially in rural and inner-city areas. So, there is now more need than ever for native-born physicians to go into primary care and to practice in underserved areas. But for that to happen, there must be greater incentives for young doctors to enter primary care fields. Meanwhile, the reliance of the healthcare system on nonphysician clinicians will continue to grow.

Nonphysician Clinicians Proliferate

The rapidly growing ranks of nonphysician clinicians, mainly nurse practitioners (NPs) and physician assistants (PAs), have significantly reinforced the clinical workforce, filling gaps as the population has grown and aged. There are now about 450,000 nonphysician clinicians in the United States, according to Weiner. Yet, despite that, and despite the growth in telehealth and alternative sites of care, such as retail clinics and urgent care centers, many people still have trouble accessing healthcare providers.

Only about 30% of NPs and 24% of PAs are delivering primary care; the rest practice in better paying medical and surgical specialties.[29] They perform an increasing range of functions in specialty practices, enabling many physicians to reduce their routine work and increase their revenues.

Debra Glasser is skeptical about this use of NPs and PAs, who are sometimes called "midlevels." Years ago, she recalls, PAs would admit patients to the hospital for orthopedic surgeons. But now they also do postsurgical follow-ups, which require a higher level of knowledge. "Midlevels do protocol medicine [i.e., follow instructions], and in some cases, that's very appropriate. But it can be problematic."

She also challenges the widespread notion that nonphysician clinicians can provide 85-90% of primary care. "That's outrageous," she says. "It takes so much training and understanding to know what's serious and what's not. Say a patient comes in complaining of burning on urination. The first thing you think of is a UTI, but you might want to have a differential diagnosis so you don't miss anything serious.

And the problem with midlevels is they don't have enough training to think broad enough or deep enough to not miss stuff."

Even if PAs and NPs can do 85% of primary care, the other 15% is "really important," notes Grace Terrell, MD, who founded a multi-specialty group in High Point, North Carolina, many years ago and still practices part time as a general internist. Christian Giordano, MD, a former PA who now practices internal medicine, wrote in *the Annals of Internal Medicine* that primary care demands significantly more knowledge and training than what PAs have. "I appreciate the expertise that quality primary care demands and personally attest that this is vastly greater than that of physician assistants."

THE DECLINE AND FALL OF PRIMARY CARE

Primary care is the most essential part of the healthcare system. But, for a variety of reasons, primary care in the United States is crumbling and has reached a crisis point that endangers the health of all Americans.

In a 2021 report by the National Academies of Sciences, Engineering and Medicine (NASEM), the authors start by summarizing the importance of primary care in our system:

> High-quality primary care is the foundation of a high-functioning health care system and is critical for achieving health care's quadruple aim (enhancing patient experience, improving population health, reducing costs, and improving the health care team experience). Primary care provides comprehensive, person-centered, relationship-based care that considers the needs and preferences of individuals, families, and communities. Primary care is unique in health care in that it is designed for everyone to use throughout their lives — from healthy children to older adults with multiple comorbidities and people with disabilities. Absent access to high-quality primary care, minor health problems can spiral into chronic disease, care management becomes difficult and uncoordinated, visits to emergency departments increase, preventive care lags, and the nation's health care spending soars to unsustainable levels. People in countries and health systems

with high-quality primary care enjoy better health outcomes and more health equity.[30]

Despite all of this, primary care accounts for only about 5% of U.S. health spending and 35% of patient visits, according to the NASEM report. The percentage of physicians who provide primary care has declined from about a third ten years ago to around 25% today.[31] From 2012-2020, one study found, only 20% of physicians trained in primary care residencies stayed in primary care; the others went into more lucrative specialties.[32]

Big Differences in Compensation

A major reason for the decline in primary care is the disparity between the compensation of primary care doctors and specialists. According to a 2023 *Medscape* survey, the average compensation of PCPs ranges from $250,000-$275,000. In contrast, many specialists make twice as much, ranging up to $619,000 for plastic surgeons, $573,000 for orthopedists and $507,000 for cardiologists. This is a crucial consideration for young doctors choosing a specialty when the average medical school debt exceeds $200,000.[33]

The lack of clinical autonomy that contributes to physician burnout is worse for employed primary care doctors, who are expected to see a certain number of patients each day and rigidly adhere to clinical guidelines. "Back when physicians were in charge of how a patient's healthcare went, we made the clinical decisions and decided who were our patients and how we practiced," Glasser recalls. "There was a locus of control that we felt we earned. Now, all of that is being taken away by the corporatization of healthcare."

This doesn't apply just to corporate- and health system-owned practices. When Glasser left her private practice to join the local VA system, she says, "I had doctors above me telling what I should do and how I should practice, and how many times I should see my patients. I said, 'You can't tell me I should see these very sick women six days a year — it's impossible. You want me to get them off opiates? I can do that, but I've got to see them.'"

Administrative burdens on primary care physicians are nearly overwhelming. "Instead of focusing on managing the health care needs of their patient populations, PCPs have found themselves spending more and more time functioning as de facto administrative assistants," says a recent piece in the *New England Journal of Medicine*. "Although administrative burdens are increasing throughout medicine, the central role of PCPs in the delivery of comprehensive care has made their escalating volume of administrative tasks especially unsustainable."[34]

Among these burdens are billing-relating documentation requirements, prior-authorization requests, and "numerous clinically irrelevant requests from non-health care entities, such as employers and schools. Taking a family or disability-related leave generates extensive paperwork for doctors." Moreover, Medicare requires face-to-face visits to prescribe durable medical equipment, and PCPs must also approve all physical therapy and visiting-nurse care plans. Electronic health records (EHRs) force PCPs, more so than specialists, to spend hours a day documenting patient visits in templates with drop-down boxes.

Diminished Respect for PCPs

In addition, Glasser notes, primary care physicians get less respect than specialists do — a fact of life that medical students and residents absorb from the outset of their careers. This is partly because most of their training occurs in academic medical centers, where specialists and surgeons rule. Knowing that primary care is considered a lesser medical profession deters many doctors from entering the field.

Terrell recalls that primary care doctors used to have a wider scope of practice than they do today. "Much of what I used to do routinely as an internist has gone to specialists now. It's become a process of screening for things and referring to specialists, because that feeds the beast of these huge health systems."

The *NEJM* article mentions an important way in which some specialists disrespect primary care physicians. When PCPs refer patients to them, specialists may require them to order tests ahead of time, communicate the results to patients and even arrange follow-up tests or visits, although these time-consuming tasks should be part of the care that the specialists provide. When imaging tests are needed, the PCP may have to get prior authorization from an insurer.

"The automatic delegation of these tasks without discussion can increase the burden on PCPs, who already tend to work in particularly busy settings with inadequate support," the authors note. "In many cases, specialists are better equipped to interpret and act on test results."

Of course, primary care doctors can refuse to do these things, but they may feel they have to in order to make sure their patient gets proper care. In addition, Terrell notes, they often believe they must refer patients to specialists for certain kinds of care that they are qualified to provide themselves. Their training predisposes them to do this, and patients may expect it.

Patient Attitudes Toward Primary Care

Many patients, especially in the Northeast, regard primary care doctors as adequate for urgent care, but prefer to see specialists for anything else. If they happen to be in a health plan that requires a PCP to refer them to a specialist, patients may view this mandate as an irritating, unnecessary barrier to seeking specialty care.

In 1980, 62% of doctor visits by adults 65 and older were for primary care, and 38% were for specialty care. By 2013, that ratio had flipped. Since then, some experts believe, it has grown even more lopsided in favor of specialists.[35] Obviously, this emphasis on specialty care generates additional costs.

In many cases, people go to specialists — or to ERs or urgent care centers — because they can't access primary care. In a 2023 article entitled "The Shrinking Number of Primary Care Physicians Is Reaching a Tipping Point," Elisabeth Rosenthal points out that people whose PCP is retiring are having trouble finding a new one. More than 100 million Americans lack access to regular primary care, twice the number in 2014. And the percentage of U.S. doctors in adult primary care is now about 25% — "a tipping point beyond which many Americans won't be able to find a family doctor at all," she writes.[36]

In a 2024 *Health Affairs* article, a trio of experts say the same thing. They estimate that almost a third of Americans didn't have a regular place to go for care, and that that number had steadily risen over the prior decade. It's getting harder to find a primary care doctor and there are long wait times for appointments, they point out.

This is a disaster for U.S. healthcare, and it partly explains why more people are delaying or avoiding care and why life expectancy is declining, they note. "Primary care plays a foundational role in an efficient, high-quality health care system. It is the only element of the health care delivery system in which an increased supply is associated with better population health and a reduction in inequitable outcomes. Studies find that continuity in primary care reduces mortality, health care expenditures, and hospitalizations."[37]

One such study shows how having a primary care doctor can improve outcomes after hospitalization. "Among patients undergoing surgery for any of 12 cancers, a primary care visit was associated with lower 90-day postoperative mortality. There were 3 deaths per 1000 patients in the study group, versus 33 per 1000 patients in the control group."[38]

The decline in primary care has been tied to poorer cardiovascular outcomes, as well. The American Heart Association set a goal of reducing deaths from cardiovascular disease (CVD) and stroke by 20% from 2010-2020. It didn't happen. Deaths decreased by only 15%, despite the many new clinical and non-clinical tools deployed against high blood pressure, heart failure, and atrial fibrillation. Now the AHA forecasts that CVD incidence and risk factors will increase.[39]

Eric Topol, MD, a cardiologist, editor and author, and Robert Califf, MD, a cardiologist and a former FDA commissioner, told STAT that the United States is losing ground in CVD. The biggest single reason? "We don't have a primary care system in the U.S. that's functional," said Califf.[40]

In a 2025 *NEJM* paper, Lisa Rosenbaum summarizes the crisis in primary care as follows:

> As the PCP's role has been hollowed out by modern medicine's dictates, new technologies, changing social norms, and exploding medical knowledge, the long-simmering primary care crisis is boiling over. Fewer trainees are entering the field, many PCPs are retiring early or cutting back substantially, and those remaining must pick up the slack until they, too, are driven out. And while clinicians struggle, patients suffer.[41]

PRIMARY CARE SOLUTIONS

We are facing a crisis of historic proportions in primary care. Even as fewer young physicians are going into the field, many primary care doctors plan to retire or leave medicine. In 2022, that included 39% of general internists, 37% of family physicians, 30% of pediatricians, and 34% of ob/gyns.[42] While the number of NPs and PAs in primary care continues to rise, they cannot fully replace physicians, as discussed above. So, at a time when Americans are getting older and sicker, and there are more of us, our primary care is slipping away,

Any comprehensive solution must address three components: 1) We have to prevent PCPs from burning out and leaving medicine; 2) We must induce more young physicians to go into primary care; and 3) We have to make optimal use of the primary care doctors we have.

These are very challenging goals, and we're not likely to reach them unless our healthcare system is restructured. But a lot of thought has been devoted to how we can address the primary care crisis within the current system. The rest of this chapter will look at proposals that concern how primary care physicians are paid. This is critical, because people respond to financial incentives, and changing those incentives can alter how medical students view primary care and how PCPs deliver care.

Primary Care Payment Reform

One caveat before I plunge into these proposals: It's important to understand that the goal of primary care payment reform is not to save money, but to improve population health.

Some studies in Massachusetts and California have shown that investments in primary care do lower overall health spending. And data from the Medicare Shared Savings Program (MSSP) shows that primary-care-led ACOs save more money than those led by hospitals.[43] However, the real value of these investments lies in their ability to create better health outcomes.

Urban Institute scholar Robert A. Berenson, MD, and two of his colleagues explained this idea succinctly in a 2023 paper:

> Some hold that a major purpose of strengthening primary care, supported with additional funding, is to reduce health spending throughout the health system. Others, including the authors, argue that primary care physicians, who receive only about 5% to 7% of overall spending and even less in Medicare, cannot readily reduce the total cost of care for purposes of spending accountability. Research shows that primary care is associated with reduced spending over the long term but not necessarily in the short term.[44]

If increasing primary care compensation wouldn't lower short-term spending, where would the extra money come from? Within the prevalent fee-for-service model, one way to do this is to shift money from higher-paid specialists to lower-paid PCPs. One reason for the pay disparity, the NASEM report points out, is the greater value placed on specialty services and procedures in CMS' Resource-Based Relative Value Scale (RBRVS). The relative-value units assigned to each type of physician work are determined by the AMA's Relative Value Update Committee (RUC). Specialists dominate the RUC, so naturally they tend to assign higher values to specialty services. One of NASEM's recommendations is that CMS lessen its reliance on the RUC in determining the relative values of medical services. Since private payers tend to follow the Medicare fee schedule, this would have a major impact across the healthcare system.

Hybrid Payment Holds Promise

The second option in the NASEM report is to blend fee-for-service (FFS) and fixed population-based payments (PBP). Known as a hybrid payment system, this approach has been tried in a broad range of public and private insurance settings with mixed results. The basic idea is to pay PCPs fee-for-service for well-defined office visits, while giving them a monthly care management fee or capitation payment for population health work. This would include care management and coordination, between-visit care, enhanced use of telehealth, and patient education. Under the NASEM plan, the combined total of FFS and PBP would exceed the amount that primary care doctors are receiving now.

Among the Medicare demonstration programs that have used the hybrid payment approach are Comprehensive Primary Care (CPC), Comprehensive Primary Care Plus (CPC+), and Primary Care First. Berenson and his colleagues noted, "These demonstrations did not notably improve quality or reduce spending, perhaps because most practices opted for participation tracks with only a small percentage of PBP and because these demonstrations did not provide the added payment needed for the models to work as envisioned."[45]

The third option on the NASEM menu is "broad risk-sharing models." Entities that may take financial risk for all or part of the total cost of care include health systems, large physician groups and accountable care organizations (ACOs). The Medicare Shared Savings Program (MSSP) was designed specifically for ACOs, and CMS has encouraged them to take on progressively higher levels of risk. An ACO that delivers high quality care and saves money for Medicare is entitled to receive a share of the savings. If the ACO is taking both upside and downside risk, and if its costs exceed its budget, it must pay back the overage to CMS.

ACOs in the MSSP have produced modest savings in total spending alongside improvements in quality and patient satisfaction, notes NASEM. ACOs with a greater proportion of PCPs perform better on cost and quality outcomes than do those that have more specialists, and physician-led ACOs outperform hospital-led ACOs. One confounding factor in measuring results in these models is that many ACOs pay doctors fee-for-service. As a result, doctors' financial incentives may be inconsistent with those of their organization, especially if it contributes only a small portion of their revenue.[46]

States Try Direct Action

The fourth NASEM option is to directly increase the allocation of spending to primary care. "To achieve this priority, policy makers would direct third-party payers to increase the proportion devoted to primary care and hold them accountable to achieving it," the report says. Rhode Island and Oregon have created programs of this type, and several other states have passed laws requiring public measurement and, in some cases, setting targets for insurers.

By forcing payers to spend more on primary care, NASEM said, this model "could have large marginal effects on the primary care sector. It also addresses the failure of private health plan negotiations or Medicare to recognize the collective social value of primary care." There are several problems with the approach, such as the difficulties of defining policy goals and an acceptable rate of primary care spending. However, since Rhode Island enacted its spending mandate, the share of commercial insurance spending that goes to primary care has risen from 5.7% to 12.3%.[47]

The direct payment approach doesn't address NASEM's concerns about the need to focus payment reform on population health management. "Primary care practices organized in response to FFS payment maximize revenue-producing in-person visits but are not configured to provide the integrated team-based care necessary to address the comprehensive preventive and chronic care needs of people and families, which must include behavioral, social, and oral health," the report noted.

NASEM concluded that the best option was the hybrid payment approach, combining a mix of fee-for-service and population-based payment with performance accountability. It also proposed substantial increases to primary care payment and reforms to the Medicare physician fee schedule.

Other Reform Proposals

Elizabeth Rosenthal, in her 2023 commentary for *Kaiser Health News*, suggested that hospitals and specialists invest some of the money they earn from procedures to support primary care staffing.

Reimbursement should also be increased across the board to reflect the value of primary care, she said. To achieve that goal, the government could enact a national primary fee schedule that commercial insurers would have to use.[48]

For policy experts who believe in value-based care, the key to sustaining primary care is to provide incentives that reward doctors for managing population health.[49] However, research shows that at least two-thirds of a primary care doctor's patients must be covered by insurance with a risk-based incentive structure before the physician will change how they practice.[50] The CPC and CPC+ programs aimed to build this critical mass by partnering with private insurers, but the incentives were not strong enough to produce real change.

A Medicare demonstration called ACO Primary Care Flex, which runs through 2029, holds real promise in this respect, say some experts. This model offers PCPs a significant pay increase, and the money is provided prospectively in monthly population-based payments. The ACOs can pass those funds through to their primary care practices in the form of capitation payments. However, the program is open only to "low-revenue" ACOs, which involve mostly independent physicians.[51]

A bill introduced in the Massachusetts legislature would extend a similar approach to all primary care physicians. Under this measure, commercial insurers would give capitation payments to all primary care practices in the state. These payments would raise their overall reimbursement by 30% in the first year. They would also have financial incentives to enhance the delivery of high-quality, team-based primary care. Depending on how much the practices invested in infrastructure and staff to improve population health, they could double their baseline payments by year three.[52]

AI to the Rescue?

Artificial intelligence (AI) has gained dominance in the U.S. technology industry and is widely expected to transform healthcare. As a result, there are now serious discussions among health policy experts, technology executives, and physician executives about the possibility of AI taking over some of the lower-level functions of primary care physicians.

In a recent article, Joseph Betancourt, MD, president of the Commonwealth Fund, and Eric Schneider, an official of the National Committee on Quality Assurance (NCQA), argue that a combination of AI and remote patient monitoring will "radically change the way primary care is delivered within the next five to 10 years."[53]

In their vision, AI will allow PCPs to "practice at the top of their license" by performing some of their less complex duties. For example, they say, AI agents can handle low-acuity problems and screening tests with minimal intervention from a clinician. They can also identify care gaps from medical records and notify patients without asking them to come in for an office visit. However, Betancourt and Schneider caution, AI and digital technologies have some risks, so smart regulation and responsible use are necessary. AI interventions must be evidence-based and must be adequately tested.

In 2025, the American Academy of Family Physicians and Rock Health, a research company that follows the digital health space, issued an AI report based partly on a national survey of 2,500 PCPs and other clinicians. It noted there has already been a positive impact from using AI scribes to take clinical notes during patient visits. In addition, the report says, "AI assistants could triage patients, summarize charts highlights, draft personalized educational materials, provide timely decision support, design care plans and flag care gaps. Offloading these tasks could free physicians to focus on complex clinical decisions and allow human members of the team to concentrate on personal elements of quality care."[54]

Whether or not the use of AI can lessen the primary care shortage is open to question. But, with nearly a third of Americans lacking access to primary care, AI is certain to be part of its future.

CONCLUSION

As we've seen, health policy experts are working hard on new approaches to rescue primary care. Unfortunately, in the unstable political climate of the mid-2020s, it's doubtful that any of these will be enacted on a broad scale in the near future. If and when that changes, primary care payment reform will have to be closely linked with larger reforms related to healthcare financing and delivery. The leading model of that today is called value-based care (VBC). The following chapter takes a deep dive into VBC, where it came from, and where it's going.

CHAPTER 3.

What Is the Value of Value-Based Care?

Although liberal politicians and some nurse and physician advocacy organizations still support Medicare for All, the consensus among policy experts and industry leaders is that the main hope for reforming U.S. healthcare is "value-based care," or VBC.

While VBC has many different definitions, the simplest and most comprehensive one originated in a 2008 article by Donald Berwick, MD, and two of his colleagues at the Institute for Healthcare Improvement (IHI). Rescuing the healthcare system, they wrote, "requires simultaneous pursuit of three aims: improving the experience of care, improving the health of populations, and reducing per capita costs of health care."[1]

Improving population health is not independent from the other goals; it is a prerequisite for reducing per capita costs and for enhancing the patient experience. But true population health management (PHM) is beyond the capabilities of most of today's healthcare providers. As we'll see, it will take a major change in how the industry is structured and financed to transform healthcare so that it delivers better population health rather than more services.

All of this has been clear to policy experts for decades. What isn't clear is how we get from here to there. Thus, VBC has become a catch phrase for a whole host of different approaches, ranging from pay for performance and shared savings to bundled payments and capitation. Moreover, the term "value-based care" has lost much of its meaning as it has been applied to anything that promises to lower cost and improve quality.

Robert Berenson, MD, a senior fellow at the Urban Institute and a former CMS official, prefers the term "value-based payment" to value-based care, because it is more specific and quantifiable. VBP can refer to paying for outcomes, paying for quality of care, or transferring financial risk to providers, he notes. But outcomes are hard to measure; the quality metrics now being used are inadequate to measure quality; and taking financial risk doesn't say anything about how well an organization delivers care. So VBP, too, is not a good indicator of value.

In any case, I will use the broader term VBC in this chapter, because it is the term commonly used to denote the overall approach or movement.

Despite the broad academic support for this approach, it is questionable whether any kind of VBC has had a significant effect on cost growth or the quality of care. For example, only a handful of the 50-plus VBC models piloted by the Center for Medicare and Medicaid Innovation (CMMI) have saved money, and some have lost hundreds of millions of dollars.[2] The Medicare Shared Savings Program (MSSP) for accountable care organizations (ACOs) saved Medicare just over \$2.5 billion in 2024.[3] When compared with the more than \$1.1 trillion spent on Medicare that year, and the \$103 billion increase in spending over 2023,[4] that amount of savings looks puny.

The data on how much VBC has saved in the private sector is less definitive, but here's one indication: Even if private insurer VBC initiatives collectively saved as much for employers and consumers as Medicare derived from the MSSP, that putative drop in private spending would have been a drop in the bucket compared to the amount by which Medicare Advantage spending per capita has outpaced costs for traditional Medicare beneficiaries.[5] It is not surprising that, in forecasting the trajectory of national health expenditures 10 years out, CMS actuaries did not even mention value-based care as a factor.[6]

Most of the MSSP ACOs have done fairly well on a brace of quality measures, but that doesn't mean that their providers have significantly improved how well they deliver care. If more people got cancer screening or controlled their hypertension, that's just a marker for quality improvement. More pertinent are data on long-term outcomes, as well as the rates of misdiagnoses and safety events.

Some insurance companies have described quality improvements in some organizations receiving VBP,[7] but their reports haven't been validated. Nearly 700 federally qualified health centers (FQHCs) that implemented a value-based "alternative payment model," one study found, had significant improvements in blood pressure control for patients with hypertension and in blood glucose control for people with type 2 diabetes.[8] That finding, at least, shows improvements in intermediate outcomes; but again, it is inadequate to prove that patients received high-quality care.

One reason for the failure of VBC initiatives to improve quality is that they place additional burdens on providers. Many primary care clinics, for example, lack the resources to put in the requisite IT infrastructure and hire sufficient care managers for population health management. As a result, they struggle to meet VBC goals for preventive and chronic care. It is also difficult to measure quality improvement because quality measures differ from one payer to another, and quality data can be difficult to collect and report to payers.[9]

HAS THE PHYSICIAN MINDSET CHANGED?

Since most physicians care for patients with multiple kinds of insurance, it is hard for them to reconcile two opposite financial incentives: the incentive to do more under fee-for-service and the incentive to do only what's necessary under arrangements that place doctors or their organizations at financial risk. Most physicians prefer to practice the same way with all patients, and, as previously mentioned, they tend to stick to their habitual practice mode when the majority of their patients are covered by fee-for-service insurance. Conversely, when the bulk of their patients are covered under risk arrangements, there is often a "spillover effect," in which doctors apply the value-based approach to their fee-for-service patients.[10]

Ezekiel Emanuel, MD, a health policy expert and a bioethicist at the University of Pennsylvania, maintains that physicians' attitudes toward VBC have changed. In his view, this shift is partly responsible for a slowing of healthcare cost growth relative to the size of the economy, which I mentioned in the Introduction. During the decade after the passage of the Affordable Care Act, he noted in a 2023 article, the ratio of healthcare spending to GDP had remained under 18%.

Why did this happen? "The mindset of American physicians and other clinicians has changed, from ignoring costs to trying to cut them," Emanuel argued. "Instead of figuring out more expensive medical tests and treatments, doctors are now asking whether a test or treatment will improve a patient's health and how a service can be performed more efficiently by shifting where and how it is administered."[11]

Berenson agrees that physicians' attitudes have changed, but he doesn't think it's related to value-based care or the ACA. "It began before the Affordable Care Act. There has been such pressure on physicians to be mindful of spending that they are now mindful of it, but it has nothing to do with the new payment models. There's a lot lower increase in utilization. At some point, there had to be a leveling off, but I don't think it's because of value-based care."

Another factor in the cost trajectory was the shift to physician employment during the decade in question. Hospital-employed primary care doctors are not being incentivized to keep people away from specialists or out of hospitals or not to order expensive tests. In addition, the amount of waste in healthcare has not declined — if anything, it has increased, Berenson points out. Studies in 2012 and 2019 found that various kinds of systemic waste formed between a quarter and a third of U.S. health spending.[12-13]

Whatever caused the plateau in the GDP-to-health spending ratio, the growth in health costs did not cease. Earlier in this book, I discussed how quickly total health costs and insurance premiums have climbed in recent years. Moreover, CMS has projected that the increase in national health spending will exceed GDP growth from 2024-2033 and that health costs will reach $8.6 trillion, or 20.3% of GDP, in 2032.[14] When the cost of healthcare rises faster than productivity, inflation or worker's wages, a progressively higher percentage of the population won't be able to afford it without government subsidies.

THE ORIGINS OF VALUE-BASED CARE

To understand where VBC is going, it is important to understand where it came from. Essentially, VBC is a descendent of the "managed care" of the 1990s. After the failure of Bill and Hillary Clinton's healthcare reform plan, employers and insurers sought to replicate the relative success of big HMOs like Kaiser Permanente in containing cost growth. The idea was to use primary care "gatekeepers," utilization review, and financial risk to slow down spending.

However, this effort was also doomed to fail. The managed care techniques developed by Kaiser and other group-model HMOs over decades were inapplicable to the fragmented cottage industry that dominated healthcare at the time. It made no sense to ask primary care physicians who knew nothing except fee-for-service to accept financial risk for all professional services. Predictably, few practices did well in this arrangement, and many of them lost money. Consumers rejected the gatekeeper model and narrow networks, and insurance companies were soon forced to offer plans with much broader networks and less control of where and how people could seek care. Costs soon resumed their upward trajectory.[15]

Searching for a new way forward, academics like Elliott Fisher, MD, of Dartmouth University hit upon the idea of the accountable care organization in the mid-2000s. The ACO is a payment and care delivery model designed to encourage groups of physicians, with or without hospitals, to focus on improving quality and avoiding unnecessary costs. A small group of researchers and policy advocates led by Fisher refined the model. The Affordable Care Act of 2010 incorporated the ACO as the foundation of the Medicare Shared Savings Program (MSSP).

The ACO was only one of many efforts in the burgeoning VBC field, as commercial payers and Medicare looked for ways to curb cost growth. But its inclusion in the ACA signaled that the government was getting serious about having providers take financial responsibility for care.

The ACA Changes the Equation

The Affordable Care Act greatly accelerated the uptake of VBC. The ACA's care delivery provisions were designed to move Medicare providers from pay for volume to pay for value in gradual steps. Essentially, this approach requires or incentivizes healthcare providers to take ascending levels of financial risk. At the bottom of this ladder is "value-based purchasing," in which providers are financially rewarded or penalized for their performance on cost, quality, and patient experience measures. This "pay for performance" program is similar to those that many commercial insurers instituted in the 15 years prior to the ACA.

The next step up the risk ladder is "shared savings," in which provider groups try to reduce the total cost of care. If they're successful, and if they meet quality benchmarks, they can share in the savings. Under an upside-only shared savings arrangement, organizations may get bonuses for cutting costs, but they aren't liable for losses if they overspend their budget. In a two-sided risk arrangement, they must pay back some of the losses they incur to Medicare.

Some healthcare organizations take financial risk under one of the ACA's bundled-payment programs. Bundled payments usually require hospitals to take financial responsibility for an episode of care such as a hospital stay plus 90 days of post-acute care. Payments to physicians and post-acute-care providers are included in the bundle.

Most of the ACA's care delivery provisions apply only to Medicare; however, this program accounts for about a fifth of U.S. health spending and is hugely influential in the private sector. So, these aspects of the ACA are a lever designed to move the entire health system. In one Medicare demonstration model focused on primary care, private insurers collaborated with CMS. Moreover, most insurers have VBC initiatives that complement those of the ACA.

Impact of VBC Hospital Initiatives

Two of the ACA's value-based programs for hospitals offer no upside but punish them for poor performance. The Hospital Readmissions

Reduction Program (HRRP) penalizes institutions that have an excessive number of readmissions. The HRRP prevented an estimated 566,000 readmissions from 2010-2015, as the rate dropped from nearly 19% to 17.5%.[16]

The ACA also levies fines for high rates of hospital-acquired conditions (HACs), such as bedsores, falls, infections, and surgical complications. This initiative, which was introduced in 2014, has also been effective. In the first three years of the program, HACs dropped by 13%.[17] However, the Hospital Value Based Purchasing Program, a pay for performance initiative, has had little effect, because too little money is at stake.[18]

The Bundled Payments for Care Improvement (BPCI) program had only a modest impact, partly because it was voluntary and relatively few hospitals joined up. While it saved some money, mainly in post-acute care (skilled nursing facilities, or SNFs, rehab centers, and home care), Medicare lost money after paying doctors and hospitals.[19]

A mandatory bundled-payment program, the Comprehensive Care for Joint Replacement Program (CJR), was tried out in 800 hospitals, and the results were more promising. Medicare payments for hip and knee replacements decreased, and nearly half of the hospitals received bonus payments for maintaining quality and reducing costs. But when the first Trump Administration cut in half the number of areas where CJR was mandatory, most of the hospitals in the other areas dropped out of the program.[20]

Berenson is skeptical of the CJR approach, partly because it didn't reduce the rate of unnecessary surgeries, which he estimates to be about 20%. And it's no accident, he says, that much of the savings in the CJR and the BPCI programs, as well as ACO shared savings programs, represent reductions in post-acute care costs. The at-risk provider group or ACO, he notes, can simply tell physicians to send patients to home care, rather than to a SNF or rehab hospital, after hospital discharge. "That's fine, but it's a one-time savings," he says.

Physician Value Incentives

The history of physician VBC programs is more complicated, because it grew out of a different law than the ACA. The Medicare Access and

CHIP Reauthorization Act of 2015 (MACRA) authorized a Quality Payment Program (QPP) for eligible clinicians, including physicians, that went into effect in 2017. The QPP includes a pay-for-performance program known as the Merit-Based Incentive Payment System (MIPS) and the Advanced Alternative Payment Model (AAPM) program. MIPS, which is mandatory, has had little financial impact on physicians, other than to increase their expenses for tracking and reporting quality data.[21] The Medicare Payment Advisory Commission (MedPAC) has recommended that MIPs be phased out.[22]

The AAPM track is a different story. Physicians who participate in an AAPM — including the MSSP, the now-lapsed Comprehensive Primary Care Plus (CPC+) program, the joint replacement program, and certain other programs — are not subject to MIPS and were eligible for annual bonuses of 5% of their Medicare revenues for performance years from 2019-2024.[23] Moving physicians into AAPMs is critical for CMS to reach its goal of having all traditional Medicare beneficiaries in "accountable care" relationships by 2030.[24]

That goal increasingly appears to be unachievable. One reason is that physicians and other eligible clinicians are walking away from the QPP. The share of clinicians who didn't participate in a VBP model or were QPP-exempt due to low fee-for-service Medicare volume or other reasons increased from 27.5% in 2017 to 38.1% in 2022. Clinician participation in MIPS decreased from 46.3% to 26.7%, again because of QPP exemptions. While the percentage of eligible clinicians participating in ACOs that took two-sided risk increased from 7.3% to 22.2%, that was counterbalanced by a drop from 17.9% to 11.7% in clinicians who participated in ACOs with upside-only risk.

In 2022, nearly two thirds of eligible clinicians did not participate in an MSSP ACO or any other APM, including QPP-exempt clinicians and those in MIPS. Some of this was due to the shift of Medicare beneficiaries into Medicare Advantage plans. That trend reduced the percentage of traditional Medicare patients in physician practices, making QPP exemptions more likely. But, regardless of the reason, the majority of doctors are not involved in Medicare's VBC programs.[25]

Pluses and Minuses of the MSSP

The ACA's most ambitious attempt to promote value-based care was its creation of the Medicare Shared Savings Program (MSSP) for ACOs. The basic idea of the MSSP is that if ACOs meet quality goals and save Medicare money, they can share in those savings. ACOs that take upside-only financial risk — meaning they share in savings but not in losses — are eligible to receive a smaller share of the savings than those that take downside risk.[26]

To share in savings, ACOs must exceed a benchmark score on three dozen or so quality measures, which are mainly the same ones as in other quality programs that physicians are accustomed to. Not surprisingly, most ACOs receive high quality scores every year.[26] However, ACOs do better on some quality scores than do similar types of physician groups, CMS said. In 2024, they scored higher than non-ACO groups on screening for depression (53% vs. 44%) and controlling high blood pressure (71% vs. 68%).[27]

In 2024, 476 ACOs covering 11.2 million people participated in the MSSP. Overall, the program generated $6.6 billion in savings, of which Medicare retained $2.5 billion. The balance that went to providers totaled $4.1 billion, a 37% increase over 2023.[28] Even more remarkable, the amount of shared savings earned by ACOs quadrupled from 2018 to 2024, while the number of MSSP ACOs declined.[29]

This achievement occurred during the same period when the prevalence of ACO risk-taking in the MSSP greatly expanded. Sixty-seven percent of the MSSP ACOs took downside financial risk in 2023, compared to 59% in 2022 and 18% in 2018. The percentage of MSSP ACOs that received shared savings bonuses grew from 63% in 2022 to 69% in 2023.[30]

Between 2018 and 2021, the number of ACOs in the MSSP dropped from 561 to 477.[31] Some of this was because of the pandemic, but the biggest reason why some ACOs quit the MSSP was because of Medicare's efforts to accelerate the adoption of downside risk.[32] Naturally, many ACOs that weren't ready to do this dropped out of the MSSP. But CMS's approach was vindicated in one respect. In 2023, ACOs that took two-sided risk were nearly twice as likely to achieve shared savings as upside-risk-only ACOs, and those taking two-sided risk saved more than the other ACOs did.[33]

Other characteristics of MSSP ACOs were consistent with earlier trends. Physician-led ACOs did substantially better than did hospital-led ACOs, reflecting the greater incentives of the former to limit hospital utilization. And ACOs with a larger share of participating primary care physicians were more likely to achieve shared savings and higher net savings per capita. In fact, the ratio of primary care doctors to specialists in the ACO directly determined the likelihood of achieving shared savings. Moreover, the performance of ACOs relative to their benchmarks for savings increased over time for the ACOs with the highest proportion of PCPs.[34]

The outperformance of primary care-led ACOs is a critical proof of concept for the reform model proposed in Part 2 of this book. It means that, in ACOs where primary care doctors have a strong incentive to manage population health, and the influence of specialists on patient care is less prominent, value-based care is more likely to lower costs.

An earlier analysis showed that ACOs participating in both the MSSP and commercial VBC contracts produced greater Medicare shared savings than those that participated only in the MSSP.[35] What this might indicate is that, where a larger portion of a provider's revenue comes from VBC arrangements, they pay greater attention to population health management. This is plausible, and it points to the need for greater cooperation on VBC between CMS and private insurers. But the opportunity for changing how care is delivered will be limited until the ratio of VBC revenue to total revenue reaches a tipping point. It has been estimated that physicians do not fundamentally change how they treat patients until 63% of their practice income is derived from risk-based contracts.[36]

WHY MANY PHYSICIANS HAVE NOT EMBRACED VBC

Currently, there is only indirect evidence of how much physician revenue comes through value-based payments. In 2023, 28.5% of all healthcare payments flowed through downside risk contracts, according to the Health Care Payment Learning & Action Network (LAN), which derives its information from insurer claims data. Those are payments for all kinds of healthcare services, not just physician work.[37]

The American Medical Association, meanwhile, found that in 2022, 69% of physician revenue was from fee-for-service and 31%, from all kinds of alternative payment models—about the same as in 2014. Among the 64% of physicians who received APM payments from any payer in 2022, pay for performance was the most common type of APM (41%), followed by bundled payments (40%), capitation (26%), and shared savings (22%). Nearly 60% of doctors worked for a practice that was part of an ACO.[38]

What this data suggests is that, even while risk contracts have slowly spread across the industry, they have hit a wall in terms of physician revenues. Why have doctors been reluctant to accept financial risk and engage in population health management?

The short answer is that physicians don't have to do this, and they face many barriers in making the leap from fee-for-service to financial risk. One key obstacle is the fragmentation of the insurance market. Because only some health plans are willing to delegate risk to providers, and because private insurers are not coordinating their efforts with those of Medicare, only a small percentage of most physicians' patients are covered under population-based payments. Consequently, most physicians are unlikely to modify their approach to patient care.

In a 2017 paper on "accelerating and aligning primary care payment models," the LAN said, "To effectively incentivize practice transformation, [primary care payment models] should be multi-payer and cover the majority of a practice's patient population." But the LAN leaves open the question of how this is to be achieved.[39]

The Center for Medicare and Medicaid Innovation (CMMI) has experimented with a multi-payer approach in its Comprehensive Primary Care (CPC and CPC+) and Primary Care First models. But these voluntary multi-payer demonstration programs did not elicit high levels of participation from commercial and Medicaid plans.

Therefore, a National Academy of Medicine (NAM) panel has urged CMMI to mandate "all-payer health-focused primary care models with two-sided risk."[40] But Medicare cannot do this without a highly implausible act of Congress.

Infrastructure for Risk Contracting

The infrastructure required to assume financial risk for the total cost of care includes care managers, allied healthcare and IT professionals, and the health information technology needed to track patient and population health and the costs of care. Most independent practices can't afford the software or the additional staff; for the most part, only large organizations have the resources and the know-how to put such a model together. However, some smaller ACOs have pulled it off, usually with the help of management services organizations (MSOs) or specialized entities that provide health IT and other support services.

Population health management depends on the availability of timely, comprehensive information on patients. The digitization of health records has provided a key element of the requisite IT infrastructure. But the various electronic health records used by different practices are still far from interoperable, and many services are delivered by outside providers, so risk-taking groups also need access to claims data.

Although Medicare claims data is available to providers, risk-taking groups and ACOs often lack access to commercial claims data that would show them what services non-Medicare patients have received from outside providers.

A full-scale PHM infrastructure also includes health IT experts, care managers, disease educators and coaches, nutritionists, pharmacists, behavioral health specialists, and ancillary providers. The use of care teams that include these professionals and clinicians is a core element of PHM. Nurse care managers typically call high-risk patients to make sure they're following their care plans and are not getting sicker. Care managers also facilitate transitions of care for patients who have been discharged from the hospital recently and may visit some patients at home.

The care team aims to optimize population health and facilitate recovery from illness to prevent avoidable ED visits, hospital admissions and readmissions. Other competencies of the care team include identifying at-risk patients, closing care gaps, and managing chronic conditions proactively. These activities are vital to managing financial risk contracts because they help at-risk entities stay within their budgets.[41]

Specialists Versus Primary Care

Many VBC programs focus on primary care, because primary care physicians hold the key to overall cost and quality in their tests, treatments, prescriptions and referrals. They are also in the best position to coordinate care. A major goal of the patient-centered medical home — an established model for improving the quality of care in primary care practices — is to enhance care coordination, and a medical home is most often a primary care practice.

Nevertheless, as Grace Terrell, MD, and Julian "Bo" Bobbitt point out in their book *Value-Based Healthcare and Payment Models*, primary care physicians and specialists must work closely together to deliver value-based care.

> Building team-based care models and properly aligning physician incentives are key drivers to success, but they are insufficient without integrating high-impact specialty care models with primary care medical homes. An integrated medical neighborhood across the continuum of care drives performance at the system level that cannot be achieved by a siloed approach of medical homes in primary care and acute care settings focused on bundled payments or episodic-based condition management.[42]

To induce primary care doctors and specialists to collaborate this closely, they must have a shared financial incentive. Such an incentive exists in prepaid group practices such as those of Kaiser Permanente, where cost and quality outcomes have a financial impact on all group members. But such groups account for only a small minority of the physician workforce. In the fragmented medical neighborhoods that most providers work in, it has been difficult for patient-centered medical homes to gain cooperation from specialists.[43] ACOs are supposed to fill this gap and knit together different kinds of specialties; it's unclear to what extent they have succeeded, but that is the goal.

Integrating Specialists into VBC

Specialty care, roughly speaking, falls into three buckets, as a 2023 *Health Affairs* article points out:

- In "whole-person health," specialists manage and coordinate the full spectrum of care for a specialized population, such as patients with end-stage renal disease or advanced chronic kidney disease. Sometimes these specialists may be quarterbacks for patients, such as those with cancer, over an extended period.
- Acute episodic care specialists, including surgeons, focus on specific, discrete interventions or events, including procedures and acute medical events.
- Many specialists collaborate over time with primary care providers to manage chronic conditions, such as serious cardiovascular conditions, diabetes, asthma, osteoarthritis, low back, and inflammatory bowel disease.[44]

Some specialists fill more than one of these buckets. For example, an ob/gyn not only delivers babies and performs other procedures for women but also takes care of many other aspects of women's health. PCPs collaborate with specialists even in "whole-person health," where they are responsible for non-specialty aspects of healthcare. And in acute episodic care, primary care doctors may help patients decide whether to have an elective procedure and may refer them to a surgeon. PCPs continue caring for patients after they're discharged from the hospital.

Physicians taking risk through group practices and ACOs have developed several different methods for integrating specialists into value-based care. These include referral steerage, gainsharing incentives, bundled payments, sub capitation, and incorporating some specialists into a primary-care-led group or ACO.

In April 2024, CMMI officials proposed that the Innovation Center deliver enhanced specialty care data to clinicians, hospitals, and other healthcare entities so that referring physicians could make more informed decisions about which specialists provide the best value. They also said they were exploring ways to create financial incentives within primary care for specialist engagement. Among other things, they considered designing new CMS billing codes for experimental models to support ongoing communication among providers who shared a patient. And they sought other ways to help primary care doctors and specialists share data.[45]

All of these are solid ideas. But, for these plans to achieve the desired effect, physicians must have incentives to change how they practice and how they collaborate with one another. So far, the evidence shows, this has been mostly lacking, because not enough revenues of either primary care or specialty physicians are at financial risk to make it worthwhile to change.

INSURERS PUSH FORWARD WITH VBC

In 2023, 21% of commercial insurance and Medicaid payments and 34% of traditional Medicare payments were made under two-sided shared savings or population-based payment contracts. But the picture was different for Medicare Advantage plans. In that part of the market, risk contracts of various kinds accounted for a whopping 43% of payments. While MA has been ahead in the VBC sphere for years, that percentage represents a significant increase from the 29% of payments to MA providers that entailed risk in 2020.[46]

Why have insurance companies focused on the MA market in their efforts to move providers into financial risk? The biggest reason is that there is so much money to be made in Medicare Advantage, although somewhat less today than in the past. For the big carriers (except for Cigna), this is their single most lucrative line of business. By aligning the incentives of providers with their incentive to lower costs, they can increase their profits substantially. Moreover, the major MA plans have gamed Medicare's risk adjustment rules to ratchet up payments for sicker patients.[47] By inducing physicians to document additional diagnoses and more severe illnesses, the plans can benefit financially.

What's in it for doctors? Much higher payments than they are accustomed to receiving from traditional Medicare. For example, about 70% of Humana's MA members are attributed to primary care providers with VBC contracts, which range from pay for performance to two-sided shared savings to comprehensive or global risk. In 2023, Humana says, its MA primary care providers earned up to 241% of the Medicare fee schedule, while specialists earned 5%-30% more than traditional Medicare fees.[48]

As noted earlier, Humana and United — which together account for nearly half of the MA business — employ thousands of their own physicians. The health plans pay these doctors more than they pay independent physicians, making it attractive for the latter to join the insurer-owned groups.[49] So United and Humana profit on both insurance and care delivery, and they can also nudge employed physicians to boost their patients' risk scores.

Humana claims big advances on some quality metrics in its MA plans. In 2023, for example, 75% of patients with hypertension who were attributed to VBC physicians controlled their blood pressure, compared to 57% of patients with hypertension with fee-for-service doctors. Similarly, the percentages were 77% versus 65% for colorectal cancer screening and 67% versus 51% for control of blood sugar among patients with diabetes.[50]

If these data are correct, it's welcome news. But the data come from Humana and have not been validated by outside researchers.

A peer-reviewed paper cowritten by some authors outside the insurance industry found that patient health outcomes under full-risk Medicare contracts surpassed those in traditional Medicare, while utilization of resources was lower. Analyzing the outcomes of care given by 15,500 physicians in 17 groups from 2016-2019, the study found that scores on 16 of the 20 measures favored at-risk MA. These included lower rates of acute inpatient admissions, lower rates of seven of nine condition-specific admissions, lower 30-day readmissions, avoidance of unnecessary ER visits, lower high-risk medication use, and higher patient adherence to a commonly prescribed class of heart drugs.[51]

Is MA Good for Healthcare?

While MA proponents argue that Medicare Advantage has improved the quality of care and the patient experience while reducing costs, critics of the program say MA doesn't necessarily provide better care than traditional Medicare does and that it has not lowered health spending. In a 2021 *Health Affairs* paper, Donald Berwick, MD, a former CMS administrator in addition to his roles at IHI, and Richard Gilfillan, MD, former CEO of the Trinity Health System and former deputy administrator of CMS and director of CMMI, maintained that "CMS consistently overpays MA plans with no demonstratable clinical benefit to patients."[52]

The Medicare Payment Advisory Committee (MedPAC), they noted, "has documented approximately $140 billion in MA overpayments over the past 12 years. MedPAC further concludes that risk adjustment overpayments are currently increasing."

Some of the payments to MA plans are spent on additional benefits for MA members, such as partial dental, vision and hearing coverage. But Berwick and Gilfillan alleged that a far greater portion of the total goes to health plan profits than to those extra benefits. There are technical arguments on both sides, but here's what MedPAC said in its 2024 report to Congress:

> In 2025, we estimate that Medicare will spend 20 percent more for MA enrollees than it would spend if those beneficiaries were enrolled in FFS Medicare, a difference that translates into a projected $84 billion. These increased payments are the primary source of funding for supplemental benefits, which include coverage of non-Medicare services…and better financial protection for MA enrollees relative to beneficiaries in FFS Medicare without supplemental coverage.

MedPAC added that "the relatively higher payments to MA plans are financed by the taxpayers and beneficiaries who fund the Medicare program…Part B premium payments will be about $13 billion higher in 2025 because of higher Medicare payments to MA plans (equivalent to roughly $198 per beneficiary per year)."[53]

The two largest factors responsible for higher payments to MA plans in recent years, MedPAC said, are favorable selection and coding intensity. Favorable selection occurs when beneficiaries who have lower actual spending than their risk scores would predict enroll in MA plans. Coding intensity is another term for the risk-adjustment gaming.

MedPAC also observed that it was impossible to measure the overall quality of care in Medicare Advantage because of poor quality reporting by MA plans. Although MedPAC didn't say this, it is also difficult to measure the impact of limited provider networks and of MA plans' prior authorization and claims denial practices on the quality of care.

More Savings, Less Return

MA plans spend 20% to 40% less on healthcare than traditional Medicare does, according to the insurers. In a 2021 *Health Affairs* paper I cowrote with David Muhlestein, then an executive at Leavitt Partners, we asked where those savings go, if they don't reduce Medicare spending. Some of the money covers supplemental benefits and reduced or zero beneficiary premiums. But that doesn't come close to accounting for all the claimed cost reductions, we calculated. What would explain the difference? Perhaps MA plans' average annual profit margin is greater than the 4%-5% that they allege.[54]

In 2023, only a few of the ACOs in the MSSP saved 15-20% of their Medicare benchmarks. Most ACOs saved 10% or less, and only 69% qualified for shared savings.[55] One reason for the relatively low savings rate is that, unlike MA plans, MSSP ACOs are not allowed to use managed care tools such as preauthorization and limited networks. In traditional Medicare, all beneficiaries, including those attributed to MSSP ACOs, are allowed to see any provider who accepts Medicare.

The managed care tools used by MA insurers enable the plans to reduce health spending more than the ACOs can. However, the savings are not lowering society's cost of providing healthcare. Instead, the MA plans apparently skim off the lion's share of the savings as profits.

At the time of this writing, it appeared that, after growing steadily for years, Medicare Advantage has reached a plateau. Major MA insurers such as United, Humana and Aetna withdrew from many counties, and seven carriers that offered MA plans in 2025 abandoned the program altogether because of escalating medical costs, stricter regulation and narrowing margins. It was projected that total MA enrollment would actually drop slightly in 2026.[56]

CONCLUSION

When it involves financial risk and population health management, value-based care can provide the foundation for effective healthcare reform. But to date, VBC initiatives have not covered enough of the population to induce most physicians to change how they practice. Fee-for-service still dominates healthcare, and doctors follow their financial incentives. As a result, they tend to maximize their revenues from caring for individual patients rather than trying to optimize the health of their patient populations.

Hospitals and health systems are also not sold on value-based care, which many of them view as a threat to their business model. Even for institutions that support the concept, VBC is a much lower priority than labor costs, staffing shortages, or the introduction of AI.

In a recent interview with *MedCity News*, Patrick Runnells, MD, chief medical officer of University Hospitals in Cleveland, Ohio, stated that VBC is not a viable business model for hospitals. In 2024, he noted, University Hospitals' ACOs earned about $50 million in shared savings, but that was less than 5% of its total revenue. Even if the system doubled or tripled that amount, he said, it wouldn't be a major source of income.

"Most [health] systems are going to be reluctant to shift their economic engine to a value-based payment mechanism that is actually going to make them less money and be less sustainable," he declared.

To change health systems' mindset, he added, they need much more downside risk or much larger shared savings incentives.[57]

Under present conditions, value-based payment methods are unlikely to replace fee-for-service. Value-based care could prevail if our health-care system were restructured in ways that would make it feasible. But several recent policy proposals offer other methods to reform the system. Some of these proposals include VBC in a supporting role, but it's not their main focus. Chapter 4 explains them all, starting with an update on Medicare for All.

CHAPTER 4.

Recent Proposals to Save Healthcare

GOVERNMENT-BASED SOLUTIONS

When my last book was published in 2020, it seemed possible that a national health insurance program like Medicare for All could finally become a reality. In 2018, six in 10 Americans favored Medicare for All, according to a Kaiser Family Foundation survey.[1] In the runup to the 2020 election, two Democratic Presidential candidates, Elizabeth Warren and Bernie Sanders, supported a single-payer, government-run system, and Joe Biden endorsed the idea of a "public option" — a government insurance plan that would compete with private health plans.

Not a word was heard about the public option, however, after Biden became President. The public, meanwhile, shifted away from Medicare for All. According to a 2023 Gallup poll, while the majority of people still believed the federal government should ensure universal access to healthcare, 53% of respondents preferred that healthcare coverage be based on private insurance. Just 43% supported a single payer system.[2]

In April 2025, Sen. Sanders and two progressive House members, Rep. Debbie Dingell (D-MI) and Pramila Jayapal (D-CA), introduced bills that, in most respects, recapitulated the Medicare for All bills that had been floated in Congress for decades.[3-4] The number of cosponsors — 102 in the House and 15 in the Senate[5-6] — was similar to the number of Democratic Representatives and Senators who had cosponsored them in previous years.

Thus, while the state of U.S. healthcare is growing steadily worse, the solution favored by most progressives seems to have less chance of becoming law than ever. Today, Medicare for All is no longer a realistic proposal that could replace the current ailing system of healthcare finance. And, even back when Medicare for All was regarded as politically feasible, it had significant problems that I emphasized in my previous book.

Critics of single payer attack the need for higher taxes, which would be offset by the elimination of insurance premiums. The most serious flaw in Medicare for All, however, is that it does nothing to change the structure or the incentives of the U.S. healthcare delivery system. So, after a onetime reduction in administrative costs equal to about 10% of overall expenditures,[7] healthcare spending would resume its upward trajectory. The same would be true for the other major source of savings: lower payments to doctors, hospitals and other providers. Even if it were possible to get providers to accept payment rates equivalent to or slightly above Medicare rates, they'd find ways to increase their incomes by performing additional services. And, if their revenues declined enough, some hospitals would close or reduce access to services, and many doctors would leave medicine.

The underlying cost growth can't be controlled without cutting the waste in the system, which is estimated to be around a third of total spending.[8] But the MFA bills ignore or downplay the need to limit the amount of unnecessary or harmful care provided. In fact, they undercut cost control by prohibiting "participating providers from accepting or entering into any arrangement for any bonus, incentive payment, profit-sharing, or compensation based on patient utilization [of services] or based on financial outcomes of any other provider or entity."[9]

Sanders' bill would establish regional Medicare offices that would devise a mechanism "to minimize both under-utilization and over-utilization and ensure that all providers meet quality standards."[10] Medicare also would establish national quality measures and medical review criteria. However, CMS has had programs like this for years, and none of them has significantly improved quality or reduced waste in healthcare.

The MFA proposals would expand Medicare benefits significantly, including coverage of institutional long-term care, which was not included in the similar 2019 legislation. There would be no patient cost-sharing, except on some prescription drugs. And all residents would be covered, including undocumented immigrants.[11]

Liberal and conservative health economists came up with very different estimates for the cost of Medicare for All under the 2019 bills. Large areas of uncertainty existed regarding how much MFA would cost compared to the current financing system, and how much taxes would have to be raised to cover the cost of universal, comprehensive health insurance.[12]

But, in the absence of delivery-system reforms, estimates of the potential fiscal impact of MFA disregard the underlying trends that continue to push up health spending, year after year. These include the fee-for-service system that rewards the volume, rather than the value, of healthcare services provided. In addition, the introduction of new medical technologies usually increases costs. Not only are the new procedures, drugs and tests often more expensive than the old ones, but in many cases, they become an alternative to, rather than a replacement for the existing technologies. For example, the advent of angioplasty greatly increased the number of cardiac procedures but did not replace open-heart surgery.

The main mechanism for cost containment in Medicare for All is price controls, or a global national budget. But there is no evidence that price controls make healthcare more efficient. If these controls were sufficiently rigorous, they would limit healthcare access and reduce quality to the point where there would be a popular outcry against the system. In other words, something has to give.

In my previous book, I proposed a restructuring of the healthcare system that would emphasize population health in the context of a regionally controlled version of Medicare for All. But since then, as the prospects for Medicare for All have faded, I have rethought my position. As will be explained in Part 2, I now see the possibility that a multi-payer financing system — albeit one very different from the current model — could be the basis for healthcare reform that includes major changes in how care is provided.

Public Option Plans

The concept of a public option — much favored by progressives — was dropped from the Affordable Care Act because of implacable opposition from health insurers. The insurance carriers viewed the public option as a step toward Medicare for All, and they weren't wrong. Since then, the public option model has faded out, although a few states have tried versions of it. The highwater mark of the public option occurred in 2018, when Reps. Rosa DeLauro (D-CT) and Jan Schakowsky (D-IL) introduced a bill embodying the Medicare for America plan of Yale health policy expert Jacob Hacker.[13]

Medicare for America would achieve universal coverage by enrolling the uninsured, people who purchase individual insurance, and those now covered by Medicare, Medicaid, and/or the Children's Health Insurance Program. Children would be enrolled automatically at birth. Large companies could continue to buy private insurance for their employees or give them the option of enrolling in Medicare for America. Employees could also leave their employer-sponsored plans and join the public option plan, aided by sliding scale government subsidies.

The Medicare for America benefits would have been nearly as comprehensive as those under Medicare for All. The plan would have been financed by rolling back Trump's 2017 tax cuts and imposing a variety of wealth, investment, Medicare and excise taxes. Hacker envisioned that a combination of employer and worker incentives would lead to Medicare for All over time.[14]

While it offers the advantage of moving gradually from a public-private system to a single payer model, Medicare for America has the same drawbacks as Medicare for All: no reform of the care delivery system, low provider compensation, and continued reliance on fee-for-service.

Medicare Advantage for All

As noted earlier, Medicare Advantage (MA) has grown rapidly in recent years, and it now covers 54% of Medicare beneficiaries.[15] President Trump and Mehmet Oz, the CMS administrator, are strong MA proponents. Despite CMS' current crackdown on overpayments to MA plans, the Center for Medicare and Medicaid Innovation (CMMI) has reportedly been ordered to draw up plans for implementing the Project 2025 goal of making MA the default for all new Medicare enrollees.[16]

If that were to happen, it would accelerate the decline of traditional Medicare. While people in MA plans can transfer back to fee-for-service Medicare, it can be more difficult for them to obtain Medicare supplemental plans, which cover most out-of-pocket expenses that traditional Medicare enrollees are exposed to. Moreover, people who enter traditional Medicare later may have to pay higher premiums for these MediGap policies, depending on their health status.[17] Since those remaining in traditional Medicare would tend be sicker and older, MediGap premiums would likely rise. So default enrollment in MA would not only expand the program more rapidly but would also heighten the pressure to stay in these plans.

The rapid growth and popularity of Medicare Advantage have led some experts to consider it as a basis for systemic reform. Stuart M. Butler of the Brookings Institution, for example, notes that MA plans offer more flexible benefits than traditional Medicare does. Moreover, he says, MA is consistent with the managed care approach of private insurance for those under age 65. And 90% of Medicaid recipients are already in managed care plans.

"Thus, for a large proportion of households, transitioning from their existing coverage to coverage more like Medicare Advantage plans would not involve a big adjustment," Butler says.

In Butler's vision, there would be a gradual transition to Medicare Advantage for All, perhaps starting with state insurance exchange plans. The subsidy system for these exchange plans could be reconciled with the tax benefits for employer-sponsored insurance, so that a similar system of government subsidies would apply to everyone. Over time, Butler projects, employers would gradually move away from sponsoring health insurance for their workers.[18]

This proposal makes sense superficially, but it places insurers firmly in the driver's seat of healthcare. Consequently, employers, workers and taxpayers would pay more for healthcare than they would in a government-run system. As noted in Chapter 3, Medicare Advantage spends about 20% more than traditional Medicare would on the same enrollees.[19] Even if it's true that care costs 20%-40% less in MA plans,[20] as some of them claim, the lion's share of those savings goes into the pockets of insurance companies.

So, Medicare Advantage for All would not be a solution to America's healthcare woes. It would worsen them by enriching profit-seeking corporations at the expense of individuals, employers and the government.

BASIC CARE APPROACH

Litan Einav and Amy Finkelstein propose a split approach, encompassing both single-payer coverage and private supplemental insurance, in their 2023 book *We've Got You Covered: Rebooting American Health Care.*[21] These experts, who teach at Stanford and MIT, respectively, believe that all Americans should be guaranteed "basic care," including the medical services necessary to restore or maintain "basic human functions." Beyond that, they say, more affluent people can buy supplemental insurance to cover other types and levels of healthcare.

This approach has similarities to bifurcated insurance systems in other countries and is also similar in some ways to the use of private Medigap plans to supplement traditional Medicare. Yet it's unclear whether the stark divide between basic and enhanced health insurance that the authors favor would fly in the United States. Of course, we already have a multi-tiered healthcare system, in which people with more money have access to more and better care. But systematizing this difference in healthcare access and quality would probably be repugnant to many people.

The authors argue that their plan would close many of the gaps in healthcare coverage that Americans now face. For example, they note, nearly a quarter of the population is uninsured at some point in a two-year period. Medicaid benefits are hit or miss: for example, coverage of pregnancy ends after childbirth, leaving new mothers uncovered for post-partum care. Gaps in Medicare coverage leave many beneficiaries with large medical bills, and about 10% of Medicare enrollees have unpaid medical debts. Because of copays and deductibles, many commercially insured people also have medical bills they can't afford to pay.

Hospitals are obligated to provide some charity care, as well as initial care for uninsured patients under the Emergency Medical Treatment and Labor Act (EMTALA). Also, they're unable to collect 90% of hospital debts owed by individuals, note Einav and Finkelstein. In addition, they point out, the government is committed to covering healthcare for certain conditions if people can't afford treatment, including COVID, TB, breast and cervical cancer, Lou Gehrig's disease, end-stage kidney failure, HIV, and sickle cell anemia. Taken together, they aver, these factors make it clear that we already have a mandate to cover everyone for certain kinds of care, but in an unfair and inefficient way.

"As long as it is an unavoidable function of government to try to provide health care for those in need, then universal health insurance is the right vehicle for fulfilling that obligation in a full and sensible manner," they state.

Furthermore, they note, universal coverage must be automatic, which wouldn't be the case if insurance premiums were charged for basic coverage. The authors also favor eliminating most copays, which pose a barrier to care for the poorest people. Research shows that few people seek healthcare unless they need it, so getting rid of copays wouldn't raise costs, they argue.

The first red flag in their proposal goes up when they present their list of medical services that can be excluded from basic coverage: Among these are infertility treatments, dental care, vision care, physiotherapy, and long-term care. Dental and vision care are for the teeth and the eyes, which are undeniably part of the human body. Physiotherapy is essential for a range of musculoskeletal ailments. Reasonable people can differ on infertility treatments, but society must find some way to cover long-term care, whether it's at home or in an institution. Today, the bulk of institutional care is covered by Medicaid.

Einav and Finkelstein also maintain that new technology is the main driver of rising health costs. It's a very important driver, accounting for

40-50% of spending growth,[22] but it's certainly not the only one. They completely miss the role of preventive and chronic care in ameliorating costs by reducing the need for hospitalization and specialty care.

This isn't surprising. Toward the end of the book, they make this astonishing statement: "We can tackle the problem of coverage — and fulfill our social contract — without tackling the problem of healthcare delivery."

Einav and Finkelstein frankly admit that going from our public/private insurance system to the universal basic coverage they're proposing would result in worse coverage for the people who now have private coverage and Medicare beneficiaries. "We suspect that many of them would purchase supplementary insurance," they suggest blithely. Well, yeah, but how about the millions who can't afford it?

Clearly, this book doesn't provide the solution to our healthcare crisis. But it does offer one worthy idea that can be built on in a different context: the concept of basic care. While Einav and Finkelstein regard this as the minimum necessary to sustain life and limb across the healthcare spectrum, one can also define basic care in a different way. That is the care that most people need most of the time, until they have a serious health emergency that requires more expensive care, such as a heart attack, a cancer diagnosis or a traumatic injury. Viewing basic care this way can provide a useful frame for restructuring healthcare.

'SOCIAL FLOOR' GUARANTEE

A trio of experts — including Katherine Baicker of the University of Chicago and Amitabh Chandra and Mark Shepard of Harvard — offer another take on using basic care to reach universal coverage. Starting with universal coverage as a goal, they describe a "social floor" of insurance that everyone would be guaranteed. Like Einav and Finkelstein, they also endorse "top-up coverage" for the more affluent that would take the form of either supplemental or replacement insurance.[23]

The authors acknowledge that the idea of a guaranteed basic bundle alongside private supplemental coverage would be controversial. Many people believe strongly in equal access to care, regardless of income or ability to pay, they note. Allowing a top-up plan means higher-income people would have access to more healthcare, which would potentially lead to better outcomes for those people, they point out.

The United States needs a government-backed social floor for health insurance, they argue, because the current patchwork system of incremental market reforms has failed to get everyone covered. But, if we want universal coverage, we must recognize that it is impossible to provide all possible care to everyone, they point out. The fairest way to proceed would be to have the government ensure basic care to all, while allowing private insurers to sell top-up policies to wealthier people.

The key questions about this social floor approach, they write, are these:

1. How do we define the scope of the basic bundle? The issue is not whether healthcare is a right, but how much healthcare we are all entitled to. Beyond a list of covered benefits, there are questions of medical necessity and what mechanisms are used to limit spending on covered services, such as global medical budgets, provider prices, capacity constraints, patient cost sharing and utilization controls.
2. Who is in charge of administering and delivering basic coverage? In the U.S. system, some decisions are delegated to private insurers, while others are subject to federal and state regulations. A more coherent system would lower administrative costs.
3. Decisions must also be made on whether and how individuals can use private funds to obtain additional coverage beyond the basic package. For example, in a population with a wide range of incomes, generous supplemental coverage could result in a wide range of health outcomes. On the other hand, the more topping up there is, the greater the incentive for innovators to invest in new tests and treatments.

Making the Basic Bundle Explicit

The current system, the authors note, already provides a floor of guaranteed coverage via EMTALA and nonemergency care in community health centers, safety net hospitals, and clinics that treat people regardless of insurance status or ability to pay. They call this the "implicit basic bundle." The United States could make it explicit "through automatic, free enrollment in some form of coverage financed by general revenues." While not being specific about what basic benefits should include, they say, "The key input into this social welfare function should be the value of the care in improving health relative to the resource cost of the care. Care with health benefits that sufficiently exceed resource costs should be included."

Care that clearly warrants its cost — such as emergency care for acute events like accidents, strokes, appendicitis, pulmonary embolisms, or life-sustaining medicines — should be covered in the basic bundle, they maintain. But lots of other services that are costly and have questionable benefits would likely be the subject of "heated" debates. Another desirable objective, they say, would be for the insurance model to encourage and support innovations in medical technologies and care delivery. They argue that public coverage of basic care won't do this, but top-up private insurance will.

Addressing the second design question about what mechanisms are used to control spending, Baicker, Chandra and Shepard dismiss arguments that we can fund universal coverage by eliminating waste, fraud and abuse, eliminating private-sector profits, or reducing administrative costs. "Aside from the limited magnitude of such potential savings, such arguments miss the inherent opportunity cost of spending on care with diminishing returns…With scarce resources, there is an inherent tradeoff between covering more people and covering more resource-intensive services."

One way to make these choices is through a centralized public process, they observe. For example, legislation could set broad guidelines to define a basic care bundle and empower a medical board or government agency to define the details. Other countries mandate basic benefits and cost sharing rules, but private insurers offer a variety of specific plans. The upside of centralized decision-making is that it's simple and has low administrative costs, the authors say. The downside is that "public entities may make suboptimal decisions."

To get away from the "one size fits all" approach, they note, healthcare providers could be capitated — that is, prepaid on a per-enrollee basis. The aim is to incentivize the providers to innovate in ways that attract enrollees while holding down costs. The authors cite the Medicare Advantage program and the ACOs in the Medicare Shared Savings Program. But these examples are like apples and oranges. They conflate the insurance risk of health plans with the financial and care delivery risk of provider-run organizations. While some MA plans capitate their physician networks, the plans themselves haven't saved money for Medicare. In contrast, ACOs led by healthcare providers have achieved savings.

Advantages of "Top-up" Insurance

Discussing the design feature of top-up insurance, the authors note that "there is social value in letting people choose a plan that fits their preferences." Moreover, top-up plans "relieve the budgetary pressure of providing a substantially large bundle of health care for everyone." Private insurance, they argue, also can help guide administration of the basic bundle by providing an "external benchmark of value." In addition, allowing a top-up supplement to the basic bundle would not require the elimination of the employer-sponsored insurance plans that now cover more than 160 million Americans.

Among the areas where the basic bundle could be supplemented, the paper suggests, are patient cost sharing, add-on services, the breadth of provider networks, and "medical amenities." The main mechanisms for supplying these extra benefits would be a wraparound supplemental plan or a replacement plan that supplants the basic program.

Most other countries with national health insurance allow supplemental plans that cover services or providers not covered by the public system. For example, U.K. residents can use National Health Service doctors and hospitals for free, but they can also purchase private insurance that covers care at private hospitals with private rooms and shorter waiting lists for nonemergency procedures. In Germany and Chile, wealthy residents can opt out of the public system and buy private plans instead. Canada doesn't allow private coverage of its

Medicare services, but Canadians can buy coverage for noncovered services, including prescription drugs.

In the United States, Baicker, Chandra and Shepard observe, taxes would have to be raised to provide healthcare to the currently uninsured without substantially cutting back on care already covered by existing public programs. But these higher taxes could be counterbalanced by lower private insurance spending. As a result, they suggest, workers might not see too much of a difference in their take-home pay.

Aside from the authors' failure to address care delivery, there is much to commend in their "social floor" approach. Any universal coverage model that hopes to gain public support must provide basic care to everyone and must give people of greater means the opportunity to buy better coverage. Other countries' experience has shown that both of these elements are necessary. The question is where to draw the line between "basic" and "supplemental." Also, how do we design a standard benefit package that meets people's health needs, even if they can't afford a top-up plan?

THE MARKET WILL FIX IT

In a deeply considered and wide-ranging 2023 book called *The Coming Healthcare Revolution: 10 Forces that Will Cure America's Health Crisis*, David W. Johnson and Paul Kusserow take no position on the best way to achieve universal coverage. Instead, they delve extensively into the flaws of the care delivery system and how to fix them. Their implicit assumption seems to be that if people became healthier and their healthcare needs were met, costs would drop and everyone would have good access to care.[24]

Before I explain their perspective more fully, allow me to introduce the coauthors. David W. Johnson is the CEO of 4sight Health, a thought leadership and consulting company that posts articles about healthcare reform on its website. A sought-after speaker and the author of three books, Johnson worked in healthcare investment banking before founding 4sight Health.

Paul Kusserow is the chairman and former president and CEO of

Amediys Health, a home care company which was recently acquired by United HealthGroup. He is also executive chairman of a women's healthcare company and another firm that supports home caregivers. In addition, he is a cofounder and chairman of Healthpilot, a "Medicare choice optimization technology company."

Johnson and Kusserow's critique of our healthcare system is spot on. They note that healthcare spending growth has reached the point where purchasers have no more to give. The high cost of private insurance, they point out, has contributed to middle class wage stagnation. Meanwhile, lower-income people with chronic conditions are forgoing care, making them sicker.

The fundamental problem of "Healthcare Inc.," they write, is that it is a sick care system focused on increasing volume and revenues rather than on improving patient outcomes. The main goal of healthcare providers in this system is to care for people when they get sick, not to keep people healthy or manage their chronic conditions. In their view, our society needs to reorder its priorities and resources to prevent people from developing chronic diseases or letting them get worse. A key component of that effort is addressing social determinants of health, which account for around 80% of the differences in the health of individuals (see Chapter 12).

Johnson and Kusserow allow that some government regulations are needed to assist in the transformation of healthcare. But their central thesis is that market trends already underway will do most of the heavy lifting to reach the Holy Grail of affordable, high quality, consumer-friendly care.

Here's a quick summary of their macro-economic trends:

1. The U.S. population is aging and growing sicker, placing increasing demands on a shrinking workforce (as a percentage of the population) to fund health costs.
2. The rest of the economy cannot continue to subsidize healthcare at an ever-increasing rate. So Healthcare Inc. will have to find a way to do more with less.

3. U.S. healthcare has not done a good job of controlling or preventing chronic diseases, which continue to afflict more Americans and cause more preventable deaths.
4. Breakthrough innovations in digital technology and biological science, including genomics, can help providers diagnose and treat diseases more efficiently and effectively than in the past.
5. Aided by growing price transparency and innovative digital apps, consumers are starting to take control of healthcare buying decisions, just as they have in other fields.

The market-based changes that authors say can address these megatrends are as follows:

1. *Whole-person health.* There needs to be a massive resource shift away from treatment to prevention and health promotion. The authors believe this shift has begun.
2. *Care redesign.* This means using technology-driven care models to deliver whole person health at lower costs with better outcomes and personalized service delivery.
3. *Care migration.* This refers to the migration of care from high-cost hospitals to outpatient care sites, including ambulatory surgery centers and the home.
4. *Aggregators' advantage.* Johnson and Kusserow cite the emergence of new health platforms that can help consumers navigate the health system while empowering them to manage their own care needs and well-being.
5. *Empowered caregivers.* Healthcare providers must be supported better so they can provide topnotch care. "Optimizing human potential builds loyalty, enriches organizational cultures, drives better results and creates market differentiation."

Moving Away from FFS

Despite their emphasis on market forces and technological advances, Johnson and Kusserow agree with VBC proponents that no real progress can be made without moving away from the fee-for-service payment system. "Healthcare's future belongs to those payer and provider organizations that can manage the care for individuals and populations under fixed payment arrangements," they state. They also maintain, "Capitated payment models are critical for balancing resource allocation between health-oriented and treatment-oriented activities."

The authors offer no guidance on how we can reach that goal. As they point out, most health systems are clinging to their traditional, volume-based business model. But they argue that competition from nimble, innovative, tech-based companies will force providers to react.

In the future, they predict, there will be fewer hospitals, and those that remain will become "focused procedure factories" and specialized "solution shops." That process has already begun with ambulatory surgery centers (ASCs), which payers favor and which many health systems are acquiring. But hospitals in affluent areas are continuing to build new wings and towers, and the demand for inpatient care has never been higher.

The authors also cite "hospital at home" (HaH). In this approach, patients with certain acute conditions are cared for at home with the help of telehealth, remote monitoring, and nurse or paramedic visits. Aided by new digital technology and a temporary Medicare waiver, HaH gained traction during the COVID pandemic, when hospitals were seeking a way to relieve pressure on their inpatient wards.

Studies show that the quality of HaH is equivalent to that of inpatient care, and its costs can be lower.[25] Yet a 2024 study found that only about 300 hospitals — 10% of those eligible — had applied for HaH waivers from CMS.[26] One reason may be that hospitals find inpatient care more profitable than hospital at home. Also, the technology needed to support HaH is expensive, and only larger health systems can afford it. Another factor is that HaH is difficult for rural hospitals to implement because of the nurse visits required; in fact, most hospitals with HaH programs are located in metropolitan areas.[27]

Meanwhile, the authors note, payers are trying to move post-acute care from skilled nursing facilities (SNFs) to the home as much as possible. At-risk ACOs also prefer home care to SNFs, and there's no doubt that this trend will continue to grow. But there's a limit to how much care can be provided at home, and CMS lowered payments to home health agencies in 2026.[28] Moreover, both HaH and home care require more unpaid work from home caregivers, nearly half of whom are already performing medical and nursing tasks usually done by clinical professionals.[29]

Consumerism and Whole Person Health

Consumers have become accustomed to performing many of their daily tasks online, Johnson and Kusserow note. That is true whether one is emailing or texting people, using banking services, making reservations for a restaurant or a vacation, or buying goods on Amazon. But, when it comes to navigating and using the healthcare system, consumers tend to rely on phone calls, in-person visits, and to a lesser extent, health system portals. By shifting as much of healthcare as possible to digital apps and tools, the authors aver, and by combining that with "whole-person health," centered around each individual's needs and preferences, healthcare can be made easier, cheaper and more effective.

"Combining whole-person health with consumerism is the path by which the U.S. can improve the overall health status of its people," they write. "Unleashing the American innovation engine to enhance outcomes and improve health status is how the U.S. can catch up and even surpass the performance of healthcare systems in other high-income countries."

Interestingly, this statement follows the authors' reference to a Commonwealth Fund report that explains why other advanced nations have much better healthcare outcomes at much lower cost than the U.S. does:

1. They provide for universal coverage and remove cost barriers.
2. They invest in primary care systems to ensure that high-value services are equitably available in all communities to all people.
3. They reduce administrative burdens that divert time, efforts, and spending from health improvement efforts.
4. They invest in social services, especially for children and working-age adults.[30]

Delivery System Woes Omitted

Johnson and Kusserow strongly endorse reducing administrative spending and increasing investments in social services. But they barely allude to the uninsured or the primary care crisis. In making their case for whole-person health, they cite the success of this approach at the Veterans Administration, a single payer, integrated system that is the opposite of the fragmented, uncoordinated health system used by nonveterans. To be sure, the foundational element of whole-person health — integrated, individualized care plans that encompass clinical care, behavioral care, activities of daily living, and social determinants of health — should be a major feature of any restructured healthcare system. But, without universal coverage, affordability, and high-functioning primary care, whole-person health is impossible.

The authors' emphasis on consumerism also has its limitations. People do want healthcare to be as easy to navigate as an ATM machine, but healthcare is orders of magnitude more complex than personal banking. Take the concept of pricing transparency, which is designed to increase competition in healthcare. In 2019, the Department of Health and Human Services (HHS) issued a regulation requiring hospitals and payers to post online the negotiated prices of "shoppable" healthcare services. After a court battle, the new transparency rules went into effect for hospitals in January 2021 and for health insurers in July 2022.[31] The Biden Administration greatly increased the fines on hospitals for noncompliance. But as of July 2023, only 36% of hospitals were in full compliance with the transparency regulations.[32] A 2025 Trump executive order sought to strengthen compliance, but the result is unclear.[33]

It's also unclear how much attention consumers pay to these hospital price lists. For starters, when a patient needs an elective procedure, they're likely to go to the hospital their doctor recommends if it is in their insurance network. Even if that hospital has made a good-faith effort to post its negotiated price for that procedure, it may be difficult for the patient to understand the medical codes in the price list, market research consultant Hal Andrews told *MedCity News*. In addition, he noted, there is no unified directory of price lists from all the area hospitals, so the patient has no basis of comparison. What's needed, he said, is something like the SABRE system used by airlines and by aggregators like Expedia and Priceline to post comparative prices for specific routes.[34]

Upstart Competitor Makes Waves

Johnson and Kusserow provide many other examples of the consumerism they allege will save healthcare. High on their list of the new companies that "get it" is Transcarent. With self-insured employers as its customers, Transcarent provides software, personal guidance, and contractual relationships that help employees find the care they need from high quality providers at an optimal price. Using a business model similar to that of Expedia, hotels.com, and other aggregators, Trancarent puts consumers in charge of their purchasing decisions. The twist is that employees are rewarded for what Transcarent regards as wise choices.

For example, the Transcarent app tells the employee which local pharmacy has the lowest price for a medication and then waives the copay if the person fills the prescription there. If an individual needs elective surgery, they can use the app to compare hospitals and clinics, some of which may be in their health plan. Assuming they select a high-quality provider based on Transcarent's advice, the visit is booked for them and they have no out-of-pocket cost. If they choose a different provider, they book the visit themselves and are subject to the copay and the deductible in their employer's health plan.

Johnson and Kusserow view the upsurge of innovative, technology-driven companies like Transcarent as a real threat to the business model of the "incumbent" health systems. Lending credence to this view, large amounts of private capital are being invested in these companies.

Transcarent is starting to gain traction in the market. After only a few years in business, it claims to have over 1,700 employer and payer clients with a total of 20 million covered lives.[35] Amazon's One Medical, which includes concierge care and an advanced primary care company, among its other services, says its clients include 8,500 organizations of various sizes.[36]

But are these companies changing how health systems do business? Johnson and Kusserow acknowledge that the incumbent healthcare providers have been very slow to change. Most systems have been reluctant to engage fully in value-based care, as noted earlier. As for dealing with the rise of consumerism, some providers have tried to improve their portals and change how they treat their customers; the authors cite Baylor Scott & White's consumer-facing app, which helps patients manage their health and healthcare in whatever care setting they prefer. The Mayo Clinic has an advanced care at home program that includes not only hospital at home, but also infusions, skilled nursing, medications, laboratory and imaging services, behavioral health, and rehabilitation services.[37] Intermountain Healthcare has a similar home care program.[38]

But these big health systems are not typical of healthcare providers. Most institutions are probably unaware of companies like Transcarent, One Medical, and Oak Street, or don't regard them as direct competition. Many systems are busy merging with other systems or are acquiring parts of the care delivery chain that they don't already own, such as ambulatory surgery centers, urgent care centers, and skilled nursing facilities.

In thinking about healthcare reform, it's always a good idea to remember how big this industry is. It takes a lot of power to turn a $5.3 trillion-a-year ship around. While market forces got us into our current plight, they won't necessarily get us out. Unless the major players can be convinced that following a more beneficial path can also be profitable, we may not be able to change course while there's still time to avoid the iceberg.

THE CONSUMER AND TECHNOLOGY WILL FIX IT

Another healthcare reform advocate who believes that consumers and technology can fix healthcare is Stephen Klasko, MD, author of the book, *Feelin' Alright: How The Message In the Music Can Make*

Healthcare Healthier.[39] The title might seem whimsical, but Klasko, a former CEO of the Jefferson Health System in Philadelphia, is also a former radio DJ who firmly believes in the wisdom and healing power of popular music. While that viewpoint lightens the introduction to each chapter, this book is full of insights gleaned by Klasko during a long career as a healthcare executive and an ob/gyn.

(Full disclosure: I helped Klasko write his book; as a result, I'm thoroughly acquainted with his thinking, but I don't agree with all of it. All the ideas in the book are his, except in the chapter that addresses the challenge of healthcare financing. I'm indebted to Klasko for his idea of a subscription model for basic care, but I created the rest of the framework myself. My concept of bifurcated financing for basic and major medical care, first proposed in *Feelin' Alright*, is explained in Part 2 of this book.)

Klasko's main thesis is that we need a consumer revolution that harnesses the power of individual preferences to bring about the necessary changes in healthcare. In his view, new technologies and entrepreneurial startup companies can give consumers the means to use their power to improve healthcare. The technologies that can make this happen range from telemedicine, remote monitoring and mobile apps to AI, genomics and drones. Private investors are supplying the necessary capital to scale these technologies to the point where the desired changes can occur, he maintains.

Klasko predicts that 90% of healthcare will eventually take place at home, and he offers the usual analogy to online banking. If telehealth reduced the need for in-person ambulatory care, and a large portion of hospital and post-acute-care services moved home, up to 60% of sick care could be provided at home, he estimates.

There are several signs that consumers are already taking matters into their own hands, Klasko notes. First, they got used to telehealth during the pandemic, and it has now gone mainstream. Most providers offer telehealth services, although they still form a small portion of patient encounters, and there are also virtual-first health plans.

Second, millions of consumers now routinely use urgent care centers and retail clinics for their minor healthcare needs. It's a whole lot less frustrating and much quicker than trying to get an appointment with a primary care doctor, he points out.

Third, many consumers are taking advantage of direct-to-consumer options ranging from concierge care and "direct" primary care to advanced primary care companies like One Medical's Iora subsidiary, ChenMed, and Oak Street, which is owned by CVS. The doctors hired by these primary care companies can give seniors in Medicare Advantage plans more individualized attention because of how they are incentivized.

Klasko also accents the rising importance of online provider reviews, which are now the most important factor in choosing a doctor. In one survey, 83% of consumers said they went online to read reviews of a physician after receiving a referral from another provider.

The book devotes a lot of attention to remote patient monitoring (RPM), which Klasko sees coming together with telehealth and AI. "To the extent that they prevent avoidable hospitalizations, decrease the need for office visits, and enable most healthcare to be provided at home, the combination of RPM, telehealth, and AI can also reduce costs," he says.

RPM is being increasingly used with some patients, but the problem of how doctors can deal with all that data on a timely basis has still been only partly solved (see Chapter 10). CMS gave a boost to RPM in 2018 by issuing regulations that reimburse doctors for using it, and some private insurers have followed suit. But fee-for-service reimbursement of RPM is a clunky compromise, and the technology is still not used widely outside of the VA system and a few big health systems like Kaiser Permanente, Geisinger, UPMC, Ochsner, and Mass General Brigham.

Self-service Healthcare

Klasko touts an approach to healthcare that he calls "health assurance," in which patients play a central role in their own care. This makes a lot more sense than the current system, in which physicians are expected to educate patients and engage them in self-care, but don't have enough time to spend with them, he says.

Following in the footsteps of Eric Topol's 2015 book *The Patient Will See You Now*, Klasko writes about a future in which continuous physiological monitoring will generate data for both patients and their care teams. The concept of the physical exam by a doctor will become passé, he says, when the patient's latest monitoring data, genomic data and information about his or her social determinants of health provide a full picture of the patient's health and what he or she must do to maintain or restore it. When the patient does see a doctor for anything other than an acute illness, the conversation will revolve around the latest monitoring data, recent developments in the person's life, and the treatment plan if the individual has a chronic disease.

There is much more in this book about the role of technology, including startups that address a variety of health conditions. But Klasko doesn't pin all his hopes for a new and better healthcare system on technology. He also devotes some space to population health management, citing The Villages Health (TVH), the outpatient health system of The Villages, a sprawling Florida retirement community. Klasko helped found this community health system and recruited its chief medical officer, Jeffrey Lowenkron, MD, when Klasko was running the University of South Florida Health System.

TVH takes full risk for its senior patients from Medicare Advantage plans, allowing its doctors to do whatever they think is necessary to keep their patients healthy. The system has formed a network of high-quality specialists to whom the primary care doctors refer patients judiciously, and it contracts with two area hospitals.

According to Lowenkron, TVH is making money on its MA risk contracts, and it's in the 99th percentile for quality of care. This shows up in the fact that only 146 per 1,000 TVH patients are admitted to the hospital each year, compared with 249 per 1,000 for all MA patients and 370 per 1,000 for traditional Medicare patients.

Lowenkron attributes a big part of TVH's success to the half-hour doctor visits that its patients get. He also credits the nurse navigators who spend time with patients who have chronic diseases between visits to make sure they're following their care plans.

Interestingly, while TVH offers its patients the option of telehealth visits, only about 10% of the patients use telehealth for primary care. TVH doesn't utilize RPM very much, because of the lack of automated decision support in RPM systems.

The system employs its own hospitalists to round on patients in the hospital. They help keep the length of stay shorter than average, while maintaining low readmission rates. The hospitals are happy with this approach, because it enables them to increase their throughput of patients and avoid CMS penalties for excessive readmissions.

TIERED USE OF TECHNOLOGY

I've discussed reform proposals based on tiered benefit structures and others that rely primarily on new technologies and consumerism to transform the system. With the rapid adoption of AI in healthcare, it is now possible to talk about a tiered use of technology, as well. Robert Wachter, MD, professor and chair of the department of medicine at the University of California, San Francisco, posits just such a model in his new book, *A Giant Leap: How AI Is Transforming Healthcare and What That Means For Our Future.*[40]

Wachter's book is an invaluable contribution to our understanding of healthcare AI and the profound changes it is starting to introduce into clinical care. In this well-researched, insightful tome, he predicts that generative AI will improve productivity so much in healthcare over the next 10 to 20 years that it will enable the health system to meet a surging healthcare demand that currently exceeds the supply of healthcare providers. Eventually, we may be able to do with fewer clinicians, he projects.

As healthcare AI continues to improve, it seems likely that this prediction will come true. But I disagree with Wachter's suggestion about how to deploy AI in primary care:

> In a world of exploding healthcare costs and massive shortages of primary care clinicians, I foresee the emergence of a tiered system, loosely analogous to our current system of concierge care, with many patients who have basic insurance plans being offered — or choosing, perhaps driven by easier access and lower copays — AI-first care. This AI would assess new symptoms, answer questions, and manage common conditions like hypertension, diabetes, high cholesterol, depression, and asthma with a human clinician providing oversight in the background and an escalation path for complex cases. In contrast, patients with more generous insurance plans, greater ability to pay, or particularly complex clinical needs will be offered human-first care — although some may prefer an AI-based option, particularly if it's more convenient.[41]

To begin with, this system is unjust. While AI chatbots may be better than no care in a world where a third of Americans lack a regular source of primary care, they are not a substitute for physicians, even if a doctor lurks in the background. According to a recent study, AI chatbots are currently no better than Google at guiding users toward correct diagnoses or helping them determine what they should do next.[42] Much of the problem stems from users' inability to fully explain their health problems to the bots; even when AI improves, the average person's understanding of how to state their issue will not. So, it's simply unfair to consign less affluent people to AI-based primary care. Wachter implicitly confirms that AI care is not — and will never be — equivalent to human care by saying that better-off people should have direct access to doctors.

We need to fix primary care, not cede it to machines. Wachter's model implies that primary care as we know it is beyond repair. I've heard something similar from other experts. But if we changed the healthcare system so that primary care physicians were given a central role in it — and reimbursement to match — I believe human primary care could be saved. It must be, or the majority of people will lose access to the humans best suited to help them.

As will be explained later, AI can be a big help in the kind of care management needed to prevent and control chronic diseases. However, it cannot direct population health management. That should be the responsibility of care teams led by physicians.

CONCLUSION

The experience of TVH and many other providers committed to population health management shows that accessible, patient-centered primary care and appropriate incentives for care providers can have a significant effect on quality and outcomes. New digital technologies have their place and will become increasingly important in the evolution of healthcare. Population health management also requires specialized software that enables providers to keep people healthy, guide them through the system when they need care, and manage their own financial risk.

In looking back over the reform proposals I've summarized in this chapter, one clear dividing line is between the ideas that are only about healthcare financing and those that are only or mainly about care delivery. It's counterintuitive, however, to think about solutions for one of these without the other. How care is delivered has a direct impact on costs. Conversely, how care is financed determines how much and what kind of care can be provided. Without dealing with both halves of the healthcare equation, reform ideas have no chance of success in the real world.

The other major theme coming out of these proposals is that, without buy-in from both the industry and consumers, no reform model can succeed. That is true first and foremost of Medicare for All, which would turn off most of the industry and would fail to provide high quality, comprehensive care at an affordable cost. Medicare Advantage for All might come closer, but only if health plans were willing to surrender a large portion of their profits. Even then, consumers are fed up with insurance companies deciding what care they can get.

The Einav-Finkelstein thesis might work for the industry players, but not for the average consumer who would be consigned to lower-quality care than the more affluent would get. The Baicker-Chandra-Shepard "social floor" plan suffers from the same defect, but consumers might accept it if the basic care bundle were sufficiently comprehensive. What's missing are any ideas about how to control spending, especially costs related to new medical technologies.

As outlined above, both the Johnson-Kusserow and Klasko books provide fascinating ideas about how consumerism and technology are changing and will change healthcare. But technological optimism is no substitute for the hard work of rebuilding the healthcare system, and leaving the solution to market forces guarantees that the profit motive will override all other considerations.

In the end, we have to look elsewhere for the solution to our out-of-control healthcare spending and the decline in Americans' health. The answer rests in the hands of physicians, who ultimately provide or supervise most of the professional care we receive. That is the core of the reform model described in the following chapters.

PART 2.

Restructuring Healthcare

CHAPTER 5.

Splitting Insurance in Half

HOW TO RESTRUCTURE HEALTHCARE FINANCING

If our goal is high-quality, comprehensive, affordable healthcare for all, we must make healthcare less profitable. If health systems and corporations continue to control healthcare and their main goal is profit, health costs will continue to rise faster than the ability of society to pay, regardless of any reform efforts.[1]

On the other hand, if we threaten to take the profit out of healthcare, the major players will rebel and nothing will be accomplished. That is the most important reason why Medicare for All is impossible. Healthcare providers don't want a big cut in their revenues, and insurers don't want to be cut out. The players must be taken care of, or effective reform will not occur.

To achieve our goal, we must thoroughly restructure our healthcare financing and delivery system. But, on the surface, relatively little would change if the model I propose in this book were adopted. Healthcare would continue to be financed through a combination of individual, employer, and government funds, rather than through a single payer system financed entirely by taxes. Employees' health insurance costs would continue to be deducted from their paychecks, just as they are today.

Insurance companies would continue to play a key role in the healthcare system. In fact, they would supply a limited form of health insurance to nearly everybody, including those on Medicare and Medicaid. (Medicare Advantage plans already cover more than half of beneficiaries, and 90% of Medicaid recipients are enrolled in private plans.) You may recall that I said just the opposite in Chapter 4, where I stated that Medicare Advantage for All would simply increase the profits of big insurers. But in this model, allowing private carriers to take over public insurance for part of healthcare would help keep them whole. By covering a smaller set of services for a larger population, they could earn most of what they do now.

Allow me to explain. In the Einav-Finkelstein and Baicker-Chandra-Shepard proposals discussed earlier, the path to universal coverage led through a division between "basic benefits," which would be guaranteed to all, and "top-up" coverage that more affluent people could purchase. I pointed out that many people would be upset about getting a lower level of benefits than they do now — especially in the Einav-Finkelstein model, which would guarantee insurance that is worse than Medicare or commercial coverage today.

I don't think that's what most Americans want from a reformed health system. What they want is high-quality care for all. So, let's redefine basic benefits. Instead of being skimpy coverage for all healthcare, basic benefits should cover the care that most people need most of the time. This would include primary care and the lower levels of specialty care, including preventive, chronic, and minor acute care. It would encompass all the tests and drugs that primary care physicians and non-hospital specialists order (up to a certain dollar level). And it would also include dental, vision, hearing and behavioral care, all up to a certain limit. Everybody would have the same basic care benefits.

No private or public insurance would be allowed for basic care. Instead, competing, independent primary care groups of a certain size would charge subscription fees that would roll up to an annual budget for each group. Similar to insurance premiums for basic care, the subscription fees would come from individuals, employers, and the government, and an employee's portion for individual or family coverage would come out of his or her paycheck. People would choose a basic care group based on its subscription fees and its published quality and patient experience ratings.

Everyone would have a basic care subscription, regardless of their economic status. In addition to employer contributions, the government would subsidize people's fees on a sliding scale, based on their income, and would cover the poor entirely. CMS would buy subscriptions for Medicare beneficiaries, and the federal and state governments would purchase them for Medicaid recipients.

As the architects of Obamacare discovered, small businesses don't want to be forced to cover their employees. So, my model would require only firms with 50 or more workers to help pay for basic care subscriptions and for the "major medical insurance" discussed in the next section. It might seem that small employers would drop their insurance if they knew the government would pay their share. But that didn't prove to be the case when the Affordable Care Act (ACA) was implemented, making coverage more affordable to small businesses and their workers. While many people were covered under the Medicaid expansion or ACA plans, there was little change in the percentage of small firms offering insurance at that time.[2]

'Major Medical' Redefined

Under my model, when a person was admitted to the hospital or went to an outpatient facility for surgery or complex chronic care, the financing of those services would transition from their basic care subscription to what I call "major medical insurance." At one time, this term referred to low-cost, low-benefit health plans, but that is not what is meant here. In this approach, major medical plans would cover all inpatient and post-acute care for a designated number of months. They would also cover outpatient services above a certain cost level. That would include procedures in an ambulatory surgery center, cancer care, and other high-cost treatments. Similarly, major medical would pay for costly tests like MRIs and PET scans, as well as expensive drugs approved by the FDA.

Major medical insurance, like ACA plans, would have standardized benefits. Of course, some people would want additional benefits, so supplemental plans would be sold to those who could afford them. These plans might give people more choice of providers, pay for amenities in hospitals (a single rather than a double room, for example), or cover certain very expensive drugs or cosmetic treatments. But they wouldn't constitute a separate tier of benefits for the well-off, as in two of the models discussed in Chapter 4.

The major medical plans, like commercial health insurance today, would have provider networks. Hospitals in each state would charge all payers the same for the same services, and most of them would have global budgets that included post-acute care but not physician services. (See the discussion of state all-payer rates and global budgeting below.) Apart from that, the insurers would be free to negotiate rates with other providers, including specialists, and their networks would be limited to contracted providers. The government would guarantee that these networks were adequate, and none of them would be exclusive; all plan members would be able to use non-network providers for an additional cost.

Like the subscription fees for basic care, major medical insurance would be universal, funded by employers, individuals and the government on a sliding scale. Whether an individual was employed or not, they'd be able to purchase one of the health plans available in their region through a marketplace similar to those for ACA plans. They would choose a plan with the help of published cost and quality-of-care rankings.

To be truly affordable, the total out-of-pocket cost of basic care subscriptions and major medical insurance would have to be limited to a certain percentage of earnings — say, 8% of household income. Low-income individuals, once again, would pay nothing. To ensure access to care, there would be no deductibles and only minimal copays to discourage unnecessary use of healthcare services.

Long-term Care Is a Challenge

What about long-term care? This is a gnarly issue because of its high expense and the difficulty that most elderly people have in paying for it. Younger people may also need long-term care if they are affected by a traumatic accident or a deadly, wasting disease. Round-the-clock care in a skilled nursing facility (SNF) can quickly bankrupt a patient and/or their family, and many people can't afford to hire a home health aide to assist with activities of daily living (ADL).

Today, Medicare pays for up to 100 days of care in SNFs and rehab facilities; after that, the patient pays.[3] As a result, Medicaid picks up the tab for the bulk of institutional care, once a patient has paid down their assets; Medicare covers only professional services for individuals who are "dually eligible" for both Medicare and Medicaid.[4] This approach is unavoidable in my model, but it doesn't contradict anything else in the model. As noted above, CMS and the states would buy basic care subscriptions for Medicare and Medicaid beneficiaries. They would also continue to cover most long-term care, while major medical would insure inpatient and post-acute care (PAC) episodes and other types of expensive healthcare.

Home care is more challenging on a conceptual basis. Today, Medicare covers only up to 100 days of skilled care in the home. This doesn't include paying a home aide to help with a patient's ADL, although Medicaid will cover that under certain circumstances.[5] Clearly, many people need help for longer than that, and they need assistance that goes beyond medical care.

There are ways to make it easier for patients and their families to cope with the cost of home care. First, there's the rapidly growing Programs of All-Inclusive Care for the Elderly (PACE), which provides home care, prescriptions, meals and transportation for mostly dual-eligible older adults.[6] Private insurers have recently partnered with some PACE operators, and the major medical plans would be allowed to do this as well.

Second, if social services and healthcare organizations worked more closely together (see Chapter 12), community health workers could help look after elderly shut-ins and ensure they got nutritious meals. Primary care doctors, of course, would also deliver basic care to these patients and refer them to specialists or admit them to hospitals. Health systems with global budgets might also assist people with certain conditions to prevent them from being readmitted, as many hospitals already do with patients suffering from heart failure.

No Self-insurance Allowed

Self-insured employers, which cover about 165 million people,[7] have their own health plans that are administered by insurers or third-party administrators. While they don't save a great deal by self-insuring, many companies do it because a federal law exempts employer-sponsored health plans from state-mandated benefit requirements and insurance premium taxes.

My model would not permit self-insurance, for several reasons. First, self-insurance would be incompatible with the subscription fees for basic care. Second, the major medical system would work only if plan benefits were standardized. And third, employees must have a choice of plans, which they usually don't have if their employer is self-insured.

The ban on self-insurance would be a boon to insurers. Today, most commercial carriers have "administrative-services-only" (ASO) contracts with self-insured employers, and those ASO arrangements are less profitable than full insurance policies are. So, between the self-insurance prohibition and the conversion of traditional Medicare to Medicare Advantage, the health insurers would be able to generate fairly decent profit margins.

Limiting Insurer Profits

Of course, we wouldn't want their profits to be too high, because that would mean higher premium costs. The remedy includes governmental interventions coupled with a dose of free-market competition.

First, the Affordable Care Act specifies that 85% of premium revenue collected by large insurers and 80% of small carriers' premium revenue must be spent on medical care, leaving the rest for administration, marketing expenses and profits. If this "medical loss ratio" (MLR) falls short of these percentages, the difference must be rebated to consumers and employers.[8] Although at least one insurer, United Healthcare, has played games with the MLR by overpaying its sister company Optum's employed doctors,[9] this approach has helped limit commercial insurance profits. In my model, I'd lift the required MLR to 90% for all insurers. One reason is that, if hospitals had global budgets, the insurers' administrative costs would be much lower.

As mentioned in Chapter 1, the concentration of insurers in local markets has increased significantly in recent years. According to a 2025 report from the American Medical Association, at least one insurer held a commercial market share of 30% or greater in 91% of metro areas, and one insurer held a market share of at least 50% in 47% of metro areas.[10] Without significant price competition, a dominant insurer could raise the cost of their plans to employers and consumers. In that case, the government might have to impose price caps on those insurers, but only in markets with minimal competition.

Weighing the positive against the negative factors for insurers, their average profit on each plan member would be lower than it is today because they'd be covering only part of healthcare and because of the higher MLR requirement. Yet, considering the major expansion of their consumer base, they'd still have a good business under this model.

MARYLAND'S GRAND EXPERIMENT[11]

As noted earlier, health systems have amassed immense market power through consolidation, and their aggregate profits have climbed faster than those of insurers. In markets where one big healthcare organization owns most or a large chunk of the delivery system, how do we prevent that system from continuing to charge exorbitantly high prices to private insurers? Even in markets divided among medium-sized health systems, what will stop some hospitals from charging much higher prices than others do for the same services?

In my view, the answer is clear: Congress should adopt a national all-payer rate setting requirement, based on the Maryland statute that helped bring down that state's hospital costs. Under this system, commercial insurers, Medicare and Medicaid all pay the same rates for the same services provided in a particular hospital.

While some observers think other states could replicate the Maryland model, we should not leave this important regulation up to the states, which might or might not adopt such laws. A federal requirement that made funding of Medicaid at current levels dependent on all-payer rate setting would induce states to implement this approach.

Besides pioneering the all-payer approach, Maryland also has led the way in requiring hospitals to adopt global budgets. Since these successive efforts are key building blocks in my reform proposal, it's worth considering their history and their results in detail.

In partnership with CMS, Maryland embarked on its rate-setting experiment back in 1977. Under its CMS waiver, the state negotiated all-payer rates with each hospital, taking into account its historical and projected costs and revenues. As a result, government payments rose and those of private payers declined, but no hospital could use its market position to play hardball with health plans.

In 2022, commercial insurers in Maryland paid hospital prices that were 11%-15% lower than the rest of the nation, on average; Medicare paid hospital rates that were 30%-44% higher than fee-for-service payments under its inpatient prospective payment system and 58%-66% higher than payments under its outpatient prospective payment system.[12]

Nevertheless, Medicare saved nearly $1 billion in Maryland from 2014-2018, following the introduction of the state's global budgeting system, and the annual savings have probably risen since then. If the earlier savings had been projected to the entire country, they would have dwarfed the cost reductions of any other CMS program at the time, including the Medicare Shared Savings Program and CMS's primary care and bundled payment models.[13]

Transition to Global Budgeting

Maryland took a while to reach this position. When the state implemented its all-payer rate setting in the 1970s, the mean cost of a Maryland hospital admission was 26% above the national average. In 2007, it was 2% below the national average. But, starting in 2000, after the state eliminated payment adjustments based on the volume of admissions, hospital volume increased rapidly.[14] By the end of the decade, the CMS waiver that allowed Maryland to operate its rate-setting mechanism was threatened, due to the rising cost of hospital care.[15]

Because the all-payer system had served hospitals and insurers well, they united behind the state's proposal to switch to global budgeting, which was approved by CMS. After trying this approach with rural hospitals and achieving some success, Maryland inaugurated the global budgeting system statewide in 2014.

Under the global budgeting model, the state's Health Services Cost Review Commission (HSCRC) and the hospitals built an annual budget for each hospital's inpatient and outpatient costs, excluding post-acute care. The budget was constructed from the hospital's revenues during a base period. Each year thereafter, the budget was adjusted, based on several variables. The HSCRC set the rates that each hospital used to bill all payers so that their total payments (based on expected utilization) would match the global budget.

The global budget established a ceiling on each hospital's revenues. If the revenues varied from the global budget, the following year the hospital either raised its rates to compensate for the amount it came in under budget or, if it exceeded the budget, lowered its rates so that payers could recoup the overage. To make it easier to navigate this requirement, hospitals were allowed to adjust their rates plus or minus 5% to stay within their budgets.[16]

Promising Early Results

A CMS-commissioned study found that from 2014-2018, Medicare beneficiaries had 2.8% slower growth in total expenditures ($975 million in savings) under the all-payer, global budgeting model relative to a comparison group. These savings were largely driven by 4.1% slower growth in total hospital expenditures ($796 million in savings) compared to the comparison group of hospitals outside of Maryland. Outpatient services accounted for the bulk of reductions in hospital spending.

The report attributed an additional reduction in total Medicare spending to "savings on professional services in hospital settings and post-acute care (PAC). Although these services were not subject to global budgets, lower spending for professional services in hospital settings is consistent with decreases both in inpatient admissions and use of some hospital outpatient department services. The reduction in expenditures for PAC was likely due to the decrease in inpatient admissions, because an inpatient stay is required to qualify for these services. It could also reflect the significant investments hospitals made in post-discharge planning and care that may have allowed patients to avoid PAC services."

Commercial plan members had a 6.1% slower growth in hospital expenditures than the comparison group did. However, the growth in total spending didn't slow among commercial plan members. This reflected other utilization patterns for the commercial population, especially increased spending on professional services that offset savings on inpatient care.

The Medicare data showed that the program's savings on hospital services were not due to cost shifting to sectors outside of the global budgets, the report said. "Hospitals were more likely to transfer patients to PAC providers following the implementation of global budgeting. However, hospital length of stay prior to a PAC transfer decreased slightly less in Maryland than in the [out-of-state] comparison group, suggesting the Maryland hospitals did not try to transfer patients out of hospital settings sooner as a result of the All-Payer Model."

Significantly, the report found, "Maryland hospitals were able to operate within their global budgets without adverse effects on their financial status." But teaching hospitals and public hospitals with a disproportionate share of low- or nonpaying patients had worse patient outcomes than other facilities did, especially in unplanned admissions and follow-up visits.[17]

Total Cost of Care Program

While hospital costs dropped, non-hospital spending in Maryland, mainly in ambulatory and post-acute care, increased by 4.1% in 2016, greatly exceeding the average national increase of 1.9% that year.[18] This rapid cost growth led to the conclusion that something more was needed to control spending growth in areas outside of hospitals' global budgets.

In 2019, CMS and Maryland launched the Total Cost of Care Model (TCOC), which set a per capita limit on Medicare's total cost of care in the state. While retaining global budgeting, this program allowed hospitals to use some or all of the savings they created for Medicare to make incentive payments to non-hospital providers that collaborated with the hospital to improve the quality of care. In addition, the hospitals could incentivize primary care physicians to coordinate care better and reduce the hospitalization rate of their patients.[19]

An analysis of the TCOC program, published in July 2021, found it was making some progress.[20] Although the pandemic impacted Maryland hospitals, they didn't perform worse during the crisis than did hospitals in other states. In fact, they weathered it somewhat better, because they weren't dependent on fee-for-service revenue.

Ezekiel Emanuel, MD, and several other health policy experts argued in a *Health Affairs* article that the Maryland global budgeting model could be successfully introduced in other states. This would not only save money, they maintained, but would also "accelerate the adoption of innovative health care services, including virtual care delivery, hospital at home, enhanced primary care services and risk-based contracting."[21]

In addition, rate setting and global budgeting would take away health systems' market power. No longer able to use their size to extract high prices from commercial payers, they would have to become more efficient and focus more on delivering high quality care. Global budgeting would work much better than some states' efforts to impose hospital rate caps[22] or the federal government's weak attempts to restrain health system mergers on antitrust grounds.[23] And it could be successful even in the most consolidated markets.

EXPANDING THE MARYLAND MODEL

Maryland's approach would work well in my reform model if some key changes were made in it. To begin with, some of the outpatient services offered by hospitals fall under the heading of basic care, which would be covered by subscription fees. So only ambulatory care services covered by major medical insurance would be part of the health systems' global budgets.

Second, while the Maryland hospitals do not take risk for post-acute care, they would in this model. One reason is that PAC is inextricably connected to acute care. If hospitals were financially responsible for the cost of PAC, they would not refer patients sooner to PAC providers and would try to ensure that the patients they did refer were not readmitted. That would incentivize health systems to send patients to higher-quality facilities. In addition, hospitals would want to reduce the cost of post-acute care wherever possible. That would encourage them to send patients home with high-quality home care where appropriate.

Overall, hospitals with global budgets would have an incentive to deliver excellent care with a minimum of resources. In essence, value-based care would replace their fee-for-service incentives. Because of that, they'd be aligned with the basic care groups that, under this model, would take financial risk for the bulk of ambulatory care.

The global budgeting model would be a win-win for insurance companies. Not only would it reduce their administrative costs, but it would enable them to lay off the bulk of their risk to health systems. As a result, they would not require prior authorization for tests or procedures. The health systems would do their own utilization management with the cooperation of their specialists and PAC partners.

ED Transition Zone

The dividing line between global hospital budgets and ambulatory care budgets is unscheduled acute care, mainly in the emergency department. In my model, emergency care is considered to be basic care until a patient is admitted to the hospital or transferred to another facility. If an individual seeks emergency care for a non-urgent problem, they are diagnosed, treated and released, as anyone would be in an ambulatory care setting.

By including ED visits in the basic care budgets, the model would discourage primary care doctors from sending patients to the ED unnecessarily. But, since most physicians would know better than to do that, the main reason for including emergency care in basic care is that it would give the basic care groups a direct way to track their patients' use of the ED. Some people use the ED for primary care and would probably continue to do so even if they had a personal physician. That doctor's care team would be informed of such visits, and they'd reach out to these patients to urge them to visit their office for primary care.

In addition, some people just don't seek medical help of any kind until it's unavoidable. Again, when these folks hit the ED, their basic care teams would be informed and could create care plans to help these patients improve their health.

One logistical problem arising from this approach is the question of who would pay the ED physicians. These doctors can't work for multiple basic care groups; the hospital is the environment in which they practice; and they need to work closely with inpatient clinicians. So, like other hospital-based physicians, such as radiologists, anesthesiologists and pathologists, ED physicians would work for or be contracted to their hospital, and their salaries would be excluded from the basic-care budget.

Other kinds of specialists would be paid either by basic care groups or insurers, depending on their specialty and the type of case. Independent specialists would continue to be paid fee-for-service, but they'd have an incentive to deliver high-value care. Both hospitals and basic care groups would be at financial risk for their portion of healthcare spending. Therefore, specialists who delivered high-quality care at a reasonable cost would likely get the lion's share of business from both parties. Hospital-employed specialists would have the same incentive on the basic care side.

Getting Hospitals Onboard

Even if all the states introduced all-payer rate setting and global budgets, it doesn't mean that all hospitals would be on board. The states could force the issue, however, by leveraging hospital payment rates. Currently, hospitals charge private payers an average of 240% of Medicare rates, claiming that they need that much to counterbalance the underpayments of Medicare and Medicaid. Experts have calculated that they could make up those underpayments if they were paid 140% of Medicare for privately insured cases. If all payers were charged the same for identical services, this would translate to about 120% of Medicare rates.[24]

Let's say that a state imposed that rate on its hospitals. If they stuck with fee-for-service, they'd find it difficult to do better than break even. But if they took financial responsibility for care, they could earn more money by delivering high quality care within their budget. So they'd have a strong incentive to accept a global budget, because that would be the only way they could produce a decent margin.

This is not to say there wouldn't be a lot of pain and protests along the way. But, over time, most hospitals would learn how to live with global budgeting, just as the Maryland hospitals have.

Hospital Report Cards

As I pointed out in Chapter 4, hospitals have been under government pressure to post lists of negotiated prices for common services but have notably dragged their feet, despite substantial fines for noncompliance.[25] If all-payer rates and global budgeting prevailed under my model, public price lists would be unnecessary, because the differences between various hospitals' rates would have no direct impact on consumers. But consumers would still want to know how the quality of care in a particular hospital compared with the quality of other hospitals in an area. In addition, basic care groups would want that information to help physicians decide where to send their patients for inpatient care. They'd also want to see similar data on skilled nursing facilities (SNFs), rehab facilities, and home care agencies.

Quality is not easy to measure, especially in hospitals and SNFs. Mortality and complication rates for procedures, adjusted for patient risk, are a starting point, but are too broad to yield much insight. Process measures, such as what percentage of patients receive prophylactic antibiotics before surgery, are too narrow a gauge. A hospital's compliance with safety measures and how patients feel 90 days after a procedure might come closer to the mark, because they show how a hospital does overall in areas that are important to patients.

For report cards on quality to be credible, they must be compiled by a neutral third party. As will be explained further in Chapter 6, regional health authorities, comprised of employer, consumer and provider representatives, would supervise the health system in each region. Among the duties that each of these authorities would delegate to an independent firm called a "health utility" would be the collection of quality data that would be used in reports on basic care groups. These health utilities would apply national, standardized metrics so that nobody could complain that the results were biased or invalid. And the health status of each patient would be factored in so that the results would be risk-adjusted for each physician group.

State agencies would create quality reports on hospitals and PAC providers. The compilation of this data at the state level would offer a better comparison of hospitals' quality measures than data at the regional level.

CMS already has similar online report cards for hospitals and PAC providers across the country. But data is missing on many providers, the measures are suspect, and only a small fraction of Medicare beneficiaries have looked at the data.[26] While it's hard to predict how much better report cards such as those described above would do, it's likely that improved quality measures, coupled with a concerted advertising campaign, would raise the report cards' profile.

Continuity of Care

While it could be argued that the model I'm proposing might harm the continuity of care, there is no reason why that has to happen. The system could be designed so that a patient passing through different stages of care, from ambulatory to acute to post-acute and back again, would receive services seamlessly, with the insurance type operating in the background.

Take somebody newly diagnosed with type 2 diabetes, for example. Perhaps the patient's diagnosis was missed for years, and they already show some severe symptoms. Their primary care doctor would work with an endocrinologist to curb the diabetes. But, if the patient's disease progressed to the point where a toe had to be amputated, they'd be admitted to the hospital. Their health coverage would invisibly switch from their basic care subscription to their major medical insurance. Everyone would get paid, and the patient wouldn't notice.

Moreover, the bipartite structure of healthcare financing would have some advantages other than that of keeping insurance companies whole. For one thing, both health systems with global budgets and at-risk basic care groups would have the same incentives to reduce waste and lower the cost of care. So, as population health improved, and as fewer people were admitted to the hospital, not only the basic care groups but also health systems would benefit financially. Additionally, it would be difficult if not impossible for physician groups to take risk for the total cost of care. It would be much easier for them to assume risk only for basic care, letting insurance companies handle the rest.

CONCLUSION

This bifurcated healthcare financing system, coupled with the budgeting of providers, would help slow health cost growth; in the long run, it could decrease overall health spending. One linchpin of the model's effectiveness would be its ability to reduce the number of people who needed hospital care. Improving basic care would lead to far fewer people being hospitalized or referred to specialists. As a result, patient outcomes would be better and costs would be lower.

The onus would be on the providers of basic care to improve preventive and chronic care and coordinate care better. Chapter 6 will explain how a system of competing, at-risk primary care groups can achieve this goal, and how such a system can be created.

CHAPTER 6.

Liberating Primary Care Physicians

PRIMARY CARE IS THE KEY

To achieve effective healthcare reform, corporate control of healthcare must be reduced, and primary care physicians must be placed in charge of basic care delivery. The formation of primary care groups capable of taking financial risk for basic care would represent a giant step toward both goals.

In Chapter 2, I cited a NASEM report about the importance of primary care. Here is a more succinct expression of the same idea, from an essay about how the lack of support for primary care has thrown our healthcare system out of whack:

> Primary care plays a foundational role in an efficient, high-quality health care system. It is the only element of the health care delivery system in which an increased supply is associated with better population health and a reduction in inequitable outcomes. Studies find that continuity in primary care reduces mortality, health care expenditures, and hospitalizations.[1]

High-quality primary care is also the linchpin of value-based care, the main hope for saving our system. However, in most health systems, primary care physicians are rewarded for production and referrals, with relatively little emphasis on quality. Insurers that employ physicians are more concerned with value, because it reduces their costs; but they are mainly in it for the money, rather than for improving long-term patient outcomes.

Accountable care organizations, which are in the vanguard of VBC, have had some success in reducing costs, as we've seen. In the Medicare Shared Savings Program, physician-led ACOs that take downside financial risk have been the most successful in that regard.[2] And, within that cohort, ACOs in which primary care predominates have outperformed: High primary care-centric ACOs generated 2.4 times as much savings as low primary care-centric ACOs from 2017–2022.[3] Let's take that lesson and use it as the basis for a radical restructuring of healthcare delivery. But first, primary care physicians must be liberated from their corporate overlords.

Corporate Practice of Medicine Laws

Most PCPs currently work for health systems or corporate entities. But, if the government wanted to pursue this reform model, there are ways to force these employers to divest their primary care practices. For example, many states have "corporate practice of medicine" laws that bar corporations from employing physicians directly. These statutes were enacted to avoid conflicts of interest between physicians' duty to provide the best care for their patients and their employers' dictates — exactly the kind of conflict in which many doctors find themselves today. Most states with such laws allow hospitals to hire doctors, however, since they're also in the business of medicine.[4]

The sole exception is California. That state's corporate practice of medicine law prohibits any non-professional organization except for a public hospital, a narcotics treatment program, or a nonprofit medical research firm from directly employing physicians. Unfortunately, the California corporate practice of medicine law has not had the intended effect. Instead of hiring doctors, private hospitals and health systems simply lease their services from "foundations" that stand in for professional corporations.

With robust incentives from the federal government, states should enact stronger laws that prohibit hospitals from directly or indirectly employing primary care physicians. The statutes should be written so that they also apply to insurance companies, private equity firms, and corporations that employ primary care doctors, such as Amazon's Medical One and CVS' Oak Street. The laws should also state that only primary care doctors are affected because they are a scarce and vital public good.

Strong Opposition Can Be Expected

Hospitals would not have to be compensated for returning primary care physicians to private practice. It's not clear that most hospitals would be worse off economically if their medical staffs were independent rather than employed. Considering that hospitals lose a median $315,358 per year per employed physician, due to rising salaries and practice expenses,[5] some hospitals would benefit financially from divesting their owned practices. The hospitals' main concern would be to prevent competitors from controlling their referring doctors. If no health system could employ primary care physicians, that wouldn't be a problem.

Nevertheless, many hospitals would undoubtedly file lawsuits — or class action suits — against their state governments. They might claim they were being unlawfully deprived of revenues that their employed primary care physicians generated in excess of what those doctors would bring in if they could refer to other hospitals, but this might be a hard case to make in court. Government attorneys would point out that hospitals cannot legally require employed doctors to refer to them. They could also observe that hospital employment of doctors has driven up health costs and, in some cases, resulted in inferior or unnecessary care.

The hospitals might also argue that they were being forced to divest their primary care practices without compensation for their intrinsic value. Most hospital-owned generalist practices, however, were acquired for little more than the value of their hard assets (equipment, fixtures, etc.) and receivables, with their goodwill loaded into employment contracts. Since most of these practices are losing money, it would be difficult to maintain that the hospitals should be compensated for giving them up. While it might be argued that some practices are more valuable because they belong to ACOs that generate shared savings, it's hard to put a number on how much more such a practice would be worth, healthcare consultant Michael La Penna says.

Based on some published sales figures,[6-7] it appears that insurers, PE firms, and primary care companies paid fairly high prices for their primary care practices. So, it would be more difficult for the states to force them to divest those practices without compensation. Perhaps some version of "eminent domain" could be used, because the PCPs are a scarce public good. If not, La Penna suggests, the federal government might create something similar to its program to pay off medical school loans for young doctors who agree to work in underserved areas. Instead of loans, the government would be paying off some fraction of a practice's fair market value over time. While this would amount to a large sum — United alone employs upwards of 25,000 PCPs — it might be justified if it helped save the healthcare system.

Other commentators have suggested using the state corporate practice of medicine laws to force companies to divest their practices. For example, in a piece about the failure of primary care as a business, Kevin Grumbach, Deborah J. Cohen, and Yalda Jabbarpour propose that these laws be tightened to avoid corporate manipulation of Medicare regulations and maybe to prohibit PE firms and insurers from owning physician practices.[8]

It's unclear whether these tactics would be legal, and, even if they were, whether all states would follow the federal directive. But if they didn't, healthcare systems in a non-cooperating state would be unable to switch to the new financing and care delivery system. That would pose a thorny problem for employers doing business in that state.

GETTING READY FOR THE NEW SYSTEM

Ironically, the consolidation of the industry has prepared most primary care physicians to form independent groups capable of delivering value-based care. Because of employment, the majority of doctors are used to working together in large groups. Also, nearly 60% of physicians work in practices that belong to ACOs,[9] and many others have had experience in taking risk from Medicare Advantage plans, participating in Medicare VBC demonstrations, or working for primary care companies dedicated to VBC. So, forming groups of primary care doctors that take financial responsibility for basic care should not be a big stretch for many physicians.

But how do we get from here to there? There are a tremendous number of practical considerations involved, and we should not expect this transition to happen overnight. Still, most of the country should be ready for the new model within five years after the project launch date. My guesstimate is that it would take about two years to prepare the primary care doctors in a variety of practice settings to come together in basic care groups, and another three years for them to form the groups, build the requisite infrastructure, and learn how to manage population health. (See Chapter 11 for my ideas on how to apply this model in rural areas, where primary care is much thinner on the ground.)

Would physicians who are now salaried employees want to make this career jump? After all, most of them now work in a comfortable corporate environment; they're familiar with their health system's or another employer's electronic health record; and, for the most part, they don't have to pay attention to the business of healthcare.

Despite those factors and the power of inertia, many employed physicians are unhappy, as explained in Chapter 2. They have little control over the conditions of their employment or how they practice, and they often feel morally compromised when they can't do what they want to for patients. Primary care doctors also know that they're supposed to refer patients to hospitals, specialists and ancillary facilities within the health system, whether or not that's good for the patient. Many physicians, particularly in primary care, are burned out and are considering retiring or leaving medicine.

So, if the question is whether a lot of primary care doctors would jump at the chance to try something new and build a better future for themselves and their colleagues, the answer is Yes. Undeniably, other doctors would prefer to stay where they are, either because they fear an independence they've never known or because they just don't like change. But in my model, they would have no choice but to go out on their own, because hospitals and corporations would be required to let them go. They could then join their colleagues in forming basic care groups or start their own practices — a daunting prospect for doctors who have always been employed.

How about primary care physicians who have their own practices and don't want to join these groups? They can remain independent if they want to. But, because no insurance for basic care would be allowed, they could accept only patients willing to pay them in cash. Some of these physicians would probably charge subscription fees for their own services, as today's "direct" primary care practices do. But all consumers would be required to buy basic care subscriptions, and most of them would not want to pay twice. So as older doctors retired, small independent primary care practices would probably fade away.

Before forming basic care groups, PCPs would undoubtedly look for colleagues with whom they felt comfortable practicing. This is not just a matter of personal relationships; doctors in the basic care groups would become business partners, and their own financial well-being would depend on how the other doctors in their group practiced. If they worked well in care teams and were wise stewards of healthcare resources, the group would benefit, and so would the physicians who owned the group.

Effects on Multispecialty Groups

Many high-functioning multispecialty groups exist today, either on their own or as part of larger entities. Mayo Clinic, Cleveland Clinic, Intermountain, Geisinger, Partners Healthcare, Baylor Scott & White, Kelsey-Seybold, Summit Medical Group, Everett Clinic, Ochsner, Advocate…the list goes on. What happens to those groups in this restructuring?

The corporate practice of medicine laws wouldn't apply to these multispecialty groups. But they would encounter the same problem that independent primary care practices would: their charges for basic care would be in addition to the subscription fees everyone would have to pay. Thus, their primary care physicians would not contribute much to group revenues, and both the practice and the PCPs would be better off if the latter joined a basic care group.

The big multispecialty groups would survive the splitting off of their primary care doctors, and they could lend technical support to local basic care groups, perhaps in return for specialty referrals. The primary care physicians leaving the multispecialty practices could also refer to their former colleagues and collaborate with them electronically.

The hardest challenge would be the Kaiser Permanente groups, some of which include thousands of doctors. Each of these groups might spin off dozens of primary care practices in their regions.

It might be argued that dividing up multispecialty groups in this manner would increase the fragmentation of healthcare providers. On the other hand, virtual integration of care teams, which will be explained in the next chapter, could get all the providers caring for a patient on the same page.

Assembling Basic Care Groups

The building blocks of basic care groups already exist. In 2022, there were more than 1,000 accountable care organizations (ACOs), of which 41% were physician-led.[10] Within the MSSP, 61 ACOs, or 11% of the total, consisted mostly or wholly of primary care doctors in 2018, the latest year for which I could find data on this. The median size of MSSP ACOs in 2018 was 315 physicians; ACOs with commercial contracts tended to be bigger.[11] So hundreds of ACOs included enough PCPs to form groups of the requisite size.

Large multispecialty groups, as noted above, could also give birth to basic care groups. In 2022, 18.3% of physicians practiced in groups of more than 50 doctors.[12] Many of these groups were owned by hospitals. If the hospitals divested the primary care physicians in these practices, they could form the nuclei of many basic care groups of the desired size.

The American Medical Group Association (AMGA), which represents mainly large groups, has 440 members. The median number of doctors in these groups is 180.[13] Assuming that a quarter of these physicians are PCPs, nearly 220 AMGA member practices include enough PCPs to form one or more basic care groups of the size needed, as explained below.

Overall, it appears that at least 1,000 basic care groups could be created out of the box. That's far short of the number of competing groups that would be required under my reform model; but six in ten practicing physicians work for hospitals,[14] and the majority of doctors participate in ACOs.[15] Therefore, it's likely that the actual number of PCPs already working together in groups of the requisite size is larger than appears on the surface.

What Kind of Financial Risk?

Over the decades since the first wave of managed care, U.S. physicians have shown themselves to be markedly risk averse. That's understandable: In the 1990s, insurance companies tried to jam the HMO style of practice down the throats of doctors across the country. They made primary care physicians into gatekeepers, which both doctors and patients hated. Some primary care doctors took full professional risk before they knew how to manage care and lost their shirts. On top of it all, a significant drop in capitation rates in California, the birthplace of HMOs, wiped out some physician groups.

Primary care capitation, which is much more common today than prepayment for all professional services, carries far less financial risk for primary care physicians. However, it doesn't motivate most doctors to practice differently if only a minority of their business is prepaid. In addition, it can incentivize some doctors to refer out to specialists more frequently than they'd do otherwise.

Many ACOs have shared savings contracts with commercial and/or government payers. For example, in the "enhanced" risk track of the MSSP, ACOs take upside and downside risk for the total cost of care for their attributed Medicare patients. These ACOs receive up to 75% of the shared savings; if they spend more than their benchmark amount, they must pay a minimum of 40% of the overage back to CMS. The upside can't exceed 20% of the benchmark, or historical spending level, and the downside can't exceed 15% of it.[16]

The two-sided risk tracks of the MSSP have gained considerable traction. In 2018, only 18% of MSSP ACOs accepted two-sided risk; in 2025, 71% of participating ACOs did.[17] Thus, most PCPs participating in the MSSP now know how to handle downside risk, and the same is probably true on the commercial side.

In my previous book, I suggested that the primary care groups in my model would need a transitional payment model to help them learn how to manage risk. I proposed a hybrid payment model, part fee-for-service and part capitation, that has been successfully deployed in CMS' Comprehensive Primary Care Plus program. As mentioned earlier, NASEM and some policy experts have endorsed this approach as a method for paying individual PCPs. But at a group level, it might be unnecessary, since so many doctors now have experience with risk.

The question is, how much risk should they take? In this model, they would be financially responsible only for basic care, as defined in Chapter 5. But should they accept 100% of that risk?

Recall that in the MSSP "enhanced" risk track, the maximum upside and downside can't exceed 20% and 15% of the benchmark, respectively. However, in CMS's ACO Realizing Equity, Access and Community Health (ACO REACH) model, a demonstration that began in 2023, some of the participants take a much higher amount of risk. ACOs that select full professional risk accept 50% of the savings or the losses, and ACOs that choose the global option take 100% of the upside and downside risk.[18] In 2023, ACO REACH participants generated $1.643 billion in gross savings and $694.6 million in net savings for CMS. Nearly 75% of participants earned net savings, including 79% in the global risk option and 67% in the professional risk category.[19]

So, these ACOs clearly were able to handle a larger amount of risk than those in the enhanced track of the MSSP. Moreover, the ACOs in the professional risk category take *full professional risk* — i.e., the cost of paying all the providers of care from primary care doctors to neurosurgeons. In my model, the basic care groups would take risk only for basic care, not for the professional or ancillary aspects of major medical care. The amount spent on basic care is a minority of healthcare spending, which is driven largely by inpatient care, higher-end outpatient care, and post-acute care. On balance, therefore, it appears that the basic care groups could take full risk for the portion of care they'd be responsible for.

How Big Would the Groups Be?

The basic care groups must be large enough to take financial risk of the kind described above. In addition, they must have the human and technological resources required for population health management. However, they can't be too large, or the groups won't be able to compete on an even playing field.

Lawrence Casalino, MD, a professor of population health sciences at Weill Cornell Medical College, told me that groups of between 10 and 30 physicians could assemble the infrastructure to do disease management (a forerunner of population health management) and measure performance. Managed care companies have fielded risk-taking groups with 20 to 80 doctors each,[20] and the Rio Grande Valley Health Alliance, a network in southern Texas, has shown that a group of 20-odd primary care doctors can successfully take two-sided risk in the MSSP.[21]

Practice sizes would also vary by region. In large metropolitan areas, where there are far more doctors, the competing groups would be larger than they would be in smaller cities and exurban areas. In rural areas, there might be only enough primary care doctors — or physicians in general — to form one or two groups. Therefore, competition could not exist in those areas, but the groups or other provider combinations could still be budgeted (see Chapter 11).

To figure out how many physicians should be in a basic care group, both the size of the local population and the ratio of primary care doctors to that population must be weighed. For example, New York City had a population of 8.48 million in 2025.[22] In contrast, 230,600 people lived in Spokane, Washington.[23] There were 114 primary care physicians per 100,000 people in the New York metro area in 2006, the latest year for which I could find data.[24] In 2014, by contrast, there were 79 primary care physicians per 100,000 in Washington State.[25]

Taking these factors into account, along with the size of the average PCP's patient panel, I estimate that groups of 50–100 primary care doctors would be the right size in the New York City area if it were subdivided into about 20 regions. In smaller markets like Spokane, groups of 25–50 physicians would suffice.

Assuming that the average group includes 50 full-time-equivalent primary care doctors, and that a PCP can comfortably manage about 2,000 patients,[26-27] between 3,000 and 4,000 basic care groups would be required to care for the entire U.S. population. Midlevel providers such as nurse practitioners and physician assistants would also have to be counted, so the numbers of physicians in these groups might be lower. If so, there could be more competing groups; however, there would still have to be enough practice owners in each group to take financial risk.

MANAGED COMPETITION

Besides giving basic care groups financial responsibility for care, my model would have them engage in a form of "managed competition." This competition would be another inducement to deliver the highest quality care at the lowest possible cost.

The Clinton Health Plan of the 1990s, it will be recalled, relied largely on Alain Enthoven's theory of managed competition. Under this legislation, which Congress never passed, health plans with standardized benefits would have competed for enrollees under very strict government regulation. The basic care part of my reform model does something similar, but with a major difference: Instead of managing the competition between health plans, it sets the conditions for competition between basic care groups. This approach places the competition where it should be: between the healthcare providers who are best situated to reduce waste without stinting on necessary care.

Such a model would be difficult if not impossible to implement under the current system. The primary care doctors must be financially at risk for all their patients to align their incentives; today, in contrast, they are constantly whipsawed between the incentives of fee-for-service and value-based arrangements of various kinds. Additionally, health plans will always interfere in medical decisions to reduce their costs. That's why, in my model, insurance is restricted to major medical care and hospitals have global budgets, allowing them and their staffs to determine how care is delivered. Everything outside of major medical and long-term care is directed by primary care physicians who take financial risk and do not answer to any payer other than the consumer.

PCPs are best suited to manage basic care because they are upstream of the major cost drivers: hospitals, specialists, post-acute care providers, and ancillary services like labs and imaging centers. Through their treatment and referral decisions, PCPs influence the cost of a case and the patient's outcome. They can appropriately manage many patients who have chronic conditions without referring to a specialist or in collaboration with a specialist. They can coordinate care across care settings, and they are well placed to interface with community-based organizations that address patients' unmet social needs.

It is difficult if not impossible to deliver this kind of whole-person care in the fee-for-service world. What makes it possible is having a budget — comprised, in this case, of the subscription fees paid by all the patients who choose a doctor in a basic care group. Within that budget, physicians and administrators who are experts in population health management can allocate resources in ways that improve patient outcomes and help people manage their chronic conditions. Ideally, the groups that devise the best approaches should have the highest quality scores and the lowest costs (see the discussion of risk adjustment below). As consumers gravitate toward those groups, theoretically, all the other groups will endeavor to raise their performance. This continuous improvement can cut waste, improve efficiency, and give clinicians an incentive to provide whatever their patients need, but no more.

One further word about the kind of healthcare budget I'm proposing: Where payers delegate risk, they determine the size of ACOs' or physician groups' budgets — whereas in this model, the groups decide that. Over time, the payers usually whittle down capitation payments or shared savings as providers become more efficient. In this arrangement, by contrast, the basic care groups themselves decide how much they must charge subscribers for physicians to earn an adequate income without setting their fees so high that they turn off consumers.

Paying Group Members and Specialists

The groups are also free to determine how to reimburse their own clinicians for the services they provide. Paying the doctors and the advanced practitioners for production (i.e., the volume of services) wouldn't work, because volume-based incentives are the opposite of those created by financial risk. Sub-capitation wouldn't make sense, either, because it's the group that would take the risk, not the individual clinician. The best way to pay clinicians in a basic care group would be to salary them. This method — used by Kaiser Permanente and other group-model HMOs — doesn't incentivize clinicians to do too much or too little for patients. Coupled with performance bonuses unrelated to production, salaries allow clinicians to focus on providing high-quality care without being concerned about personal financial consequences.

Basic care groups also must figure out how to pay and negotiate with specialists. In most cases, they would pay them fee-for-service, because sub-capitating specialists is challenging and ultimately self-defeating. The PCPs referring patients to specialists don't want them to stint on care; they just don't want them to overuse or misuse services.

Bargaining with specialists on rates could also be a challenge. Independent specialists would want to cooperate with the basic care groups and not overcharge them if they hoped to get referrals. But specialists working for a health system might charge high prices to basic care groups to generate extra revenue outside of the system's global budget. If that happened, the basic care groups could refer patients to other specialists, including those working for rival health systems. Knowing that this could have a negative impact on its bottom line, the health system would not want its specialists to charge the groups unreasonable fees.

This description of the financial relationships between PCPs and specialists reveals that the possibility of business conflicts between the two is very real. Who would resolve these conflicts, and who would deal with the many other questions arising from this novel model of providing basic care?

Regional Health Authorities

Because of the local nature of healthcare, it would make sense to administer the basic care system on a local or a regional basis. (Major medical insurance and global hospital budgets, on the other hand, would be administered by the states.) Organizations that I call "regional health authorities" would supervise basic care in districts that included a certain number of people. Densely populated metro areas would be divided into multiple districts.

Although the regional health authority would have an official legal status, it would not be a government agency. Instead, it would function as an independent council or board. Among its members would be representatives of the consumers and employers who would pay part of the subscription fees, as well as the federal taxes that would fund the balance. The basic care groups supported by these fees would also be represented. Since each of these stakeholder groups has somewhat different interests, the opportunity for all of them to provide input into the decision-making process should help clarify the issues. The authority's supervision would also guarantee a degree of citizen control over the healthcare system.

The regional health authorities would delegate operational responsibility for managing the local basic care systems to what I call "health utilities." The health utilities, which would be private companies something like third party administrators, would run the day-to-day operations of each system and manage the competition among physician groups. They would be highly regulated, and their fees and functions would be strictly limited by federal law. Each regional health authority would contract with a health utility for a specified period — say, two years. At the end of that time, the council would look at the health utility's performance and decide whether to renew the agreement.

The basic care groups would pay the health utility for necessary functions, including patient enrollment, the collection of subscription fees, claims processing and payment to outside providers, performance measurement, and the posting of public report cards. Each health utility would have claims data for most of the specialty and testing services provided to referred patients, and a national claims database would be automatically cross-checked to pick up claims generated outside each group's network. This information would be available to the basic care groups to help them track the costs that they were financially responsible for.

PROVIDER REPORT CARDS

The competition between the basic care groups would be driven by the consumers who received that care. The key to this competition would be group report cards posted on the health utility's website. Before selecting a primary care doctor in one of the competing groups, consumers could compare the groups on cost, quality and patient experience. The quality rankings would be risk-adjusted to reflect the differences in the average health status of the patient populations served by each group. The relative costs would be the subscription fees, which would not be risk-adjusted because they'd be set by the groups. While this method would not fairly compare the efficiency of the different groups, consumers would be interested only in the cost to them of enrolling in a particular group.

The employer, consumer, and government contributions to subscriptions would give each individual access to sufficient funds to sign up with any of the available basic care groups. An individual's or a family's income and their choice of a basic care group would be the only factors determining how much they'd have to pay for a subscription. If they picked one of the lower-cost groups, their part of the subscription fee would be reduced. People who earned too little to contribute to subscriptions would get some kind of bonus for choosing lower-cost or higher-quality groups.

A similar system was used in the 1990s in Minnesota's Patient Choice program, which allowed employees of large, self-insured companies to choose among competing "care systems." In that experiment, workers paid a smaller percentage of the insurance premium if they enrolled with a lower-cost group, and their employers made up the difference. Giving employees "skin in the game" led to enrollment gains for the least expensive care systems, as well some moderate-priced groups with high quality ratings.[28]

Some people would undoubtedly select groups with lower subscription fees, regardless of quality. Not everyone would be able to find a doctor in a low-priced group, because physicians in those groups could care for only a certain number of patients. Yet the system would still incentivize the groups to offer high quality care at a reasonable price.

The Problems with Report Cards

There have been numerous attempts over the years to enlist consumers in improving quality by publishing provider report cards. Health insurers, employer coalitions, multi-stakeholder community groups, and the federal and state governments have all published ratings in the hope that consumers would choose higher-quality, lower-cost physicians and hospitals.

Most of these efforts have come to naught. Over the past quarter century, studies have consistently found that consumers were largely uninterested in these report cards and rarely used them to pick providers. Here's what RAND researchers found in 2002:

> Although evidence from surveys and focus groups suggests that consumers want more information about the performance of their health care providers, few individuals are apparently influenced by the information in their decision making. According to the surveys, consumers' choice of hospitals relied more on anecdotal press reports of adverse events than on the comparative assessments that were available.[29]

Similarly, a 2012 paper based on a survey of and interviews with experts on report cards stated, "Public reporting to date has been disconnected from consumer decisions about providers."[30] A 2014 consumer survey by the Kaiser Family Foundation found that about 10% of Americans said they had seen comparative quality information on hospitals or doctors. But of those who had viewed the information, just 4% used it to select a hospital and 6% to choose a doctor.[31]

A 2018 study of provider ratings found that in 2015, there were only 5.3 million unique page views on Medicare's Physician Compare and only 3.7 million unique page views on the Hospital Compare site. These were small numbers in relation to the number of Medicare beneficiaries. Other public report cards also had relatively low readership, the researcher found.[32]

Some physician report cards measure the quality of groups rather than individual doctors. The California Department of Managed Care's website posts cost, quality and patient experience ratings of physician groups and IPAs.[33] The Wisconsin Collaborative for Healthcare Quality posts detailed quality information for group practices and health systems in Wisconsin,[34] and Minnesota Community Measurement, a private, nonprofit organization, rates clinics, medical groups, and hospitals.[35] There are no data on how widely viewed these sites are.

A 2021 consumer survey found that online reviews and star ratings were the most important factors in choosing a new healthcare provider. In selecting a new primary care doctor, 51% of consumers said they went on the Internet first; 24% sought a referral from another healthcare provider; and 4% got their information from an insurer or a benefits manager. Provider report cards were not mentioned. The leading online destinations were a hospital or a clinic site, WebMD, HealthGrades, and Facebook. Eighty-three percent of respondents said they went online to read reviews of a physician *after* receiving a referral from another doctor.[36]

Why Report Cards Aren't Used More

Observers cite several reasons for the public's unenthusiastic response to provider report cards. First, many people are simply unaware that they exist. Second, some patients trust their own doctors to refer them to the best specialists and hospitals. Third, even when consumers do look at comparative data on physicians and hospitals, they often find them hard to understand, inconsistent, and lacking the pertinent information they need to make decisions.[37]

The literature on this topic suggests that most consumers don't have a compelling reason to consult report cards. One obvious reason is that most people are healthy at any point in time. Sick people, being vulnerable, tend to depend on their doctors' guidance. Also, since most provider scorecards don't include out-of-pocket costs for particular services or procedures, there is no financial incentive for consumers to use the report cards.

There are a couple of hints that cost information might move this needle. One study found that, when presented with a combination of cost data and easy-to-understand quality data, consumers were more likely to choose lower-cost, higher-performing providers than higher-cost, lower-performing providers.[38] And in the 2012 paper based on interviews with experts, representatives of consumer and quality organizations said that cost data should be included in provider report cards.[39]

CONCLUSION

Primary care physicians are well qualified to manage basic care, and giving them that role could help break the vicious cycle of ever-increasing costs and ever-decreasing quality of care. If that were to happen, overall spending growth would slow and possibly reverse over time. The savings that this virtuous cycle would produce could also stop the decline of primary care. Not only could PCPs earn more than they do now, but they'd also be able to practice up to the limit of their professional qualifications. That, plus being able to give patients the care they need, should lure many more young doctors into primary care.

Before we reach this promised land, however, basic care groups must build the infrastructure and the financial reserves they need to execute their plans. In addition, they must learn how to cut waste by following evidence-based guidelines, reducing overtreatment, taking more time with patients, and coordinating care with specialists. The next chapter describes how they might achieve these challenging goals.

CHAPTER 7.

How To Organize Basic Care Groups

A BLUEPRINT FOR CARE DELIVERY

Liberating primary care physicians from corporate control is just the first step in creating the basic care system I envision. After becoming independent, the doctors would have to form groups of the right size. For the purposes of discussion, let's assume that those groups will include an average of 50 doctors each, as proposed in the last chapter. In some large employed groups and ACOs, there may be multiples of that number of PCPs. Those physicians, if they wanted to practice with their colleagues, could form their own basic care groups. Other doctors could join other groups or could be the nucleus of a group that would attract other physicians.

No money should change hands when the primary care physicians establish basic care groups. The majority of the doctors were previously employed, and the value of their practices dropped to zero when they left their health systems or companies. The practices of independent doctors will lose most of their value when insurance for basic care disappears. So the physician owners of the basic care groups will come together with the same amount of equity in the enterprise.

The process of group formation should begin while the employed doctors are still with their health system or company. They must be allowed to communicate freely with the other PCPs in their enterprise so they can plan their next steps. Besides setting up their new group, they must also decide how to build the group's infrastructure. To start with, that includes administrators, staff, offices, and an EHR. In addition, the physicians must figure out how to finance their new groups' infrastructure.

Creating Regional Health Authorities

While the basic care groups are being formed, the federal government will establish the insurance regions and the regional health authorities. Next, employers, consumers, and providers in each area will select the members of these boards. In their first meetings, the authorities will put out bids for the health utility contracts.

Once the health utilities have been chosen, they can begin to help the basic care groups get on their feet. For starters, the health utilities can offer centralized IT assistance to all the basic care groups in their region. They can certify that the groups have enough doctors, but not too many. They can help arrange financing for the groups and/or help them locate infrastructure vendors.

Another major challenge for the new basic care groups will be to ensure that most of their doctors' existing patients stay with them so their physicians can get paid. Therefore, a principal early objective of the basic care groups must be to contract with the insurers that cover each physician's patients. Traditional Medicare and Medicaid will be no problem. But private insurers, including Medicare Advantage plans, might throw up barriers to block the switch to the new system. To prevent this, the government must require insurance companies to let their members' coverage follow them to the basic care groups. Of course, that insurance will go away when the groups start charging subscription fees.

It will be difficult for the groups to figure out what to charge at first, because their historical data on healthcare costs will be limited. But, based on their initial claims data from Medicare, Medicaid and private insurers, the health utilities will be able to help each group establish a benchmark it can use to set an initial subscription fee. At the start, this benchmark will be mostly guesswork, but it can be refined after the first year of operating in the new system. To address the possibility of errors in the original estimate, the groups could set their fees higher than they think is necessary. It would be better if the budgets were too high and had to be reduced later than if they were too low and some groups started off at a deficit.

Transition to Financial Risk

The ability of individual basic care groups to assume financial risk will vary considerably. As stated in Chapter 3, less than a third of primary care physicians belong to ACOs that take two-sided risk in the Medicare Shared Savings Program. If Medicare Advantage and commercial plans were included, the ratio would probably be somewhat higher. Still, the basic care groups will have to go through a shakeout period during the period before the inception of the new system. During that period, some groups will continue to rely mainly on fee-for-service.

Nevertheless, their goal should be to assume as much risk as they can handle as soon as possible. The groups can immediately start taking primary care capitation from private payers, and Medicare should also make this option available to basic care groups. This isn't something CMS has done up to now, except in its ACO Primary Care Flex model and earlier, in the Comprehensive Primary Care (CPC and CPC+) demonstrations. But to support the transition to the new model, it would make sense for CMS to do so more broadly. The groups should strive to have two-thirds or more of their patients in some kind of risk arrangement by the time they're ready to switch to basic care subscriptions.

INFRASTRUCTURE REQUIREMENTS

To support population health management and risk management, the basic care groups will need software for data aggregation and analytics, as well as applications for automating a wide range of PHM functions. In addition, they will need care managers, social workers, and other nontraditional care team members to help keep patients out of the hospital and other expensive care settings. Before the launch, they must contract with medical specialists, as well as dentists, audiologists, eye care centers, labs and imaging centers. They will also require substantial financial reserves to hedge against higher-than-expected healthcare costs.

Of course, hardly any of this will be in place on day one. But most of it should be ready by the time the subscription model commences and the groups begin taking risk for all basic care.

Clearly, physicians can't directly fund this infrastructure. Wealthy physicians with outside financial backing provide the bulk of the initial investment in many ACOs, but that means they own the majority of the ACO's equity. It's unclear whether this arrangement incentivizes the other ACO members to work hard to reduce costs and improve quality.

A study of physician-led ACOs in the upside risk-only track of the Medicare Shared Savings Program (MSSP) found that they had a variety of funding sources, including physician contributions, loans, venture capital, and investments by founders. ACOs not financed by larger companies, the study found, had a limited ability to make upfront investments in health IT, and their data analytics infrastructure was very basic. Their clinical relationships with specialists and hospitals were also limited. For the most part, these ACOs just tried to coordinate care well enough to get some bonuses from the shared savings program.[1]

The basic care groups must function at a much higher level than that to provide excellent care within a budget. The physicians can learn how to do this; but, without a larger entity behind them, they will have to find another way to attract or generate sufficient resources.

Raise Capitation Rates

The transition of the basic care groups to financial risk and population health management could be supported by switching them to capitation payments that are higher than their fee-for-service revenues. Some experts have long endorsed this idea, and a primary care investment bill that would do just that has gotten pretty far in the Massachusetts legislature, as noted in Chapter 2. Under this measure, year one capitation payments from commercial insurers would increase PCP revenues by 30%, enabling the practices to invest in practice transformation. By year three, practices could double their baseline payments, depending on how much they invested in specified "transformers."[2]

Considering that primary care receives only about 5% of the healthcare dollar, these higher payments would not increase overall spending by very much. And, if this idea were applied to our basic care groups (with Medicare included among the payers), it would give them a leg up on building the infrastructure they'd need to succeed. As one reference point, primary care practices that try to offer PHM as patient-centered medical homes need 1.57 more full-time staffers per full-time physician than traditional practices do.[3] This is where some of the money from enhanced payments could go.

A related approach to financing the infrastructure of the basic care groups would be to have the government fund it by setting Medicare and Medicaid primary care payments high enough to cover the cost. The government could recoup its investment over time from its share of the groups' savings.

The Health Care Payment Learning & Action Network (LAN), a collaborative network of public and private stakeholders established by the Department of Health and Human Services, advocated a similar approach in a white paper on primary care payment models (PCPMs). In their recommendations on how to transform primary care, the LAN authors said:

> Prospective payments [i.e., capitation] should be in excess of historic primary care payment amounts to support the infrastructure of the clinical team that will be held accountable for greater coordination of services and for bending the total health system cost curve….PCPMs should use prospective payment to fund the necessary investments by primary care organizations in practice infrastructure to result in more efficient delivery of health care.

The report's authors envisioned that payers' additional spending on primary care would be recouped through "savings from reductions in the utilization of unnecessary care outside the primary care setting… In return for accepting increased payment rates, primary care teams will create additional value for the healthcare system, consumers and purchasers."[4]

Infrastructure Vendors

The government is not the only potential source of infrastructure funding. It's likely that many basic care groups would contract with "infrastructure vendors" that provide population health management software, and, in some cases, coaching and other PHM services. Some of these vendors provide their software and services in return for a percentage of an ACO's shared savings. The accompanying sidebar lists some of these companies and what they do.

Lightbeam

This company's product line includes data aggregation and analytics that measure care gaps, stratify the population by health risk, and track cost, financial risk, and productivity. Lightbeam also offers a health information exchange, referral management, automated patient messaging, and care management software, but the firm does not supply care managers or other personnel.[5]

Privia Health

Based in Arlington, Virginia, Privia manages ACOs, other VBC networks, and primary care-centric groups in 15 states and Washington, D.C. It furnishes population health management infrastructure, performs billing and collection, and provides other services. Privia is backed by private equity investors.[6]

Aledade

Aledade describes itself as "the nation's largest network of independent primary care. Our Accountable Care Organizations (ACOs) help practices and health centers improve patient outcomes and generate sustainable revenue." Aledade supplies population health management software and delivers a range of on-the-ground services, including practice transformation coaching and contracting. Aledade also draws on venture capital investments.[7]

Arcadia

Arcadia features "population health for the enterprise." The firm aggregates and analyzes clinical and claims data, identifies care gaps, does patient outreach, provides reports on quality and utilization, coaches providers, measures performance, negotiates contracts, and advises ACOs on care management and other aspects of population health management.[8]

Innovaccer

Innovaccer presents itself as "The AI Cloud for Healthcare Performance." Its software platform for large health systems is said to enhance VBC performance and reduce administrative costs. Its population health management suite features a comprehensive view of patient data, predictive and prescriptive analytics, financial contracting and risk management, patient engagement, and performance and quality tracking.[9]

Elligint Health

Elligint offers a comprehensive PHM solution for "mid-market" ACOs, including care management, utilization management, case coordination, and disease management. The company also provides "expert advisory services that equip payers and ACOs with strategic insights, operational expertise, and data-driven guidance..."[10]

Health Catalyst

Targeting health systems and ACOs, Health Catalyst sells "solutions for data-driven improvement." Among other things, the firm tackles "rising risk and health disparities by identifying and engaging key populations with tailored interventions that close care gaps and improve health outcomes." Health Catalyst's apps also help manage financial risk contracts and reduce waste in healthcare delivery.[11]

Farzad Mostashari, MD, CEO and founder of Aledade, an infrastructure vendor that works with ACOs, told me that his company provides "population health as a service." Because the firm takes 40%-50% of its ACOs' shared savings, however, it might also be regarded as a management services organization (MSO). Some ACOs have an even closer relationship with MSOs. Partners in Care (PIC), a New Jersey-based ACO and clinically integrated network (CIN), is majority-owned by an MSO called Continuum Health.[12]

MSOs have a long, checkered history in healthcare. Back in the 1990s, some MSOs funded by private equity rebranded themselves as "physician practice management companies," or PPMCs. Companies like Phycor, MedPartners, and PhyMatrix bought practices, often partly or wholly for stock, with the aim of pumping up their valuations and going public. But their business model was faulty; even with capital infusions, they weren't able to increase practice revenues enough to justify their management fees. Eventually, eight of the 10 largest PPMCs went bankrupt, leaving their physician investors with worthless stock.[13]

There are signs that private equity is back to its old games. Some current MSOs aggregate PE-owned medical groups, negotiate payer contracts, and facilitate corporate investment. Increasingly, PE firms, insurers, and other corporate entities are using MSOs to bypass state prohibitions on the corporate practice of medicine.[14]

Infrastructure vendors, however, are a different breed. To begin with, they're not run by venture capitalists, even if they have private equity backing, and they're not interested in buying practices. Their financial interest lies in ensuring that their ACOs save money and generate shared savings that they split with the vendor. Aledade, as noted above, manages and supports the population health management activities of its ACOs. It shares in the ACOs' earnings but not in the other revenue streams of member practices. Nevertheless, it's important to remember the lessons of the PPMC apocalypse.

Although private equity could be vital to providing the capital for infrastructure vendors, investors should not be allowed to buy and sell basic care groups. To prevent business collapses and to ensure they can pursue their healing mission, the basic care groups must always be under exclusive physician ownership. However, PE firms might be allowed to invest in basic care groups without taking an equity interest.

Another Take on Venture Capital

In a 2024 *Health Affairs Forefront* article, I explored the idea of inducing private equity firms to invest in value-based-care-oriented entities. After summarizing the long litany of PE abuses in healthcare, I pointed out that there is a fundamental mismatch between the classical PE business model and the requirements of patient care. A PE firm will typically hold onto an acquisition for a few years and then try to flip it or take it public. In the meantime, the PE firm will cut costs and raise prices, frequently loading the acquired company with debt and taking exorbitant management fees.[15]

Applied to healthcare, these strategies have proved to be a disaster in many cases. As noted earlier, however, some PE firms have invested in infrastructure firms as well as VBC-oriented companies such as Iora, Oak Street, ChenMed, and One Medical. While this model can take time to bear financial fruit by reducing hospital admissions and emergency department visits, some PE investors have had paydays when their client firms were acquired. Iora, for example, was bought out by One Medical,[16] which was later acquired by Amazon. Similarly, the investors in Oak Street made a big profit when CVS acquired Oak Street.[17]

Because of the well-publicized problems in some PE healthcare investments, several proposals have been made to limit the ability of PE companies to invest in healthcare. David Cutler and Zurui Song, for example, suggest changing tax policy so that PE firms would have to hold healthcare assets for a longer period (say, 10 years instead of three years) to qualify for the lower capital gains tax rate when they sell their hospitals or nursing homes. They'd also have to set aside money in escrow accounts to cover losses in case their business strategy fails.[18]

Emily Stewart and Jim Baker would create joint liability for private equity firms and their portfolio companies. This would prevent PE firms from making huge profits while saddling healthcare entities with debt. They also want Congress to close tax loopholes used by private equity.[19]

Sen. Edward Markey (D-MA) has proposed legislation requiring PE firms to get licenses from the Department of Health and Human Services (HHS) before acquiring healthcare entities. The bill would also mandate that they establish an escrow account to cover operating and capital expenditures for five years in the event of a facility closure or reductions in healthcare services. HHS would also have the authority to review, and if appropriate, to stop sales of healthcare properties to real estate investment trusts.[20]

What I suggested in my article is that, if Congress passed these or similar proposals, investments in VBC-oriented entities such as primary care groups, ACOs or infrastructure vendors might be exempted from the requirements. While this approach wouldn't allow PE investors to make quick profits, they might earn more in the long run if they could take a cut of rapidly rising VBC revenues.

Would this work for basic care groups? I don't know, but it seems to be worth a try. Some PE firms, as mentioned above, already have experience with VBC-oriented entities. In a radically changed environment where the basic care groups were the cornerstone of the healthcare system, this might look to investors like an attractive proposition. Moreover, if the model could cut waste and improve health to the degree I believe it could, investors stand to earn back their investment many times over in the long run. And if they wanted to get their money out sooner to invest in something else, their investment in VBC would prove to be a very saleable asset.

FINANCIAL RISK

Beyond building an infrastructure, the basic care groups would have to learn how to handle financial risk and how to protect themselves from insolvency. Even primary care capitation can be a risk if utilization isn't managed, but the risk is limited to the services of the physicians themselves. Therefore, every group, as soon as it was fully organized, could be prepaid for primary care. Upside risk for the total cost of care, similarly, doesn't threaten groups with insolvency. If they don't reduce healthcare spending enough to garner shared savings, they are only on the hook for the cost of their infrastructure.

But taking two-sided risk for a percentage of the total cost of care is completely different. While not as perilous as global capitation, which transfers 100% of the downside risk to the provider group, a far lower amount of risk can threaten a group or ACO with insolvency if they don't have financial reserves or stop-loss insurance.

For this reason, CMS requires ACOs in the MSSP's two-sided risk tracks to maintain financial reserves equal to 1% of total per capita Medicare Parts A and B spending for the beneficiaries assigned to them.[21] The basic care groups in my model would also need reserves to hedge their risk. How large those reserves would have to be and where the groups would obtain the funds are the questions we now turn to.

How Much Risk Is Too Much?

Paul Keckley, a healthcare strategic adviser and a former Navigant and Deloitte executive, says that CMS's 1% reserve requirement is insufficient. If an ACO or group is taking a significant portion of risk for the total cost of care in the MSSP, he estimates, it should maintain reserves of between 1% and 4% of total annual spending.

In determining how this might apply to basic care groups, we should remember that, because of their age, Medicare patients — the population of MSSP ACOs — have much greater health risks than the population as a whole. Moreover, our primary care groups are taking risk only for a subset of services; when a patient needs more expensive care, their coverage slides over to major medical insurance. In contrast, MSSP ACOs take up to 15% of the downside risk for the total cost of care (TCOC), including all Medicare Part A and Part B services.[22]

Based on CMS data, it appears that the total cost of personal care in the United States was roughly four times greater than the amount spent on basic care in 2023.[23] Assuming this is true, 15% of TCOC would be less than 100% of basic care costs. But, considering that Medicare patients 65 and older account for almost three times the spending of the average working-age person,[24] the downside risk of the MSSP ACOs would still be significantly higher than that of the basic care groups.

Let's stipulate that the proper reserve percentage for a group taking risk for basic care is 1% of its benchmark. In 2023, the average cost of personal healthcare was approximately $14,570 per person.[25] If basic care were a quarter of that, the benchmark of a basic care group would average $3,642 per capita. Using that number, a basic care group with 50 doctors and 100,000 patients would need reserves equal to 1% of $3,642 times 100,000, or about $3.6 million.

It would not be out of the question for a 50-doctor group to fund a reserve of that size through personal savings or borrowings. An infrastructure vendor could also finance it.

Aledade funds the reserves for its small ACOs with venture capital, Mostashari notes. But Keckley cautions that some infrastructure vendors may not remain stable in the long term. So ACOs should perform due diligence on their vendors before letting them provide reserves. The same would apply to the basic care groups in our model.

KEY MEASUREMENTS

Attribution

Patients must be attributed to individual primary care physicians to determine which group is responsible for their care. Attribution is the prerequisite for calculating the cost of basic care, as well as for risk adjustment and benchmarking.

In my model, each person would have to choose a primary care physician or another provider in one of the basic care groups. By doing so, in effect they'd be choosing that doctor's group as their care system. If they didn't select anyone, they'd still have to buy a subscription for basic care, and they'd be assigned a physician or an advanced practitioner.

Consumers would elect to stay with their doctor or choose another physician prior to the start of each calendar year; in some cases, this would entail moving to a different group. The enrollment process, which would be conducted by the health utilities, would be similar to the process of enrolling in a health plan today. The system would have to keep track of people who signed up for the first time in the middle of the year or died during the year. Nobody would be able to switch groups until the next year's enrollment period. So groups would know which patients they were responsible for at all times.

Risk Adjustment

In the current system, capitation payments and benchmarks for the total cost of care are risk-adjusted for each patient's health status. CMS and private payers have developed sophisticated risk-adjustment techniques that depend on claims data.

In my model, the basic care groups would, in effect, take insurance risk for their own patients. Claims from specialists and other outside providers would be submitted to the basic care groups and processed by the health utilities. As noted earlier, the health utilities would use that claims data and other information to risk-adjust each group's quality scores, but the subscription fees would not be risk-adjusted.

Benchmarking

In the MSSP, benchmarking is the key to the equitable payment of shared savings for the total cost of care. Supported by patient attribution and risk adjustment, benchmarks can be based on the historical claims experience of an ACO, the experience of all providers in the region, and/or the national experience of ACOs.

Under the historical benchmarking method, efficient ACOs are punished financially because their performance is compared to their own previous claims experience; therefore, they have to work harder than inefficient ACOs to generate savings. In the MSSP, the disincentive to low-cost ACOs has been further compounded by rebasing their benchmark at the beginning of each contract period.

CMS now combines historical with regional benchmarking, which makes the benchmark of a particular ACO partly contingent on the performance of other ACOs in the same region. Thus, if the ACO is more efficient than its peers, its benchmark is raised to somewhere between its own claims experience and that of the other ACOs in the area. This makes it easier for the ACO to achieve shared savings in relation to the benchmark.[26]

More Room to Maneuver

The basic care groups would set their own benchmarks, which they'd use for internal purposes and to build subscription rates. As they became more efficient, they'd find it more difficult to beat their own past performance, just like the ACOs in the MSSP.

However, they'd have more room to maneuver than the ACOs do. For one thing, they could charge whatever subscription fee they wanted to, as long as they stayed within the range of fees set by competing groups. Also, waste reduction and quality improvement would create larger savings over time as the groups became more adept at population health management (see Chapter 9). While better preventive and chronic care don't necessarily result in short-term savings, they are bound to cut costs in the long run because patients will be healthier.

It is important to understand the key difference between shared savings schemes based on the total cost of care and the direct savings that the basic care groups would generate. These groups would not share their savings with anyone — except, perhaps, for infrastructure vendors. Whatever savings they created would drop to their bottom line, and they could decide whether to distribute those funds among their owners, invest them in infrastructure, or use them to reduce their subscription fees. Because they'd be taking risk only for basic care, they wouldn't share in downstream savings, such as those from lowering hospital and specialty care use. Those savings would go to society in the form of decreased overall healthcare spending.

CONCLUSION

Although the primary care groups would be responsible only for the cost of basic care, the clinical decisions of their doctors and their processes for keeping their patients healthy would have a direct effect on the appropriateness and cost of downstream care. Even within the realm of primary care, they'd be able to generate savings by doing as much as possible for patients instead of referring them out unnecessarily. Similarly, the basic care groups' approach to high-risk and rising-risk patients would reduce costs at the basic level, regardless of whether some of these patients were eventually hospitalized.

The next two chapters will explore these two topics: how to cut waste and how to manage the health of a population in a way that maximizes health and minimizes the need for more advanced types of care.

CHAPTER 8.

Waste Not, Want Not

Vertebroplasty is a surgical procedure designed to alleviate severe, disabling back pain caused by a compression fracture in a vertebra. Unfortunately for patients with this condition, there is no solid evidence that vertebroplasty is effective.

In 2009, a pair of randomized controlled trials of vertebroplasty were published in the *New England Journal of Medicine*.[1-2] These studies found that one month and six months after the procedure was done, there were no significant differences in the amount of pain reported by patients in the study and control groups. A similar study published in 2018 in the *BMJ* reported the same results through a year of follow-up.[3] A 2018 review paper by the international Cochrane Collaborative stated, "High-quality evidence shows that vertebroplasty does not provide more clinically important benefits than placebo."[4]

Despite these findings, surgeons frequently perform vertebroplasties — as well as a related procedure, kyphoplasty — "because they are highly profitable," says Grace Terrell, MD, the former CEO of the Cornerstone Health Care Group. Claire Neely, MD, president and CEO of the Institute for Clinical Systems Improvement (ICSI) in Bloomington, Minnesota, which has created a statewide clinical practice guideline for low back pain, agrees that vertebroplasties are overused.

This is just one example of the huge waste that permeates the U.S. healthcare system.

In a 2012 paper, Donald M. Berwick, MD, who had just stepped down as acting CMS administrator, and Andrew D. Hackbarth, a RAND Corp. researcher, estimated that healthcare waste, including unnecessary treatments, overpriced drugs and procedures, and the underuse of preventive care, represented 34% of U.S. health spending. The coauthors stated:

> In just six categories of waste — overtreatment, failures of care coordination, failures in execution of care processes, administrative complexity, pricing failures, and fraud and abuse — the sum of the lowest available estimates exceeds 20% of total health care expenditures. The actual total may be far greater.[5]

Looking at the same categories of waste, a 2019 paper by William H. Shrank and his colleagues estimated that the annual cost of healthcare that did not improve health could be nearly $1 trillion.

> The estimated cost of waste in the US health care system ranged from $760 billion to $935 billion, accounting for approximately 25% of total health care spending, and the projected potential savings from interventions that reduce waste, excluding savings from administrative complexity, ranged from $191 billion to $286 billion, representing a potential 25% reduction in the total cost of waste.[6]

Administrative complexity is the biggest source of waste. For example, just think about all the people whom hospitals employ to bill insurers and all the people employed by insurance companies to deny those claims. In my model, most of that administrative complexity would go away. Basic care groups would not deal with health plans, and they wouldn't have to micromanage the specialists they contracted with; if the specialists wasted resources and didn't treat patients well, the primary care doctors could just refer them elsewhere. As for health systems, hospitals with global budgets based on all-payer rates would have minimal contact with insurers. So they'd be paying far fewer administrative staffers, and administration would be much simpler. For instance, there would be no revenue cycle management, which today is a big industry.

OVERTREATMENT AND UNDERTREATMENT

Compared to administrative waste, waste in care delivery is much more difficult to deal with, because it's harder to identify and to prevent. This kind of waste includes overuse, misuse and underuse of services, safety issues, poor care coordination, and a lack of adherence to best practices.[7] The PCPs in the basic care groups would be ideally positioned to reduce clinical waste within their sphere, but they would have to make a concerted effort. Among other things, they could follow evidence-based guidelines to avoid low-value care, while doing as much as possible for their patients before referring them to specialists.

The full extent of overtreatment in U.S. healthcare is unclear; however, landmark research by Elliott Fisher, MD, the father of the ACO, and his colleagues at Dartmouth Medical School showed that nearly a third of Medicare spending pays for services that don't improve health. Medicare costs in the most expensive areas of the United States, the researchers found, were about 60% higher than those in the least expensive areas,[8] but the extra spending didn't improve patient outcomes. Patients hospitalized in the low-cost areas for hip fracture, colorectal cancer, and acute myocardial infarction had outcomes that were just as good as those of similarly ill patients in the high-cost regions.[9]

While rates of major surgery didn't vary greatly across the country, one of the Dartmouth studies found, patients had more tests and more minor procedures in the high-cost areas. The paper concluded that regional differences in Medicare spending "are due almost entirely to use of discretionary services that are sensitive to the local supply of physicians and hospital resources: more frequent physician visits, greater use of specialists, and greater use of the hospital and intensive care units as sites of care."[10]

Some of these services are provided despite clear evidence that they don't help and may even harm patients. One study of geographical variations in healthcare found "significant levels of inappropriate use: 17% of cases for coronary angiography, 32% for carotid endarterectomy, and 17% for upper gastrointestinal tract endoscopy."[11]

The McAllen Syndrome

In a famous *New Yorker* article published in 2009, Atul Gawande, MD, explored the overutilization of healthcare in McAllen, Texas. Although McAllen was one of the poorest cities in the country, it was the second most expensive market in the country for Medicare. The relatively poor health of McAllen area residents wasn't to blame; El

Paso, Texas, had similar health statistics, yet half as much was spent on Medicare patients in El Paso as in McAllen. Doctors also received similar training in both cities.[12]

One surgeon interviewed by Gawande attributed the high costs in McAllen to overutilization of procedures. For example, surgeons operated right away on gallstones rather than waiting to see if the pain went away. Patients with chest pain were immediately catheterized. So the difference in costs between McAllen and other areas of the country appeared to be at least partly linked to differences in practice patterns.

Similar relationships between practice patterns and costs have been observed in other parts of the United States. One study found that those patterns were principally responsible for the difference in annual Medicare costs per beneficiary between Miami ($13,596) and Minneapolis ($7,998).[13]

In a follow-up *New Yorker* article in 2015, Gawande reported that between 2009 and 2012, McAllen's health costs had dropped by almost $3,000 per Medicare recipient. Inpatient visits had decreased by 10%, and home health spending had declined by 40%. In total, these changes saved Medicare half a billion dollars, Gawande said.[14]

The national focus on McAllen because of his first article had something to do with this, he wrote. Federal prosecutors had cracked down on fraud in the market, and a local hospital had launched a campaign to reduce unnecessary care. But the major reason for the change, Gawande said, was that local primary care physicians changed their practice patterns to garner bonuses from Medicare Advantage plans. One top-performing doctor, for example, built a team around his patients, including cardiologists and surgeons. He selected specialists who didn't order low-value care and persuaded his patients to shift to them.

Another factor driving up costs in McAllen was home healthcare. The area had hundreds of home health agencies, some of them owned by physicians. One local primary care-led ACO, the Rio Grande Valley Health Alliance (RGVHA), used data analysis to determine that some non-ACO physicians were ordering home care at a rate far above the national average and that many of these orders failed to meet Medicare requirements. By persuading these physicians to provide better care coordination, RGVHA cut its home care costs by 41% over two years, said Victoria Farias, the ACO's program administrator, in a *Group Practice Journal* article.[15]

Underuse of Services

Besides overtreatment, underuse of recommended services also generates waste. For example, the failure of some physicians to provide appropriate preventive and/or chronic disease care can lead to preventable ED visits and hospital admissions. Patients also may be harmed because of underuse. Cancer diagnoses, for instance, may be delayed when patients aren't screened in a timely manner. Similarly, patients with diabetes who don't receive timely care and don't manage their condition may become severely ill and may have limbs amputated in extreme cases.

It's difficult to measure underuse because it consists of potentially beneficial services not provided to patients.[16] But an often-cited study by Elizabeth McGlynn and her RAND colleagues found that U.S. adults received only 55% of recommended acute, preventive, and chronic care services. Adherence to these care processes ranged from 52% for screening tests to 59% for follow-up care. There were wider variations in adherence among different health conditions.[17]

Overall, the researchers found underuse to be a greater problem than overuse. For example, patients with hypertension received 65% of recommended care. High blood pressure is linked to increased risk for heart disease, stroke, and death, and poor blood pressure control contributes to over 68,000 preventable deaths annually, the paper noted. Although the study didn't look at financial costs, the underuse of recommended care for hypertension undoubtedly drives a lot of avoidable ED visits and hospital admissions.

QUALITY ISSUES AND MISDIAGNOSIS

Medical errors — estimated to cause upwards of 98,000 deaths per year in hospitals alone[18] — also account for a significant amount of waste in the system. To prevent these errors, a hospital must develop a "safety culture" as part of its quality improvement efforts, says Kedar Mate, MD, founder and CMO of Qualified Health-gen AI and former president and CEO of the Institute for Healthcare Improvement (IHI).

"In safety culture, the causal pathway to increasing value is through the avoidance of defects," Mate says. He draws an analogy to the continuous quality improvement process used by Japanese auto manufacturers to improve their cars and to prevent errors and slowdowns on the assembly line. "If you prevent defects, you avoid rework, which is where the true cost to the system lies," Mate notes. "Safety culture helps avoid the rework that is a source of waste and a source of bad outcomes for the individual patient."

Besides increasing complications, readmissions and other kinds of rework, the lack of a safety culture also leads to inefficient processes and a lack of reliability, Mate says. One example is poor planning of the patient flow in a hospital. "Failing to achieve hospital-wide patient flow — the right care, in the right place, at the right time — puts patients at risk for suboptimal care and potential harm," states an IHI white paper.[19]

IHI has found that when cost data are supplied to nurse supervisors and physician leaders in a hospital, they tend to tackle the sources of financial waste, Mate observes. "In many cases, we're seeing 20%–30% reductions in the cost basis of service delivery in these units," he says. "That's a combination of changing consumables [drugs and supplies], improving locums tenens utilization, and improving patient flow and throughput."

Hospitals are concerned about this kind of waste because it directly affects their bottom line in Medicare diagnosis-related groups (DRGs), which limit the amount Medicare pays for each case. When it comes to low-value care, however, many hospitals have a different attitude. For example, Mate says, healthcare resources are often wasted on inappropriate hospital admissions.

"I'm an inpatient physician and I've seen plenty of people admitted to the hospital who could have easily been managed in an outpatient environment and were thereby exposed to the harms and risks of being hospitalized. And this becomes even more of a factor as patients age. We tend to hospitalize folks who have relatively minor ailments that can be treated in an outpatient setting."

Misdiagnosis is Prevalent

Misdiagnosis — including missed, delayed, and wrong diagnoses — leads to an estimated 371,000 deaths in the United States each year, and to 424,000 permanent disabilities, according to a 2021 study.[20] "Diagnostic error is the single largest source of deaths across all care settings linked to medical error," the study said. "It exceeds estimated death from all other patient safety concerns combined." According to the study, nearly 40% of serious harms or deaths due to misdiagnosis stem from five conditions: stroke, sepsis, pneumonia, venous thromboembolism (blood clots in the veins), and lung cancer. Stroke, the most commonly misdiagnosed condition, was missed in 17.5% of cases.

"We're not missing strokes when somebody is paralyzed on one side and can't talk," explained David Newman-Toker, MD, PhD, lead author of the study and a professor of neurology at Johns Hopkins Medicine, in a 2024 interview with WebMD. "We're missing stroke when it looks like something else, such as inner ear disease, where the patient presents with dizziness or vertigo, or has headaches that look like migraine."

Misdiagnoses are especially dangerous in the hospital, where patients are the sickest. More harm-causing misdiagnoses happen in primary care offices than in hospitals, but those clinics also have far more visits. The overall diagnostic error rate for all diseases is about 5%-10% across care settings, Newman-Toker said.

In the fee-for-service system, there is no financial penalty — other than a possible malpractice suit — for misdiagnosing a patient's health issue. Most health systems do not prioritize the improvement of diagnostic accuracy, and physicians are not rewarded financially for low misdiagnosis rates. Instead, they are rewarded for production, which leads to shorter visits and may result in missed diagnoses.[21]

Value-based care incentivizes physicians to take more time with patients, explore their health issues, and try harder to reach the correct diagnosis in every case. When a patient's problem is misdiagnosed, and the care for their actual disease is delayed, the costs of caring for them rise. That kind of waste can wreak havoc with the budget of an ACO or a basic care group. So, in theory, VBC should reduce the incidence of misdiagnosis. While I'm not aware of any studies that prove this to be true, it's something the basic care groups should bear in mind.

CARE COORDINATION

Chronic diseases generate most healthcare spending. Hence there is a need for healthcare providers to build an infrastructure that can provide the full complement of services required by people with chronic conditions such as heart disease, diabetes, and asthma. Yet this is the exception rather than the rule, the Institute of Medicine pointed out in its landmark 2001 book on the state of U.S. healthcare, *Crossing The Quality Chasm*:

> Physician groups, hospitals, and other health care organizations operate as silos, often providing care without the benefit of complete information about the patient's condition, medical history, services provided in other settings, or medications prescribed by other clinicians.[22]

Twenty-five years later, not much has changed. And it isn't just health information exchange that's still inadequate; there's also a lack of coordination and teamwork across care settings. Hospitalist physicians and ambulatory care physicians don't usually have close working relationships,[23] and community doctors often don't receive discharge summaries before the patient makes a follow-up visit.[24] Primary care doctors count themselves lucky when they receive a report from a specialist they referred a patient to, and specialists frequently don't understand why patients were referred to them.[25] Ambulatory care coordinators are rarely employed except in practices that take financial risk, belong to ACOs, or qualify as patient-centered medical homes.

In Berwick and Hackbarth's paper on eliminating healthcare waste, failures of care coordination were estimated to cost between $25 billion and $45 billion in 2011 — a relatively small sum compared to other major sources of waste. Yet inadequate care coordination, the authors noted, can lead to complications, hospital readmissions, and a decline in patients' abilities to function on their own.

A bigger driver of waste, according to Berwick and Hackbarth, are failures of care delivery related to "poor execution of known best care processes, including, for example, patient safety systems and preventive care practices that have been shown to be effective. The results are patient injuries and worse clinical outcomes."[26]

Good primary care can improve care coordination. In a 2017 study, Commonwealth Fund researchers compared primary care coordination of adults in 11 advanced countries. Poor coordination was defined as having at least three of five gaps in the coordination of care. Across all the countries, the average rate of poor coordination was 5.2%. In the United States, which has the weakest primary care system, the average rate was 9.8%.

Coordination was less likely to be subpar, the study noted, if a patient's PCP knew them well, knew their medical history, spent sufficient time, involved them, and explained things well. A continuous relationship between a patient and his or her physician enhances care coordination, improves medication adherence, and reduces hospitalizations, the authors pointed out.

However, programs to improve care coordination are difficult to implement in this country, they added. The main barriers are PCP shortages, health professional workloads, the underfunding of primary care, the fragmentation of the healthcare system, and the burden of disease in the population.[27]

GUIDELINES AND MEASURES

To promote the use of best care processes, specialty societies have created thousands of clinical practice guidelines. Healthcare systems and regional quality improvement organizations often tweak these guidelines for local use and/or develop their own guidelines for certain conditions, tests, and treatments. Currently, there is no up-to-date national database of guidelines. The Trump Administration defunded the National Guidelines Clearinghouse, which had been maintained by the Agency for Healthcare Research and Quality (AHRQ).

At one time, practice guidelines were based largely on expert opinion. Today, they're much more likely to be based on the best available evidence from clinical trials. The Institute of Medicine defines practice guidelines as "statements that include recommendations, intended to optimize patient care, that are informed by a systematic review of evidence and an assessment of the benefits and harms of alternative care options."[28]

This sounds reassuring, but in fact there are still large areas of ignorance and many gray areas in medicine. Solid, high-grade evidence justifies less than 50% and perhaps as little as 15% of what doctors do.[29] This is partly because there is no money to fund certain kinds of randomized clinical trials — the gold standard of medical evidence. In addition, there may be ethical issues involved in performing sham versus real surgery. Also, as former ICSI Executive Director Gordon Mosser, MD, told me many years ago, there are any number of decisions that doctors make for which there is no protocol, such as how to respond when a patient says they have an odd pain in the right side of their chest.

Even where there is good evidence, expert opinions still play a role in guidelines. "It is difficult to produce clinical practice guidelines that are completely evidence-based," Earl Steinberg, MD, and Bryan Luce, MD, stated in a 2005 *Health Affairs* article.[30]

Guidelines are still often based partly on expert opinion and community consensus, notes Ken Cohen, MD, executive director of translational health for Optum Health. He recalls how his former group, New West Physicians of Denver, selected guidelines. Wherever possible, he says, New West chose guidelines based on large randomized controlled trials and large meta-analyses of studies. Specialists convened by New West then examined the evidence and made whatever changes to each guideline that they felt were necessary. Even after that, he says, the physicians could follow a guideline for only about 85% of their relevant patients; the other 15% required clinical judgment outside of the algorithm.

Quality Measure Challenges

A big problem with the quality metrics used to measure adherence to guidelines is that they're more about processes than outcomes. In other words, physicians are being judged on measures like the percentage of their patients with diabetes who got annual eye exams rather than how well the patients controlled their blood sugar by following the regimen prescribed by their doctor.

Process measures don't reveal much about the quality of care and don't capture whether patient symptoms improved; therefore, they shouldn't be used in the report cards on the competing basic care groups. Nevertheless, some process measures might be valuable for internal quality improvement and for identifying outlier physicians.

Measures of intermediate outcomes reveal more than process measures do about how well patients fare as a result of treatment or preventive care. Examples of such measures include the percentage of diabetics with a value of 7% or less on an HbA1c test or the percentage of patients with hypertension who have their blood pressure under control. However, intermediate outcomes measures are available for only some chronic conditions and may not reflect patients' current symptoms.

Outcome measures like mortality and hospital readmissions are important, but they depend on a range of factors that may or may not be under a physician's control. Physiological measures such as the sustained virologic response in a patient with hepatitis C or HIV can show how well a treatment has worked within a certain time frame; however, the patient perspective provides a more holistic interpretation and a more comprehensive assessment of a patient's long-term outcomes.[31]

To obtain this long-term perspective, some healthcare organizations rely on patient-reported outcomes measures (PROMs) that "use validated questionnaires to turn a symptom into a numerical score."

PROM surveys, which can be general or disease-specific, measure functional status, health-related quality of life, symptoms and symptom burden, personal experience of care, and health-related behaviors such as anxiety and depression.[32]

Many validated functional status surveys exist, although they aren't used widely. Organizations such as Mass General Brigham (MGB) in Boston have found them to be useful in tracking recovery after procedures and the response of cancer patients to radiation therapy. MGB also uses angina and dyspnea surveys to measure patient outcomes after cardiac catheterizations.[33]

Physician Resistance to Guidelines

Even if a systematic literature review or a large, well-conducted clinical trial shows that a particular technique or drug is superior for treating a certain condition, the majority of physicians may not adopt it for many years. Among the reasons for this are inadequate dissemination of the data, poor educational methods, and a resistance to change. In some cases, physicians don't believe that their patients will accept certain treatments. This might explain why they were so slow to embrace antibiotic treatments for ulcers. It also explains why many doctors are reluctant to prescribe diuretics as the first-line treatment for hypertension, although these drugs have results equivalent to those of more expensive medications.

Physicians have good reasons for disbelieving the results of some clinical trials, based on the affiliations of the researchers with drug companies and other interested parties. Also, the subjects of clinical trials may not resemble the patient sitting in front of a doctor in an exam room. For example, researchers often exclude certain patients from a study because they have a comorbid condition in addition to the condition being studied. Yet the patient in the exam room may have one or more comorbidities.

Many clinical trials exclude people over 65. Consequently, the physician has no way of knowing whether the study's results apply to a Medicare patient. The same problem applies to children; pediatricians can't assume that because a particular medication worked in adults, it will help their patients. Women and minorities have long been underrepresented in clinical trials, Grace Terrell notes.

It's also impossible for practicing physicians to keep up with the literature. With more than 150,000 new studies being published each month,[34] doctors can only skim the surface of new knowledge. Online services that search the medical literature and boil down the most pertinent research — including UpToDate, DynaMed, the Cochrane Collaborative, and specialty-based "journal clubs" — help fill this gap. But high subscription costs deter many physicians from using these services.

Still, there are good evidence-based guidelines that cover many of the conditions that doctors diagnose and treat day in and day out. Why don't clinicians consistently follow these guidelines to reduce the amount of inappropriate and useless care they deliver?

One reason is that the guidelines are extremely long and detailed. Doctors aren't going to browse through a 30-page or a 100-page guideline to figure out how best to manage a patient who has a condition they have been treating for years. Moreover, they may not want to apply what they regard as "cookie cutter" guidelines to individual patients.

Malpractice concerns also affect how doctors approach guidelines. An old country doctor, asked why he didn't use a well-established rule to determine whether a patient had an ankle fracture without X-raying it, responded, "It's the patient's ankle, but it's my ass. I would rather X-ray 100 sprained ankles than go through the hassle of defending a single missed fracture in a malpractice suit."[35]

Performance Measures

Parts of many guidelines have been compressed into clinical quality measures. Specialty societies, CMS, and other parties are the stewards of these metrics. The National Quality Forum (NQF), a nonprofit organization, convenes multi-stakeholder committees that recommend submitted measures for endorsement. CMS has been using selected NQF-endorsed measures in its quality programs since 2011. Today, about 300 of these metrics are used in more than 20 federal public reporting and pay-for-performance programs, as well as private-sector quality initiatives. The measures are related to clinically reported outcomes, patient-reported outcomes, intermediate outcomes, processes, efficiency, and cost/resource use.[36]

One might expect that these measures — especially when they're imbedded in EHRs — would spur greater adherence to best practices. But there is little evidence of that. Studies of insurer pay-for-performance programs failed to demonstrate that they moved the needle on quality.[37-38] Similarly, the average quality scores of ACOs in the Medicare Shared Savings Program (MSSP) were 95% in 2012 and didn't vary much after that if one accounts for technical changes in 2022. This fact suggests that many clinicians were simply "checking off the boxes" to meet MSSP requirements for getting a portion of shared savings.

That's exactly the problem in today's value-based-care programs, says David Nash, MD, founding dean emeritus of the School of Population Health at Thomas Jefferson University in Philadelphia. "Even though we're on the road to redemption with value-based care, the measures to get us there are blunt instruments — mostly process measures. It becomes a check-the-box mentality: did you order the mammogram, did you get the cholesterol checked, rather than a set of measures such as whether we're preventing hospitalization and self-reported measures of health."

Measuring Outcomes

Patient outcomes are notoriously hard to measure, notes Cohen of Optum Health. "Intermediate quality outcomes are easy to measure at a primary care level: what's the hypertension control of your population, the diabetes control, cancer screening rates. When you get to specialists, it becomes incredibly difficult to measure outcomes. The only way to do it is through what are called PROMs: patient-reported outcomes measures. How is the patient actually doing a year or two after a back operation? The vast majority of providers in this country are not measuring that."

Aside from the fact that there is no financial incentive for providers to measure long-term outcomes, many physicians are skeptical about the validity of patient reports. Moreover, if patient-reported data is to be used to measure outcomes, it must be integrated with electronic health records, probably through patient portals connected to EHRs. While this is feasible,[39] it isn't clear how patient-reported data could form the basis for outcomes measures.

In any case, physicians are already overwhelmed by a proliferation of quality measures from myriad private and public payers. As Nash quips, he's not sure how well he'd score on all these metrics after having been in practice for 30 years. "There's no way to effectively keep up with the checklists."

Other physicians agree. In addition to having to pay attention to a variety of tasks that are not germane to the reason for a patient's visit, they must also document everything they did in the EHR — a very time-consuming chore. This is one reason around half of physicians say that EHRs reduce their efficiency.

In the current environment, physicians tend to view the emphasis on quality improvement as an onerous assignment that does not actually improve quality but does reduce their time with patients. "Physicians want to provide our patients with the best care possible, but today there are confusing, misaligned and burdensome regulatory programs that take away critical time physicians could be spending to provide high-quality care for their patients," commented Robert M. Wah, MD, then president of the American Medical Association, in 2014.[40]

New Approach to Reporting

The basic care groups in my model would not have to cope with confusing or burdensome requirements for quality reporting. To start with, the basic care groups would have a single set of measures that would vary only by the age, sex and condition of their patients. Those metrics would follow national guidelines, although the groups would have the ability to make changes through the health utilities, if all the groups in that region agreed on them.

These quality metrics would not include process measures other than cancer screening. They would emphasize intermediate outcomes metrics and long-term, self-reported outcomes measures. Intermediate outcomes would include control of diabetes, asthma and hypertension, as well as hospitalization rates.

For the most part, the data on these measures would be collected automatically without the need for physician input. The home use of digitally connected blood pressure cuffs, for example, would provide daily information on patients with hypertension.[41] Similarly, digitally connected blood glucose meters could send data on patients with diabetes directly to physicians' offices, and the data would also be available to the patients.[42] Technical staffers in the practice would analyze the data, perhaps with the aid of artificial intelligence, and escalate it to the physician's attention if it was concerning.

Because remote patient monitoring provides the values needed for some quality measures, there is no reason for the physician or their staff to collect data from the EHR. So, no additional work is required to harvest this data for quality reporting.

Similarly, patients with serious chronic conditions and those recovering from surgery or a medical hospitalization can fill out online questionnaires at set intervals to measure their long-term outcomes. Financial incentives can be used to raise the response rate. Even if some people do not provide accurate responses, the survey results can give a good read on the long-term outcomes of people with particular conditions.

CHOOSING WISELY

In our fee-for-service system, the wise stewardship of resources is not at the top of many priority lists. In fact, just the opposite is true for many providers. As noted earlier, a great deal of unnecessary and inappropriate care is being provided, and some physician leaders are concerned about it. In 2012, the American Board of Internal Medicine (ABIM) Foundation teamed with *Consumer Reports* to create a mechanism to inform doctors and patients about treatments and tests that specialty societies view as low value. The Choosing Wisely campaign encompasses more than 80 specialty societies that have made more than 700 recommendations regarding unnecessary services. Choosing Wisely also has created dozens of patient handouts to inform discussions between doctors and patients.[43-44]

The Choosing Wisely recommendations cover a broad range of situations. For example, one patient handout notes that some physicians place blood clot filters in patients who don't have leg clots but are at high risk for getting them. But filters don't prevent clots — only blood thinners can do that, the handout notes. Also, the filters present health risks.

Another patient resource discusses bladder catheters that are placed in patients in hospitals and nursing homes when they have problems with bladder control. The handout notes that antibiotics should not be given to these patients unless they develop urinary tract infections. Indiscriminate use of antibiotics can lead to complications and more pathogen resistance.

Choosing Wisely also recommends against whole-body scans to screen for cancer, noting that these scans rarely find cancer in asymptomatic people and that many of these tumors would never cause a problem if left alone. Whole-body scans create health risks and can cost from $1,000 to $4,000.[45]

Impact of Choosing Wisely

Frontline physicians recognize the problem of low-value care. In a 2017 survey, the ABIM Foundation found that three of four U.S. physicians said the frequency with which doctors order unnecessary medical tests and procedures is a serious problem for the health system. Sixty-nine percent of respondents said the average physician orders unnecessary tests and procedures at least once a week.[46]

Yet studies suggest that there has not been a significant drop in the use of low-value or unnecessary care since the Choosing Wisely campaign began. For example, a 2017 study found there had been only a 4% decrease in low-value back imaging two and a half years after the program was launched.[47] Another study showed that of seven services that Choosing Wisely had recommended against, only two had showed a modest decrease in usage.[48]

Other research based on data from a large commercial insurer found that the growth in spending on five low-value services decreased an average of 1.7% annually from 2014 to 2016. However, the drop was less than expected. Among the low-value services in the study were vitamin D screening tests; PSA tests in men over 75 years old; unnecessary testing and lab work prior to low-risk surgery; imaging for uncomplicated low back pain within the first six weeks after onset; and the use of brand-name medications when generics were available.[49]

The ABIM survey showed that while doctors were aware of the problem, they were not necessarily disposed to change their own practice patterns. Just 59% of the doctors exposed to the Choosing Wisely campaign said they were likely to have reduced the number of times they ordered a test or a procedure after learning it was unnecessary.

Seventy-five percent of the primary care physicians aware of Choosing Wisely agreed with the statement that the campaign had empowered them to reduce the use of unnecessary tests and procedures. When that figure is compared to the 59% of all doctors aware of the campaign who decreased the use of low-value care, it can be deduced that specialists are less likely than primary care doctors to heed these recommendations.[50]

Patient Demands

While some doctors are concerned about not ordering tests or medications that patients expect, Richard Baron, MD, immediate past president and CEO of ABIM, downplays that issue regarding the Choosing Wisely recommendations. For example, he notes, many patients with upper respiratory infections expect to receive an antibiotic prescription, even if it they don't need one. "But some doctors extend that assumption to other patients who don't have that wish at all," and prescribe antibiotics to everyone with that condition.

Nevertheless, he notes, some patients distrust the motives of insurance companies, ACOs, and providers that take financial risk. When a doctor tells them something is unnecessary, he says, "Patients ask, 'are you doing that because an insurance company or administrator wants you to — somebody who doesn't care about me but does care about the bottom line?'"

Choosing Wisely provides a strong argument against that viewpoint, he notes, since the recommendations come from specialty societies. Still, when a doctor says that something isn't necessary, some patients are surprised and suspicious.

Recommendations Not Made

One study of the campaign's impact notes that the specialty societies tended to omit services that physicians frequently performed and to target services that were performed infrequently.[51] For example, vertebroplasty is not the subject of a Choosing Wisely recommendation.

Ken Cohen of Optum lists some other low-value procedures that have been left out of the database, including carotid endarterectomy in asymptomatic carotid artery stenosis, the aggressive treatment of low-risk prostate cancer, the overuse of lumbar spinal fusion, and the overuse of arthroscopy for osteoarthritis of the knee. In his view, Choosing Wisely is moving in the right direction but hasn't gone far enough.

Berwick agrees. "Choosing Wisely is a very good step in the right direction. I agree with the observation that a lot of the tests and procedures that were involved in Choosing Wisely don't represent the mainstream activities of these professions. It's a good first step, but should be bolder."

Baron doesn't deny that some societies have pulled their punches in making recommendations; but he says that some of them *have* addressed services that generate a lot of income for their members. The society of radiation oncologists, for instance, has recommended against proton beam therapy in most cases, he notes.

"The value of Choosing Wisely was that it got a lot of people into the value-based conversation, and it engaged a lot of professional societies in that conversation," he concludes. "It gave consumer organizations credible information to convey to patients about how to think about low-value care. And it created some tangible tools for people to use when they wanted to put these conversations forward."

PRIMARY CARE SCOPE OF PRACTICE

Primary care physicians can control the amount of unnecessary and harmful care provided to patients, but only up to a point. That point is reached after a patient is referred to a specialist and that doctor orders tests, performs procedures, or refers the patient to a surgeon or other specialist. So the basic care groups should have protocols that guide PCPs when they decide whether to refer patients to specialists.

Both for the good of the patient and to conserve the group's resources, PCPs should provide whatever care they are competent to provide before making those referrals. Today, this approach is less common than it used to be decades ago. Many people, especially in the Northeast, go directly to specialists for a wide variety of complaints. At the same time, primary care physicians have become prone to refer their more complex patients to specialists, even if they could handle some of these cases themselves.

Robert Berenson of the Urban Institute recalls that when he needed surgery for spinal stenosis, all his primary care physician did was clear him for surgery. "He compared my new EKG to the old EKG and said it's abnormal, but it's always been abnormal. He's very well trained, but he's made it clear he doesn't want to get involved in the more challenging diagnoses. Chronic back pain? Not his problem. He's happy to refer me."

Not all physicians welcome this turn of events. As recently as 15 years ago, says retired family doctor David Boles, if a patient had a minor laceration, he'd take care of it in the office. If he were still in practice now, however, he'd refer the patient to a specialist. There also are orthopedic practices with nurse practitioners who do primary care orthopedics, he notes. That takes away the strains and sprains that his practice used to handle.

The economics of primary care largely explain why generalist physicians refer out so frequently. "It's related to the rat-race factor: you have to see a certain number of patients each day to survive," says Boles. "It takes the physician less time to fire off a consult [with a specialist]."

Over time, this deference to specialists has resulted in primary care doctors losing skills and confidence in their ability to provide complex care. For one thing, PCPs no longer follow their patients in the hospital; hospitalists and specialists do that now. Even services that family physicians were trained to provide, such as sewing up minor cuts and setting simple fractures, seem more daunting when they haven't done them in a long time.

"When I trained in primary care, you were trained to feel like you should be able to handle a lot of stuff, and only refer patients when you couldn't," says Lawrence Casalino, MD, of Weill Cornell Medicine. "The main reason that PCPs refer out today is the pressure to see a lot of patients each day. And then gradually it becomes a habit and they lose confidence."

Considering that this is the background that the doctors in basic care groups would be coming from, it's likely that many of them would need remedial training. Medical school professors would be useless as trainers; most of them are specialists, and they don't understand the demands of value-based care. My prediction is that the physicians who'd show their colleagues the ropes would come from ACOs and other groups that had been successful in taking financial risk. It's not that the basic care group doctors would not know how to freeze off a wart or set a bone, but most of them would never have done it in practice before.

In some cases, physicians would "work up" patients further than they were accustomed to before referring them to a specialist. For example, say that a patient had lower back pain and might benefit from physical therapy coupled with a pain reliever. The primary care doctor would start with this kind of conservative therapy and ensure that the patient had been properly vetted as a candidate for surgery before she or he was referred to an orthopedist, Cohen notes. "By the time the orthopedic surgeon sees these patients, there's a much lower likelihood that they will be subject to low-value care, because the PCPs have done a good job of working with those patients prior to referral."

CONCLUSION

Doctors in basic care groups would have a strong financial incentive to avoid low-value care, to do as much as they could for their patients, and to be careful about referring them to specialists. When patients went to see specialists, the PCPs would try to retain some control by insisting that the specialists send them timely reports. But ultimately, the primary care physicians would have to develop trust with the specialists they commonly used. A close working relationship between PCPs and specialists is essential to care coordination and to delivering good outcomes for patients.

By reducing waste, basic care groups could lower health spending, stay within their budgets, and generate savings that could increase their doctors' earnings. The other main goal of basic care groups would be to enhance the health of their patient populations. To do that, they would need to engage in population health management, the subject of the next chapter.

CHAPTER 9.

Population Health Management

MAKING THE POPULATION HEALTHIER

Rio Grande Valley Health Alliance (RGVHA), a small primary care ACO in south Texas, saved $9.8 million in 2018 in the Medicare Shared Savings Program (MSSP). The ACO was in a two-sided risk track of the MSSP, meaning it could receive up to 75% of what it saved Medicare. Since its quality rating was 93 out of a possible 100, its gainsharing percentage was reduced to 70%. At that ratio, the McAllen, Texas, ACO garnered $6.8 million in earnings. Even after accounting for the ACO's expenses, its 21 primary care physicians made out very well on their participation in RGVHA.

They had done well in the MSSP for several years. The ACO had achieved much of its success by reducing certain kinds of waste, such as the over-ordering of home care by area physicians. In addition, notes Bo Bobbitt, a North Carolina attorney who helped start RGVHA, the ACO had the advantage of starting with a very high MSSP benchmark because of the unusually high Medicare costs in the area. This benchmark — in effect, an annual budget for the total cost of care — made it relatively easy to achieve savings, at least initially.

But the not-so-secret-sauce of RGVHA is the ACO's commitment to population health management (PHM). With strong physician support, RGVHA invested in the requisite PHM infrastructure, including health IT. It also hired five nurse care managers who provided telephone support to the 15% of the ACO's patients who had chronic conditions and were likely to become sicker. RGVHA also had field nurses who looked after the sickest 5% of patients.

Meanwhile, the ACO used PHM software to stratify its 6,100 MSSP patients by health risk and to compile lists of patients with gaps in preventive care and chronic disease care. The physicians tried to make sure these patients got the recommended care when they came into the office, and their practices reached out to patients who were overdue for the necessary services. All this not only bolstered the ACO's quality scores in the MSSP but also improved patient outcomes. For example, the ACO reduced unplanned hospital admission rates for its patients with diabetes and congestive heart failure.[1]

Planned Care

Population health management, as noted in Chapter 3, requires healthcare organizations to optimize the health of their patients. Rather than focus mainly on diagnosis and treatment, providers must also try to prevent patients from getting sick or sicker. They must do this as efficiently as possible to conserve the limited amount of healthcare resources. And they must do it with consistency. In other words, population health management is planned care.

Group-model HMOs such as Kaiser Permanente and large integrated delivery systems like Intermountain Healthcare and the Geisinger Clinic have long deployed major components of population health management. Today, an increasing number of ACOs and risk-bearing physician groups use PHM to manage financial risk. The main tenets of this approach include:

- An organized system of care.
- Care teams that include physicians and allied health professionals.
- Coordination across care settings.
- Easy access to primary care.
- Centralized resource planning.
- Continuous care provided both during and between office visits.
- Patient self-management education.
- A focus on health behavior and lifestyle changes.
- Interoperable electronic health records.
- Electronic registries that track patients by disease state.
- A focus on social determinants of health.[2]

Of course, population health management didn't come out of nowhere. Following in the footsteps of the group-model HMOs, many health insurers adopted various forms of "disease management" in the 1990s. Patient-centered medical homes (PCMHs) were the next major effort to coordinate care and to ensure that patients received ongoing, appropriate care for their chronic conditions. Some health-care organizations have adopted the PCMH model as preparation for more extensive forays into value-based care, including ACOs.

Some group-model HMOs also pursued disease management using what was known as the Chronic Care Model. Pioneered at Group Health Cooperative in Washington State, this model attempted to integrate care for patients with chronic diseases across care settings and over time. This approach required the resources of large groups or health systems; it could not readily be implemented by smaller groups or ACOs. As noted earlier, PHM is beyond the capabilities of most of today's healthcare providers, although some ACOs have taken it pretty far. Big health systems could do it, but most of them don't see it as in their interest.

Rio Grande Valley Health Alliance showed that a smaller group could do this under very favorable conditions, with the help of automation, and taking partial risk for the total cost of care. My basic care groups, which are two or three times the size of RGVHA, would take full risk for basic care, which means they could not profit by decreasing hospital admissions or the amount of home care delivered. So, their approach to PHM would be somewhat different than that of MSSP ACOs, although fewer hospitalizations would improve their quality scores.

Training Doctors in PHM

As stated earlier, financial risk changes how doctors practice, but not until it forms about two-thirds of their practice. Few primary care practices get that much of their business from risk contracts. Moreover, most of today's primary care doctors are employed, meaning they may not even be aware of their organization's health insurance arrangements.

"Most employed doctors aren't participating in the conversation about the scope of the downside risk," notes David Nash. "This is what the suits do, and the doctors are typically not part of it. Outside of some busy, large practices — of which there are not many left — I don't know how many doctors could tell you how much they are at financial risk for their clinical decisions."

In fact, he adds, not many physicians or their staffs are even aware of their practice's participation in ACOs or what that entails. (However, the success of physician-led ACOs in the MSSP indicates they must have some engagement with these organizations.) So, while far more doctors are engaged in population health management than was the case a few years ago, most of the PCPs in the basic care groups would need a lot of PHM training and support. That is part of why I envision a transition period of at least three years after the formation of the basic care groups before they could start taking significant financial risk.

So, where would the trainers come from? Back when I wrote my first book on healthcare reform and the competing primary care groups in 2006, I thought insurance companies could supply the trainers, because they were the experts in managed care. But I now believe that people coming from a clinical background would be more appropriate. While we want primary care doctors to be efficient, the most important thing to teach them is how to provide excellent care as part of a care team.

An obvious source of trainers would be ACOs. The primary care nuclei of those ACOs could seed several hundred basic care groups. In addition, primary care companies like Oak Street, ChenMed, and Medical One would contribute all their PHM-trained primary care physicians to the basic care groups. Another source would be doctors from the physician divisions of insurers such as Optum and Humana, which have trained doctors in PHM. Groups with deep managed care experience, such as Kaiser, Geisinger, and Intermountain, could furnish many more trainers. And infrastructure vendors, as earlier noted, could also provide some coaching.

PRIMARY CARE SHORTAGE REDUX

The primary care shortage is not going to go away when primary care physicians form basic care groups. And as discussed earlier, the additional production of advanced practitioners has not and will not solve the underlying problem. In the long run, if PCPs earn more money and receive more respect as members of basic care groups, more young doctors will go into primary care. But that wouldn't change the equation for at least a decade after this model was introduced, because it would take that long to fill the pipeline with new primary care doctors.

So, a knotty question arises: How does the current number of primary care practitioners meet the demand for primary care, especially when they're expected to deliver better, more comprehensive care?

One answer comes from Thomas Bodenheimer, MD, a longtime advocate for the reorganization of primary care. Bodenheimer, professor emeritus of family and community medicine at the University of California in San Francisco, has described advanced primary care teams that include a core team or "teamlet" and an extended team. The core team consists of a physician or a midlevel practitioner and one or more medical assistants. The extended team may include any of the ancillary clinical and social work professionals mentioned earlier. These professionals work with all the providers, and patients receive care from the teamlets and the extended teams. Everybody works to the limit of their license: Medical assistants may provide routine diabetes services, for example, and RNs can change medication doses under standing orders.[3]

In another study, Bodenheimer and his colleagues explored the implications of a delegated team model of primary care for determining appropriate panel size. The researchers first estimated the amount of time it would take for a primary care physician to provide all the recommended preventive and chronic care services. Then they looked at how much of this work could be automated or safely delegated to lower-level clinicians in an advanced care team. The researchers concluded that with maximal delegation, primary care doctors could provide high-quality care to more than twice as many patients as they could if they tried to do all this work themselves.[4]

This study has significant implications for the basic care groups. First, the use of advanced care teams such as these could make the groups more efficient. Second, it would allow them to provide higher-quality care. And third, at a time when the primary care shortage continues to worsen, it would help them stretch their physician resources. The same kind of delegated care model could support a nurse practitioner or a physician's assistant, making it possible for these midlevel practitioners to be counted as primary care providers in the groups.

This model could be adapted to population health management. But, despite Bodenheimer's calculation, it's unclear how much adoption of his care team model would offset the additional work required to ensure that appropriate preventive and chronic care was delivered to most people. An earlier-cited study by Elizabeth McGlynn and her RAND colleagues found that U.S. adults received only 55% of recommended acute, preventive, and chronic care services.[5] That leaves a big hole for care teams to fill in this model.

To raise significantly the percentage of patients receiving appropriate care, physicians and advanced practitioners would have to provide longer appointments, especially at the outset, to fill care gaps. Online notification of missing care could be automated, but there would also be more follow-up care than is usually provided today. For example, if a visit or remote monitoring revealed that a patient with hypertension or diabetes wasn't controlling their condition, a nurse care manager would have to follow up with them, and a physician might have to be consulted.

So, even if under the ideal conditions described by Bodenheimer, a primary care physician could handle up to twice as many patients as he or she does today, the increased demands of population health management would reduce that number. There are too many factors involved to estimate what the correct number would be, but it would amount to fewer patients than what Bodenheimer predicts.

Back to the Future

Another potential piece of the solution loops back to the early days of managed care. In the mid-1990s, when insurers were focusing on primary care and shedding specialists from their networks, some internal-medicine subspecialists expanded the primary care portion of their practices or switched entirely to primary care. Among the specialties most likely to transition to primary care were allergists, non-invasive cardiologists, endocrinologists, infectious-disease specialists, and rheumatologists. Some gastroenterologists and pulmonologists also did this, although surgeons generally didn't.

Here's why this stab from the past is relevant to my model: Risk-taking basic care groups would select specialists carefully and would do more for their patients than they do now. As a result, many specialists would see a decrease in referrals; some would not be able to stay in business purely as specialists. Under those circumstances, they too might become generalists.

Some specialists today — as was also true in the '90s — provide some primary care to their patients as "principal physicians." That's fairly natural for an oncologist who sees people regularly for their cancer, or for an endocrinologist who cares for patients with diabetes on an ongoing basis. But these specialists can't provide the full range of primary care. Even though they once studied general internal medicine, they don't necessarily remember all that they were taught decades earlier, and they haven't kept up with the field. Their ability to handle patients with a rash, a headache, or a sore throat varies, and they may not feel comfortable treating a patient complaining of chest pain.

Nevertheless, they can be retrained. Here's how I described the retraining of specialists in my *Medical Economics* article on this subject in 1996:

> Subspecialists can learn how to do primary care fairly quickly, but only if they receive the right kind of training and support, says general internist Michael D. Baldinger, president of Chicago's Sage Medical Group. "They'll do well if they work in a group environment where they get a lot of feedback and a lot of help,"

he observes. "Certainly, within six months to a year, someone who's smart and has a good background can learn to function very efficiently as a generalist."[6]

THE MANY SIDES OF AI

In Chapter 2, I alluded to statements from experts and physician leaders about the ability of artificial intelligence to perform some primary care tasks. To recap, Commonwealth Fund chief Joseph Betancourt and NCQA executive Eric Schneider predict that AI will allow PCPs to "practice at the top of their license" by performing some of their routine clinical functions so that they have more time to treat patients with complex problems.[7]

For example, they say, AI agents can handle low-acuity problems and screening tests with minimal intervention from a clinician. Additionally, they can identify care gaps from medical records and notify patients of them. A recent report from the American Academy of Family Physicians (AAFP) and Rock Health states that, "AI assistants could triage patients, summarize charts highlights, draft personalized educational materials, provide timely decision support, design care plans and flag care gaps."[8]

What's the Evidence?

The evidence to date is mixed but promising. There already is compelling evidence, for example, that AI "ambient scribes" can reduce physicians' workload and mitigate their tendency to burn out by documenting patient visits.[9] Another study found that clinical notes generated by ChatGPT are on a par with those written by senior internal medicine residents.[10]

In a study of AI's assistance in diagnosis, the researchers found that using AI to augment a doctor's work made little difference in diagnostic accuracy, compared to the doctor alone, but the AI chatbot alone was more accurate than physicians. On the other hand, a review article on the topic noted, "Clinical diagnosis is both an art and a science, and is more challenging for AI to optimize than visual diagnostic interpretation, such as radiographic and pathologic diagnosis."[11]

The authors point out that physicians often make diagnostic errors, some of which could be caught with AI backup. Moreover, AI can scan a patient's medical record much faster than a doctor can, helping the clinician to reach a diagnosis sooner. Nevertheless, they note, AI can be acting on inaccurate information in the EHR or on an incomplete physical exam. Also, patient histories are naturally subjective, and experienced doctors may be more skillful than an AI chatbot in teasing out the salient features of what the patient is describing.

An AI agent is only as good as the information available to it, and here the lack of interoperability between health IT systems can create serious problems. Although the ability of a provider's EHR to ingest coded data from other systems is improving, vital data may be missing from the record that the AI is perusing when it suggests a diagnosis.

In addition, AI chatbots sometimes "hallucinate." Researchers at New York's Mount Sinai Health Network recently found that "when fictional medical terms were inserted into patient scenarios, large language models [i.e., AI agents] accepted them without question — and went on to generate detailed explanations for entirely fabricated conditions and treatments. Introducing just one false medical term, such as a fake disease or symptom, was enough to prompt a chatbot to hallucinate and produce authoritative-sounding — yet wholly inaccurate — responses."[12]

Despite these drawbacks, optimism is high about the potential of AI in primary care. "AI doctors can already augment the capabilities of primary care providers, assisting in diagnosis, treatment planning, and patient education," said physician executive Steve Charlap in an October 2024 article. "By leveraging vast amounts of clinical data now part of emerging large language models and machine learning algorithms, these systems can offer personalized care tailored to individual patient needs, reducing diagnostic errors and improving outcomes."[13]

On AI, David Nash belongs to the glass-half-full camp. "When we get to agentic AI, which is coming close, you'll take the medical advice you're given, and a day later, you'll put in your remote vital signs and your new update, and the agentic AI will be smart enough to tell you,

'Woops, wrong antibiotic,' or 'woops, change in therapy,' or 'you've got to go to the doctor.' I think that's a year or two away. We're going to have a lot of improvement in that area quickly."

Clinical Work Versus PHM

To make sense of the emerging evidence, it helps to separate the use cases for AI agents into two buckets: clinical work that directly impacts the well-being of the patient, and work that helps to organize and facilitate the system of care. Until we can validate the AI agent — which is largely not being done today — and until we can be assured that the AI is operating with the best available information, it is too soon to rely on it to diagnose and treat patients. But AI could play a major role in population health management right now.

For example, the AAFP/Rock Health report mentioned the use of AI to identify care gaps and notify patients about them. Well, as it turns out, there are already apps for both of those tasks; on some PHM platforms, the apps are part of a suite, along with other capabilities. What AI could do is to orchestrate the work of these disparate apps, analyze remote monitoring data, facilitate patient portal communications, and perform many other tasks related to PHM.

When a patient is discharged from the hospital, for example, the AI agent could direct the patient portal to contact the patient to remind them to schedule an appointment with their primary care doctor within a week. The AI chatbot could also scan remote monitoring data from a patient with congestive heart failure to detect weight gain or irregular heartbeats. Could clinicians do this as well? Of course. But an always-on intelligent agent could do it better and could take over routine, repetitive tasks that are a poor use of the clinician's or the staff's time.

Some developers of AI-based solutions are starting to move in this direction. For example, Stanford Health is working with a company called Qualtrics to develop AI agents "that interact directly with patients and care teams in proactive ways — such as targeting missed appointments and automatically arranging transportation, or detecting language barriers and then routing patients to interpreters or bilingual staff."[14]

In addition, they plan to use AI agents "to alert care teams to medication delivery support needs. To reduce the likelihood that a patient receives conflicting instructions, AI agents will scan communications for consistency and accuracy and help address social determinants of health by linking patients to housing, food and transportation resources."

AI agents can also synthesize and organize population health data, according to a report by the California Healthcare Foundation. They can also analyze patient data in the context of risk models to determine how best to deploy healthcare resources. And, as will be explored further in Chapter 10, AI agents can help clinicians monitor patient symptoms and medication adherence by integrating patient-collected data from wearable devices or apps into the EHR.[15]

There are already many digital health platforms that automate population health management, and they don't necessarily use AI. Tom Carmouche, MD, executive vice president of Lumeris, a PHM infrastructure vendor, writes that "flashy AI tools won't fix health care without real infrastructure." His company, he notes, has "focused on solving the hard, structural problems — data quality, system connectivity and workflow integration — because without those elements, AI becomes just another layer of complexity. It may look impressive, but it doesn't meaningfully change how care is delivered or experienced."[16]

AI has a distance to go before it becomes a major factor in healthcare diagnosis and treatment. Nevertheless, AI already has the potential to reshape PHM and to greatly reduce the amount of human work that this complex undertaking requires.

PHM INFRASTRUCTURE

Population health management depends on the availability of timely, comprehensive information on patients. But EHRs are still far from interoperable, as noted above, and providers often don't have access to vital information about the care that their patients received elsewhere.

Providers must also have access to insurance claims data to form a full picture of a patient's health and the care they've received. But, as noted earlier, many health plans are reluctant to share that data with providers; even if they do provide it, the data can be three to six months old by the time a physician sees it. However, this should not be a problem for the basic care groups, which will have immediate access to their own claims data.

Specialized software is also required to analyze claims and clinical data so that it can be useful in population health management. The ability to aggregate disparate kinds of data and map them to a standard format is especially important in ACOs where practices use different EHRs — which is to say, most ACOs based on physician networks. This would also be true initially for basic care groups formed by physicians from multiple healthcare organizations. In the long run, however, these groups would adopt a single EHR.

Among the common types of data analysis for PHM are:

- Risk stratification, which classifies individuals by their level of health risk.
- Care gap identification, which shows which patients have not received recommended preventive and/or chronic care services.
- Provider measurement, which shows how well individual providers perform in delivering evidence-based care and managing the utilization of healthcare resources.
- Utilization of services, broken down to primary care and specialist physicians, hospitals, and post-acute care providers.
- Reports on out-of-network care.

Many ACOs and physician groups have implemented software that is used to automate the routine aspects of PHM. One example is patient outreach software that automatically contacts patients when they're overdue for preventive or chronic care services and that can even make appointments for them. Automation software also can be used to electronically send tailored educational materials and alerts to healthy patients and people who are in the early stages of a chronic disease such as hypertension or diabetes.

A PHM infrastructure should also include health IT experts, care managers, disease educators and coaches, nutritionists, pharmacists, and other ancillary providers. The number of these care team members varies with the size, resources, and philosophy of a healthcare organization. But the use of care teams itself is a core principle of population health management.[17]

HIGH-RISK VERSUS WHOLE POPULATION

A healthcare organization that invests in PHM infrastructure needs to see a return on that investment. The organization can get this return fastest by focusing on high-risk patients who have conditions that are already bad and likely to get worse. Often known as "super-utilizers" or "frequent flyers," these patients may see several different specialists for multiple chronic conditions. An ACO can reduce spending quickly by coordinating their care and keeping them out of the hospital, by handling their discharges appropriately, and by dealing with their mental and behavioral issues.

Supporting this viewpoint is the fact that the sickest 5% of patients account for about 50% of health costs.[18] Only 30% of the high-risk patients, however, were in that category a year earlier;[19] and by the time an organization knows they're high risk, there is a limit to what it can do for them. So ACOs and risk-bearing groups also must manage the next group of patients in the risk hierarchy. Known as "rising-risk" patients, these people form another 15% of the population. High-risk and rising-risk patients generate about 80% of health spending.[20]

The patients in these two categories are the central focus of RGVHA's population health management efforts. But the ACO also tries to ensure that its physicians fill as many care gaps as possible for all their patients. In addition, the practices contact people who are overdue for recommended services.

"It's really hard to manage patients under care coordination if they already have a malignancy," RGVHA manager Victoria Farias told me. "We know there's not a lot of impact we can make, unfortunately.

So, we want to target a step down from that and we want the physician offices to help us with the patients in the lower-risk categories."

A basic care group would try to keep their patients healthy and out of the hospital; but, from a financial viewpoint, good management of rising-risk patients would provide their biggest bang for the buck. These patients are less likely to be hospitalized than high-risk patients, and their conditions can often be stabilized or mitigated. The earlier their primary care doctor can intervene with them, the less likely they are to be referred to a specialist, and the less advanced care they will need. This is good not only for the patient, but for the group's bottom line.

Ultimately, a survey of several groups shows, the most effective approach to PHM is one that aims to engage everyone in the population, from the healthiest to the sickest individuals.[21] By providing online health education and trying to get people to improve their health behavior, a basic care group can nip minor health problems in the bud and prevent them from blossoming into serious conditions that require expensive forms of treatment.

CONTINUUM OF CARE

A key part of PHM consists of managing the care of patients with a chronic disease from its early stages to exacerbations of the illness, hospitalization, and post-acute care. In conjunction with specialists, the basic care physicians would direct chronic disease care up to the point where a patient was hospitalized or needed expensive treatments such as cancer care. And, although hospitals and health systems would take financial responsibility for the initial phase of post-acute care, primary care physicians would pick up outpatient care as soon as possible after hospital or PAC discharges or during prolonged episodes of home care.

Most of the PHM process was worked out decades ago, albeit in the context of large groups. The Chronic Care Model, which I alluded to before, was designed to "reduce fragmentation while at the same time improving health outcomes at an acceptable cost to the healthcare system." The core elements in the Chronic Care Model are "mobilizing community resources, promoting high-quality care, enabling patient self-management, implementing care consistent with evidence and patient preferences, effectively using patient/population data, cultural competence, care coordination, and health promotion."[22]

Studies of the Chronic Care Model have shown consistently positive results for patients with conditions such as diabetes, asthma, chronic obstructive pulmonary disease, depression, and HIV.[23-24]

For the purposes of this discussion, let's focus on the Chronic Care Model's care coordination piece. According to the Group Health Cooperative Institute, "Referrals and transitions work best when all parties — patients, primary care providers, and consultants — agree on the purpose and importance of the referral, and the roles that each will play in providing care."

Among the issues and expectations that should be included in agreements between specialists and patient-centered medical homes (PCMHs) — care teams led by primary care doctors — are the following:

- Types of patients referred — many specialists have developed criteria for the patients they prefer to see;
- Information provided at time of referral;
- Notification of the PCMH of ED visits and hospitalizations;
- Testing to be completed prior to referral;
- Availability for "curbside consults";
- Consultation report content and timeliness;
- Post-ER or post-hospitalization care expectations;
- Specialist-to-specialist referrals — many PCPs do not want specialists to refer their patients to other specialists without first consulting with the PCP.[25]

In a multispecialty group that has adopted the Chronic Care Model or another disease management approach, the PCPs and specialists must agree on the practice guidelines they will follow. It's not easy for physicians to agree on clinical protocols, even if they're in the same specialty and the same group. Yet the PCPs in the basic care groups could get specialists to sign on to nationally recognized guidelines that both parties have tweaked, if those protocols would result in better care.

Under the basic care subscription model, however, the specialists would face an additional challenge related to the competing primary care groups. If each group had its own set of practice guidelines, the specialists would have the same problem that doctors now have with multiple insurer guidelines and quality measures. Therefore, it would be advantageous for the basic care groups in a particular region to sit down with specialist representatives and agree on the guidelines they wanted to use. A precedent for such a regional concord is provided by the Institute for Clinical Systems Integration in Minnesota, which has developed guidelines that physicians across the state have agreed to follow.[26]

Modified Gatekeepers

Another point of contention between PCPs and specialists is the "gatekeeper" role that some health plans have assigned to primary care doctors. The requirement of HMOs that patients see a primary care physician before going to a specialist — and the consumer backlash it sparked — was one of the reasons for the failure of the first managed care wave.

Today, HMOs cover about 13% of Americans covered by employer-sponsored insurance plans.[27] Typically, HMOs require PCPs to approve referrals to specialists, as their predecessors did. A 2018 study of commercial HMOs and PPOs in Massachusetts found that HMO insurance was associated with lower rates of new specialist visits than PPO insurance, which usually had wider networks and fewer restrictions on specialty care.[28]

As noted earlier, my reform model would require consumers to choose a primary care doctor in a basic care group. But patients wouldn't be prevented from seeing specialists on their own or going to out-of-network specialists. Their PCPs would encourage them to see one of their group's contracted specialists and might show them that doctor's quality scores. If a patient insisted on being referred to a different physician, however, the PCP would accommodate him or her. Because out-of-network specialists would charge the group significantly more than those in network, the patient might have a copayment if they saw a non-contracted specialist.

Due to the basic care groups' power over referrals, specialists would tend to cooperate with PCPs in caring for patients with chronic diseases. Ideally, the specialists would operate as part of the basic care team. Not only would they follow the same guidelines as the primary care doctors, but they'd work closely with the PCPs to coordinate care, avoid duplicate tests or contraindicated medications, and try to ensure that patients followed care plans. The question is, how would the groups pick the right specialists?

Ken Cohen, MD, former CEO of New West Physicians in Denver and currently an official at Optum, recalled in a 2015 article that the risk-taking group chose specialists based on their quality and efficiency. In selecting physicians for its network, he wrote, the group first made sure that all the specialists it was considering provided high-quality care. However, that was just the price of admission. "Inherent in our model was the recognition that high-quality care afforded only small improvements in efficiency," Cohen wrote. "We recognized that cost of care was not linked to quality of care and that excessive care was both costly and dangerous to patients."

If a chosen specialist still provided a significant amount of low-value care, he added, a group medical director would meet regularly with the doctor. "By repeatedly feeding information back to our specialists and by orienting referrals to the specialists who are doing the best job, over time you quickly gain alignment on optimal care."[29]

PATIENT ENGAGEMENT

Population health management involves patients; without their cooperation and engagement, nothing useful can occur. Therefore, the basic care groups would have to devise and follow strategies designed to engage patients. Among other things, people must be persuaded to follow their doctors' care plans, adhere to medications, and improve their health behavior. In addition, physicians should involve patients in important care decisions wherever possible.

It has been estimated that 40% of deaths in the United States are caused by modifiable behavioral issues, such as smoking and obesity. People with chronic diseases take only 50% of the prescribed doses of medications, on average. Fifty percent of patients do not follow referral advice, and 75% do not keep follow-up appointments.[30]

Many patients are unaware of their risk factors because they have not received recommended screening tests. For example, when a group of 4,000 people was screened for high cholesterol, a government study found, only 40% of those with this condition were aware of it. Adherence to drug prescriptions is also low. Even among heart attack survivors, adherence to medications prescribed to them ranged only from 36% to 49% in one study.[31]

Occasional visits to physicians by patients with chronic illnesses and people with risk factors for chronic diseases are insufficient to address this compliance problem. "Sporadic contact (such as every six months) with a healthcare provider is often inadequate to maintain and reinforce complicated lifestyle modifications and pharmacologic regimens," noted Thomas Pearson in a paper on the prevention of cardiovascular disease.[32]

How to Effect Change

There is substantial literature on engaging patients in their own healthcare. Among other things, studies have shown that patients who are active participants in their own care have better health outcomes and measurable cost savings.[33]

But it isn't easy to activate some patients, either because they're depressed or because they don't believe they're up to the task. One study, for instance, showed that only 30% of seniors felt they had the motivation and the skills to participate fully in their own care.[34]

Activation strategies include using care managers or coaches to increase patient awareness of the need for change; having care managers help patients build confidence in their ability to change health behavior; and persuading patients that they need to improve health behavior to avoid negative outcomes.[35-37] However, the barriers to patient engagement go beyond the willingness of patients to take responsibility for self-care or to follow doctors' orders. These include social and economic factors, cultural factors, a lack of health literacy, and poor access to healthcare.[38]

Many patients do not have a regular primary care doctor, as observed earlier. Even if they do have one, it may be difficult for them to secure an appointment, take time off from work, or find transportation to see the doctor. Some patients can't afford the tests or medications their doctor orders, especially if they have a high-deductible health plan or lack insurance. A fuller discussion of these issues can be found in Chapter 12.

Patient Outreach

Continuous care that encompasses the periods between visits to a healthcare provider is essential to PHM. While most patients care for themselves between visits, providers can send them online educational materials or prompt them to seek information about their condition on reliable websites. If the patients have a chronic disease, they may also receive phone calls from care managers. Whatever their health status, they should also be alerted about their preventive and chronic care gaps.

Maintaining contact manually with every patient in a practice is beyond the means of even large organizations, and care managers are an expensive resource. So, the basic care groups will have to use the kind of automation software described earlier. Using data extracted from EHRs, these programs build patient registries and use clinical protocols to trigger messaging to patients who have care gaps.

Risk stratification software can be used to track how sick a patient is and what type of interventions they require. The information that these programs use comes from EHR and claims data. In addition, patients can fill out health risk assessments to provide a richer pool of data.

But many people are disengaged from healthcare. This is especially true of young people, some of whom imagine themselves to be immortal. It's also true of people who can't take time off from work to go to the doctor and parents who take their children to the local urgent care center when their pediatrician is unavailable. Busy people may want to stop at the retail clinic in a CVS or a Walgreens on their way to pick up some items at the store.

This is not necessarily bad if the person is treated properly and if the clinicians in the urgent care center ask the patient who their primary care doctor is and send that physician a report on the visit. Unfortunately, this doesn't happen very often today. So, to begin with, the basic care groups should establish connections with the alternative primary care sites in their area. They should also offer evening and weekend hours to cater to people who need to be seen then. They should offer walk-in appointments and figure out how to shorten the wait for a regular appointment.

Social Determinants of Health

Population health management requires that providers address their patients' social determinants of health (see Chapter 12). Healthcare accounts for less than a quarter of health differences among individuals. Genetic factors, health behaviors, social and economic factors, and physical environmental factors explain the rest.[39] Therefore, it is incumbent upon the basic care groups to engage with patients and community-based organizations (CBOs) to mitigate the unhealthful effects that the conditions of some patients' lives can have on them.

Unlike big health systems, relatively small basic care groups can't do much to help meet their patients' social needs by donating money for food and shelter or getting involved in local programs that help the destitute. So, the groups' efforts in this regard will be largely dependent on the financial strength of CBOs. However, PCPs can and should consider the circumstances of their patients when they treat them. For example, if they know that a patient is struggling to make ends meet, they should prescribe a generic drug rather than a brand name medication. Groups should employ social workers to help patients with unmet social needs. And they should refer patients to community-based organizations that can help them, such as food pantries, housing services, and social services.

CONCLUSION

The basic care groups must learn how to manage population health to improve the overall health of their patients and stay within the budgets they set for themselves. As this brief summary indicates, there are a lot of moving parts in PHM, and the primary care physicians in these groups can learn a great deal from colleagues who have already been there.

In the discussion about how to ensure a sufficient supply of primary care, I touched on the role that AI might play in population health management. But AI is only one of the digital technologies that are currently being used to improve patient outcomes. Telehealth, mobile health apps, remote monitoring and e-visits are all getting increased attention, and they'd be essential tools for basic care groups that took financial risk. The next chapter explains how these technologies are being used in healthcare, and Part 3 also explores the ramifications of my model in other areas.

PART 3.

Ramifications

CHAPTER 10.

Technology in Healthcare Reform

Technological innovations have led to a boom in various forms of consumer-oriented digital healthcare. For example, the use of telemedicine mushroomed during the COVID pandemic. It has since fallen far from its peak, but telemedicine appointments are far more common than they were before the pandemic.

Meanwhile, e-visits using secure patient portals have vastly increased in number and impact. Physicians complain about all the time they must devote to responding to portal messages. They don't get reimbursed much, if at all, for this work under fee-for-service. But, within the budget of a basic care group, e-visits become another tool in the toolbox that doctors can use to improve patient care.

Digital healthcare is not just about communications. The invention of the smartphone spawned a vast industry of digital health apps. While most of the many thousands of mobile health apps help consumers obtain health information or support their wellness activities, there are many — including a growing number on smartwatches — that can be used in chronic disease care.

Remote patient monitoring (RPM) has finally begun to expand beyond pioneering healthcare organizations such as Kaiser Permanente, Geisinger Health, and Mass General Brigham. While RPM still has limitations, AI promises to help overcome some of them.

Here's a brief summary of these developments and how they're changing patient care.

TELEHEALTH CAN BE A LIFELINE

After soaring during the pandemic, the usage of telehealth (also called telemedicine) fell substantially, but it is still much more widespread than it was before COVID.[1] As a percentage of all healthcare claims, telehealth services remain in the single digits,[2] and telehealth visits — while still much more frequent than before the pandemic — represented only 4% of outpatient visits in 2023.[3] On the other hand, many physicians use telehealth at least occasionally,[4] and nearly 40% of behavioral health sessions take place during telehealth visits.[5]

In 2023, 19% of Medicare beneficiaries living in rural areas received a telehealth service, compared to 27% of urban Medicare patients, according to a Kaiser Family Foundation study. The difference was partly attributed to the paucity of broadband access in rural areas.[6]

For a long time, Medicare covered only rural telehealth services of certain types. During and after the pandemic, the program authorized telehealth use by all Medicare-participating doctors everywhere, and it gradually expanded coverage to other types of providers. Crucially, Medicare patients are allowed to have telehealth visits at home instead of having to go to physician offices to have video consults with specialists. The government pays doctors at the same rate for telehealth visits that it does for in-person encounters without facility charges.[7]

Telehealth visits raise short-term Medicare costs because they expand access and lead to more follow-up visits than in-person encounters do.[8-9] Therefore, Congress has been reluctant to make these telehealth expansions permanent. Every year or two, it has extended the pandemic-era relaxation of telehealth rules; the most recent extension is set to end December 31, 2027.[10]

According to the Department of Health and Human Services (HHS), many commercial insurers have broadened telehealth coverage since the pandemic, and most health plans now offer some kind of coverage. Medicaid reimbursement varies from state to state.[11]

There is no doubt that physicians and patients would like to keep telehealth as part of healthcare. In a recent survey, 83% of physician telehealth users said they prefer that virtual care remain a permanent part of their clinical practice. Nearly all telehealth patients surveyed said that the quality of virtual care is equivalent to or superior to in person care, and 78% indicated that telehealth visits improved their access to healthcare services.[12]

"Greater use of telehealth has improved convenience, decreased travel time, and led to small but meaningful improvements in health care quality, particularly for underserved groups such as lower-income patients and racial minorities," health policy experts Ateev Mehrotra and Jared Perkins recently wrote. "Not surprisingly, most beneficiaries want telehealth to be an option, and telehealth has received broad congressional support."[13]

What It's Used For

Telehealth is most commonly used for routine follow-ups, prescription refills, mental health therapy, and minor acute conditions like colds and flu.[14] But some physicians said in a recent survey that they also use it for chronic disease care and complex cases. The specialties most likely to use telehealth for ongoing care management are endocrinology, urology, gastroenterology, rheumatology and neurology.[15]

Nearly two-thirds of the responding doctors said that telehealth visits improved patient outcomes. This means that, in the long run, the additional cost of telehealth might be outweighed by the decreased cost of caring for healthier patients. And it also means that, if physicians did not have to depend on face-to-face visits for most of their revenue, the use of telemedicine might grow substantially.

The enhanced access provided by telehealth is critical for some patients. Aside from rural patients who use virtual visits to see physicians remotely, there are many elderly and disabled patients in more populated areas who have difficulties in getting to a doctor's office, particularly if they don't own a car. In a recent letter to Congress from 350 healthcare organizations, the signatories said, "Access to telehealth services serves as a lifeline to Medicare beneficiaries across the country, allowing access to critical health care services even when they have barriers to accessing in-person care."[16]

If telehealth continues to expand, the technology is likely to be used increasingly in conjunction with remote patient monitoring (RPM).

Both technologies, for example, are fundamental to hospital at home (HaH), which has been expanding steadily since the pandemic. A patient who chooses HaH, which is available for selected conditions, is treated at home in a hospital bed connected to monitoring equipment. Besides speaking with the nurses or paramedics who visit the patient one or more times a day, HaH patients can connect via telehealth with clinicians in a hospital command center.[17] The same legislation that extended Medicare coverage of telehealth did the same for hospital-at-home, but for a five-year period.[18]

A related trend that has emerged more recently is at-home emergency care. In this scenario, which has direct applicability to our basic care groups, patients are referred to at-home emergency care if they don't have life-threatening illnesses or injuries. Services deploy paramedics or nurses to check vital signs, draw blood and take x-rays with portable imaging devices. Emergency physicians supervise the visits via telehealth. Patients can later be referred to their PCP or sent to an emergency department. Many private insurers reimburse for this service, but Medicare and Medicaid do not.[19]

Telehealth also plays a large and growing role in rural healthcare. For example, Texas Health Resources, a health system based in Dallas, has developed a robust telehealth capability to serve its rural communities in several ways. For one thing, virtual visits have cut the long waiting times for behavioral healthcare appointments. THR also offers hospital at home to patients needing acute care and those recovering from procedures.[20]

E-VISITS IMPROVE ACCESS

Another channel of digital communication that is used much more frequently than telehealth is the patient portal attached to EHRs. Patients can utilize the portal to ask questions about their condition, their treatment, or their medication, and to access lab results. Care managers can use this channel to keep track of how their patients with chronic illnesses are doing.

These asynchronous "e-visits" offer patients some of the same advantages as telemedicine visits: improved access, greater convenience, and reduced or eliminated travel time. "Interactions that are more frequent but shorter than traditional visits, such as weekly check-ins using telemedicine or portal messaging, may result in better outcomes for patients with chronic illnesses, including reductions in avoidable hospitalizations," noted Julia Adler-Milstein and Ateev Mehrotra in a 2021 article.[21]

During the pandemic, CMS and private payers began reimbursing providers for e-visits. An increasing number of practices and health systems now bill for electronic messaging, especially when it requires substantive medical decision making. In a survey, 43% of clinicians said they had used e-visit billing codes.[22]

However, billing for e-visits entails some difficulties. An e-visit can be billed to Medicare only if the visit was initiated by the patient, patient consent was obtained, and a clinical decision was made. So those elements must be documented. In addition, patients who previously received these services for free now have a copayment, which some may resent.[23] Perhaps for that reason, billing for patient portal messages led to a modest decrease in message volume in a large health system, a study found.[24]

As with all the digital "touchpoints" described here, this billing conundrum would not concern the basic care groups, because their reimbursement would not be fee-for-service. Physicians and care teams could use any digital modality to communicate with patients or measure their vital signs, and it would be covered under their group's subscription fee.

Burden on Clinicians

However, there are other questions about how to respond to electronic messages and whether this is the best use of a physician's time. According to a 2023 *JAMA* commentary on e-visits, "There is evidence that electronic messaging between patients and their care teams is associated with improved outcomes, adherence [to care plans], and experiences of care." Yet these exchanges have placed an extra burden on physicians, requiring them to spend more time answering messages in addition to their EHR documentation tasks. This is especially challenging for primary care physicians, who receive five times as many patient messages and 15 times as many prescription messages as surgeons do.

Electronic messaging has also changed the work of ambulatory care teams, "who now must be trained to triage and respond to messages related to appointments, clinical concerns, prescription refills, and other issues," the authors note. "Yet at present, our health care system is not adequately designed for the delivery of high-quality, asynchronous, EHR-based care delivery, and the fee for service paradigm that underlies much of US health care does not reimburse for the time spent on EHR-based communication. Consequently, physicians and other clinical staff try to perform this work in the crevices of their time or, less commonly, in designated time slots within a broader clinical schedule."

The authors recommend that non-physician members of the care team handle most of these tasks, except when the answer to a message requires a doctor's expertise. If a patient needs to speak with a clinician, they could be "seamlessly transitioned to either virtual or in-person visits, depending on the complaint." Even better, they suggest, "AI-powered solutions could help filter and direct messages and answer straightforward questions prior to a message being directed to a care team member."

In recent studies, they continue, AI agents "have been shown to craft empathic responses to patient messages and to appropriately answer questions related to clinical knowledge." Even if the AI chatbots don't actually write the responses, they can categorize patient messages and suggest responses or relevant information to physicians.[25]

As I noted earlier regarding the uses of AI in primary care, the technology should be viewed as augmenting rather than replacing the work of primary care providers. AI can be a powerful tool, but it cannot replace the physician in the physician-patient relationship.

MOBILE HEALTH APPS IN PATIENT CARE

Digital health apps, which may be paired with wearable sensors, have had a significant impact on consumer involvement in their own healthcare during the past decade. However, it is unclear what effect these apps have had on health or on how physicians care for patients.

In 2019, according to a consumer survey by Stanford Medicine and Rock Health, one in three respondents owned a wearable monitoring device, and one in four wearable owners used it to manage a health problem. Just over half of the respondents who tracked their health in some way discussed their tracking data with a physician or other medical professional. Among those who used digital health tracking tools, 75% discussed the data with a clinician.

Forty-four percent of people with a chronic disease used one or more digital health tracking tools, the survey found.[26] But that result gives a false impression about how digital health apps are being used overall.

In 2021, there were roughly 350,000 digital health applications on the market — about twice as many as in 2015. Approximately half of smartphone users had downloaded at least one of these apps, according to a literature scan by the Canadian Agency for Drugs and Technologies in Health (CADTH).[27]

The CADTH report noted that digital health apps generally fall into one of four categories: informational, diagnostic, disease management, and fitness tracking. "A survey in 2017 found that for individuals who frequently use mobile health apps, 64% monitor physical activity, 41% monitor nutrition, 36% monitor weight, 36% monitor sleep, and 19% monitor sport performance," the report said. In other words, most downloaded apps were used for something other than chronic disease management.

Smartwatches Cue App Use

Nevertheless, the spread of smartwatches and other wearables that include health-related functions has implications for chronic care. According to the CADTH report, Fitbits, Garmin watches, Samsung watches and Apple watches can measure heart rate, blood oxygen saturation levels, activity levels, sleep quality and quantity, electrodermal activity, and skin temperature. Today's Apple watches also can detect atrial fibrillation.

CADTH describes the kinds of apps available for a few chronic conditions. For example, people with diabetes can choose among about 1,000 apps, some of which are also for reducing weight. "These apps provided patient monitoring through information regarding weight management and diabetes management, reminders for medications or diet, feedback for diet and test results, and supportive and motivational remarks."

Among the functionalities of digital health apps for self-management of hypertension are self-monitoring, automatic feedback on the readings, reminders regarding blood pressure measurements, appointments and medications, communication with health providers, and exportation of data to providers. A few apps claim to be able to use the smartphone directly as a medical device to measure blood pressure by using the phone's camera.

Although positive data exists for some of these apps, there is a "lack of clinical evidence to support claims made by app developers about their efficacy," the CADTH report points out. "The descriptions in apps routinely state medical expertise and backgrounds that are not supported by the application content or development process. There are limited apps that have been tested in clinical studies, and of those that have been tested in studies, the results are not supportive of their efficacy or there are limitations in their study designs."

Many Doctors Recommend Apps

Despite these drawbacks, roughly a third of U.S. physicians advise some patients to use digital health apps, says Joseph Kvedar, MD, a professor of dermatology at Harvard Medical School, the editor in chief of NPJ Digital Medicine, and a longtime proponent of digital health. Considering that most apps are about engaging patients in improving their health behaviors, he notes, physicians don't have much to worry about when they recommend these apps.

As for digital health apps that address chronic conditions, Kvedar could think of only two categories that have really gained traction among doctors: apps and devices that detect atrial fibrillation, such as the Apple Watch, and continuous glucose monitoring apps. The latter have two important features, he says: First, they provide feedback that helps people understand how certain behaviors trigger swings in their blood glucose so they can adjust those behaviors accordingly. Second, some apps can be connected with insulin pumps that adjust patients' insulin levels as needed. In Kvedar's view, this connectivity between monitoring apps and insulin pumps represents a revolution in diabetes care.

How reliable is the data from digital health apps overall? Except for the two types of apps described above, Kvedar says, the quality of data from these apps is not medical grade. So physicians might not pay too much attention when a patient brings this kind of information to their attention. However, he notes, the apps "are not meant to be medical grade. They're usually about healthy behavior."

Health Assurance Approach

In the previously cited book by Steve Klasko (see Chapter 4), he emphasizes a new model of disease management that he calls "health assurance," which integrates digital health apps with other technologies. Klasko predicts that, as digital technology increasingly empowers consumers to take charge of their own health, what the healthcare system can do for them will become secondary. Instead of being the prime source of healthcare, he says, physicians will act as coaches and as backups when patients get severely ill.[28]

One example of the health assurance approach is a company called Livongo. Formed by a serial entrepreneur named Glen Tullman and now owned by Teladoc, the company offers a one-stop shop for helping patients with diabetes manage their condition. As the book notes,

> Livongo provides these patients with unlimited test strips, a smart meter, and personalized tips and coaching, all paid for by self-insured employers and health plans. The meter uploads blood sugar readings to the patient's secure account in the cloud through the Livongo smartphone app. AI-powered analytics are applied to the data, learn the patient's metabolic patterns, and tailor health advice to that person. The app provides real-time, 24/7 tips and insights after every blood glucose check. A Livongo

> coach calls the patient if a reading is out of range, and users can contact a coach at any time. The meter also reminds the patient when they need to order supplies.[29]

The key advance of Livongo, Klasko writes, is that it helps patients manage their condition by giving them instant feedback and guidance 24/7 — something that no physician or practice can do, but that available technology can accomplish. As a result, the service reduces the frequency of physician office visits and the likelihood of medical emergencies. And it requires little of the patient, other than paying attention to the app's advice.

Other health assurance companies cited by Klasko have taken a variety of approaches, including Mindstrong (depression), Mindful (well-being and performance), Glooko (diabetes and other chronic diseases), Noom (weight loss, stress and anxiety, hypertension, and diabetes), and B. well (a range of healthcare conditions). What they all have in common is that, in some way, they automatically coach and guide patients to take better care of themselves.

Undoubtedly, the digital health app market will continue to evolve, and digital health companies will keep innovating. Billions of dollars in venture capital have been invested in these entities, and consumers will continue to download and use apps they think can make them healthier. But the question is which apps can actually do that. Some have been shown to help people, but many more are simply vaporware.

REMOTE PATIENT MONITORING GROWS

Some health systems utilize medical-grade digital health apps and devices in chronic disease management programs. For example, the Medical Center of the University of Alabama uses remote patient monitoring (RPM) to extend care to patients with chronic diseases who have difficulties in traveling to see a doctor. The hospital has deployed devices in patients' homes to monitor diabetes, high blood pressure and other chronic illnesses.[30]

Southwest Community Health Center in Bridgeport, Connecticut, also uses RPM to track the blood pressure and other vital signs of its patients with hypertension. With about 1,000 patients enrolled, the hospital says it has seen a more than 30% improvement in blood pressure control.[31]

Although Medicare and some private payers cover the use of FDA-approved RPM systems, the reimbursement has declined and future payments are uncertain. There is also a steep upfront investment for the setup, making it difficult for individual hospitals and physician groups to provide RPM. A monitoring program for 1,300 patients with diabetes at the University of Nebraska Medical Center, for example, cost $4.3 million to implement and $1.2 million annually to operate.[32]

Despite the cost, some health systems persevere. Several years ago, UCHealth in Denver launched an RPM initiative that initially focused on diabetes and is now part of UCHealth's Virtual Health Center. In the diabetes program, enrollees received an app that paired wirelessly with their glucometer via Bluetooth. Patients took their blood glucose readings twice a day, then transmitted the values back to UCHealth. When technicians noticed a worrisome blood sugar spike, they would contact the patient to identify the problem, such as a high-carb meal or a missed medication.

In a 2022 UCHealth article, a nurse leader commented, "We're able to provide better outcomes when we have these continuous touchpoints rather than seeing patients once every three months, then making a change and having to wait another three months to see if that change had an impact."

At the time, she said, patients enrolled in the program had stayed with it an average of 135 days. During that period, their HbA1c levels declined, on average, from 10.3% to 7.7%.[33]

Continuous Glucose Monitoring

There's a lot to know about how to set up an RPM program. Patients with diabetes, for example, can be monitored by using Internet-connected blood glucose meters, as described above, or continuous glucose monitoring (CGM) systems.

A continuous glucose monitor includes a sensor (a filament inserted into the skin) and a transmitter attached to or imbedded in the sensor.

The transmitter sends glucose data to a reader or a smartphone app. In some systems, as previously mentioned, data is sent to an insulin pump to enable the adjustment of insulin delivery. All systems have smartphone apps, enabling users to access data at any time. In some cases, data is sent to third party data management sites.

Some glucose meters have software that can be installed on a computer in a medical office; others have Bluetooth connectivity to an app. Data logs can be downloaded as PDF files and scanned into an EHR system or uploaded to commercial sites for review. Practices can also purchase accounts to access data from third-party platforms such as Glooko and Tidepool.[34]

The CGM systems, in particular, transmit a massive stream of data. Even if a practice or health system had some way to integrate that information with its EHR, technicians would have to keep checking the data to pick up unfavorable trends or use some other method. But there are those who argue that AI could once again come to the rescue.

In a 2024 *New England Journal of Medicine* article, Geoffrey S. Ginsburg, Rosalind W. Picard, and Stephen H. Friend said that the sheer volume of data generated by wearable sensors was one of the biggest challenges in remote monitoring. However, they added, "Approaches to sorting and analyzing data efficiently, deriving insights, and making them clinically useful are evolving (particularly since the advent of AI)."[35]

Multistage Transition to AI

Kvedar says the nascent use of AI in remote monitoring is the latest stage in efforts by healthcare providers to deal with the firehouse of data coming out of RPM devices. Ten or 15 years ago, he recalls, he and his colleagues at Mass General Brigham (then known as Partners Healthcare) would go into an RPM program and adjust alarm thresholds. Physicians would be alerted, say, when a patient's blood pressure went above or below a certain level, or, in the case of heart failure, if their weight exceeded a certain level.

The next stage was pattern recognition. The software would tell clinicians that a reading for a particular patient was "correlated with them going to the ER or having a bad outcome," he relates. "And more and more, this is being integrated into the software that vendors use for remote monitoring. So the data still goes into the record, but it's not incumbent on the doctor or the nurse to look at every single data point. Rather, you have the software cull out the meaningful results and detect a trend or make a suggestion.

"AI just makes better predictions," he points out. "It's better pattern recognition, and all of a sudden it can talk to you — which is the magic part, although it's just statistics, too."

Patient-Facing Dimension

Another perspective is offered by Amanda Bury, the chief commercial officer at Infermedica, which markets an AI-driven "symptom checker and virtual triage" package. RPM data is just as overwhelming and hard to understand for patients as for providers, she told *Health IT News* recently. AI-driven tools, she declared, can transform this data into personal insights that are easy for patients to understand.[36]

Kvedar believes that the patient-facing side of AI-powered remote monitoring has "huge potential." In the earlier phase of RPM, he recalls, he and his colleagues did studies on how exposure to monitoring data affected health behavior.

"In one case, we gave everyone a pedometer, and half of the study subjects had access to a virtual coach called Karen, which was informed by their step counts from the pedometer. Whenever they'd engage with Karen, she'd tell them how to do better with walking and so forth. Those people were far better at meeting their step goals than the controls were. The other study we did was with patients who had type 2 diabetes. We fed their multiple different behaviors that they would share or that wearables would record into a rule set and would send them highly personalized messages twice a day. And their A1c went down significantly more than the control group."

Outcomes Versus Savings

RPM has been shown to improve health outcomes in a series of studies, Kvedar says, and the data on that is "quite solid. What we haven't been able to demonstrate is cost savings." He argues, however, that various types of telehealth — including telemedicine and RPM — shouldn't be held to that standard. "For nearly every other technology that comes along, we ask, 'Is it going to improve care?', not 'will it save money?' But people keep asking that question, and we haven't proved it yet."

Even if it can't be proved, he adds, providers have been getting paid for RPM that meets certain requirements since 2018, when billing codes for it were introduced. As a result, he says, an increasing number of health systems are billing for RPM. While that may or may not mean that more of them have launched RPM programs, they might see some return on investment, depending on the health condition involved. "With heart failure, if we keep some people out of the hospital, that helps the patient flow and reduces overcrowding in the ED, and we can get paid for it," he points out. "That one tips people over the edge [of accepting RPM]."

This use case was thoroughly documented back in 2012, when the Geisinger Health System showed that a heart failure RPM program reduced readmissions by 44%. A 2014 follow-up study of patients with the same condition, using Bluetooth scales with an interactive voice response solution, lowered readmissions and saved more than it cost, according to Geisinger.[37]

Many RPM programs continue to target patients with heart failure. But there are now also programs for many other health conditions, including hypertension, diabetes, coronary artery disease, COPD, chronic kidney disease, sleep apnea, cancer, obesity, perinatal care, post-surgical recovery, and neurological disorders.[38-39] What this suggests is that healthcare providers have gone beyond seeing RPM mainly as a way to reduce readmissions and now view it as part of population health management.

FUTURE VISIONS, CURRENT REALITIES

The basic care groups in my model would use telehealth and e-visits to complement in-person visits when it made sense to do so. And, because of the flexibility afforded by operating within a budget, care teams could use whatever combination of communication methods worked best in chronic disease management. One goal would be to help patients manage their own conditions to the greatest extent possible. They would still come into their doctor's office for regular check-ups; but, with the help of technology, they would have more frequent contacts with their care teams than most patients do today. Some of these contacts would be initiated by patients and others by clinicians, depending on the patient's health status and other circumstances.

Physicians and advanced practitioners would also recommend certain digital health apps to patients if they thought it could help them improve their health or manage their chronic disease. While more of these apps should be validated, clinicians can learn from experience about which apps actually help patients. They might not want to receive data from the apps and related devices, however, except in areas like continuous glucose monitoring, where the data has proved to be reliable.

Most remote patient monitoring would be too expensive for the basic care groups. They wouldn't be able to afford the equipment or the personnel required to make such programs effective for large numbers of people with chronic conditions. But the hospitals taking financial risk for inpatient and post-acute care could use RPM programs to improve follow-up care and prevent readmissions. Forward-thinking health systems might also share this data with the local basic care groups.

The advent of AI offers both immediate and long-term opportunities. At some point, AI agents could use RPM data, coupled with the patient's medical record, to identify patterns and make recommendations or send out alerts to clinicians and patients. These analyses would be far more personalized than what has been available up to now, and a chatbot might use them to guide the patient through self-care in a manner similar to Klasko's "health assurance" approach. But, even if this kind of automation were validated, a clinician would have to oversee it to ensure that no harm befell the patient.

How Much Will Patients Take Over?

In *The Patient Will See You Now*, the prescient 2014 book by Eric Topol, MD, the founder and director of the Scripps Translational

Research Institute envisions a future in which each person has all their own medical data and the computing power to process it, and most care is provided at home. Here's how he describes the result:

> The doctor will see you now via your smartphone screen without an hour of waiting, at any time, day or night. It might not be your primary care doctor, but it will likely be a reputable physician who is conducting part of his or her practice through secure video consults. And those consults will involve doing parts of the standard physical examination remotely. More importantly, they will incorporate sharing your data — the full gamut from sensors, images, labs, and genomic sequence, well beyond an electronic medical record. We're talking about lots of terabytes of data about you, from the womb to the tomb, in your personal cloud, stored and ready for ferreting out the signals from the noise, even to prevent an illness before it happens.[40]

We seem to be well on our way toward creating this kind of future with the help of an artificial intelligence that was just starting to emerge when Topol wrote his book. But the ability to do this may be several years away — if not a decade or more. And, even when it arrives, the level of patients' use of these technologies will be determined by each person's willingness and ability to participate and to stick with it.

In the meantime, the basic care groups could benefit their patients and themselves by taking advantage of as much digital health technology as they could afford. And, with the help of AI, they could increasingly personalize care. This would facilitate insights into each individual's health and the expected trajectory of their chronic disease, if they had one. It could also help clinicians understand the person's genomic makeup and how that might affect their condition, the medications prescribed to them, and many other parameters.

Of course, this prediction applies to all medicine of the future, not just the kind of healthcare that would be possible if my model were adopted. But it is especially relevant to a primary-care-oriented reform model that seeks to lower costs by reducing waste and improving health. The more precisely and efficiently the basic care groups deliver care, while optimizing outcomes, the more likely they are to thrive and their patients to do well.

CHAPTER 11.

Saving Rural Healthcare

The policy recommendations I made earlier in this book apply only to urban and suburban areas. Because my model is based on competition among large primary care groups, it would not work in rural areas where there aren't enough primary care doctors to form such groups. In addition, the shaky financial condition of many rural hospitals requires a different approach to stabilize and augment local healthcare resources.

While my reform model must be revised to match the conditions of rural healthcare, that tailored solution should be based on the same values and goals that underlie the model elsewhere. All rural residents — who comprise about 20% of the U.S. population — should have access to quality healthcare at an affordable cost, and the required benefits should be the same for every individual.

Above all, rural healthcare should be planned rather than left vulnerable to market forces. This means a much greater degree of government intervention than is now the case. Regardless of how small or isolated a community is, its residents are entitled to receive the national standard of care. It will not be possible to provide all the resources that people have in more populated areas. For example, not all counties have hospitals or even physicians. But, with the technologies now at our command, and with greater financial support for the hospitals and clinicians that deliver care in rural areas, there should be a way to ensure that rural residents have the same chance at long, healthy lives that their non-rural counterparts do.

Today, that is not true. For example, rural individuals have higher rates of dying from heart disease, cancer, unintentional injuries, chronic lower respiratory disease, and stroke than urban residents do.[1] With a growing number of hospitals closing their labor and delivery units, there are now large "maternity deserts" in many states, leading to an increased risk of maternal mortality.[2] In recent years, cervical cancer incidence has been 25% higher and cervical cancer deaths have been 42% greater in rural than in urban counties.[3] Over the past 20 years, the death rate for working-age people has increased in rural areas, while the mortality rate for this age group has decreased in urban areas.[4] Overall, the average life expectancy of people living in rural areas is nearly two years less than that of metropolitan residents.[5]

Meanwhile, the impending cuts to Medicaid and the expiration of Obamacare subsidies pose a major threat, not only to the health of rural residents, but also to the financial solvency of rural healthcare providers. For example, researchers for the Commonwealth Fund estimate that net operating income for the 300-plus rural hospitals in Medicaid expansion states could drop by 24.5% to 28% because of new Medicaid work requirements that will start in 2027.[6] That could be a death blow for the many rural hospitals that are on the brink of bankruptcy.

What all of this means is that rural healthcare is likely to get much worse before it gets better. And it will only get better if it operates under a new model that guarantees universal healthcare and that strengthens the rural workforce.

RURAL HOSPITALS ON THE BRINK

Since 2010, 153 rural hospitals have closed.[7] The Commonwealth Fund study says that more than 700 rural facilities are at risk of closing, and that more than 300 of them are imminently threatened.[8] The at-risk facilities represent more than 30% of the country's rural hospitals.[9]

There are two schools of thought about why so many rural institutions are in trouble. Some experts say that the hospitals' woes are mainly the result of inadequate reimbursement from commercial health plans. It's more expensive to deliver healthcare in rural areas, and private plans pay lower rates to rural hospitals than to larger urban health systems that have negotiating power. This is especially true of Medicare Advantage plans, which pay less than Medicare rates after figuring in the cost of dealing with their aggressive prior authorization policies.[10] With MA plans now claiming about 40% of rural Medicare beneficiaries as members,[11] this is a growing problem for rural hospitals.

Another explanation for the parlous state of rural hospitals — one embraced by the Medicare Payment Advisory Commission (MedPAC) — is that many of them don't treat enough patients to remain financially viable. In the 10 years preceding the closure of 40 rural hospitals that MedPAC looked at, the annual number of their admissions dropped to a mean of 488 per hospital from 1,045 at the start of the period — a decline of 53%. Since rural populations didn't dwindle overall, it's likely that some people preferred to go to larger regional hospitals.[12]

However, the population *has* dropped in some rural areas. According to a Pew Research Center report, the populations of urban counties have grown at roughly the average national rate since 2000, while those of suburban and small metropolitan areas have grown faster. Rural counties have lagged, and half of them have fewer residents now than they did in 2000.[13]

Jack Westfall, MD, a family physician who works part time for a critical access hospital in Yuma, Colorado, attributes the poor financial condition of his hospital to both low payment rates and low utilization of the facility in relation to its fixed costs. He notes the CAH has 20 beds but only three or four patients in them at any given time.

One thing that's certain is that many rural hospitals are facing serious threats to their survival. Nearly half of rural hospitals are in the red, and in some states, the rate is much higher. In Kansas, 87% of rural hospitals are losing money, followed by Washington (76%), Oklahoma (70%), and Wyoming (70%).[14]

A recent paper on the predicament of rural hospitals blames "large decreases in demand for care, driven by declining populations, a shift toward ambulatory care, and a tendency for patients to seek care outside of their local area. Low patient volumes limit revenues at rural hospitals and make it difficult for hospitals to cover the fixed costs of delivering care."[15]

The paper also notes that Medicare, which funds more than half of inpatient days in rural hospitals, pays less than commercial insurers do for the same services. Medicaid, which covers roughly a quarter of rural residents,[16] pays nearly a third less than Medicare, on average.[17] And the percentage of uninsured patients is higher in rural than in urban and suburban areas.[18]

CMS provides additional support to rural healthcare by paying "critical access hospitals" — which comprise about 60% of rural hospitals[19] — on a cost basis. This means that they receive higher payment rates from Medicare than urban hospitals do. However, Medicare Advantage plans are not required to pay critical access hospitals (CAHs) on a cost basis; so, as these plans spread, CAHs suffer.[20]

Not surprisingly, many rural hospitals have eliminated some services to stay afloat. For example, more than 290 rural hospitals dropped obstetric services between 2011 and 2023. Partly as a result, "maternity care deserts" now stretch across about a third of the country. Many facilities that still have maternity units depend on a patchwork of federal grants. Rural maternity wards are difficult to maintain because of high physician recruitment costs, a payer mix that skews toward Medicaid and the uninsured, the threat of legal liability, and the declining rural birth rate.[21]

Rural Emergency Hospitals

The CAH program, one of several federal programs that support rural hospitals, has not been sufficient to stem the tide of hospital closings. So, in 2021, the federal government launched the Rural Emergency Hospital Program to preserve rural outpatient and emergency care while downgrading inpatient care. Critical access hospitals with no more than 50 beds are eligible for this program. If they agree to close their inpatient units and maintain their emergency departments 24/7, they receive about $3.3 million a year in facility payments and are paid 5% more than Medicare's hospital outpatient rates for emergency services.[22-23]

While this may sound like a good deal, as of August 2025, only 42 hospitals had enrolled in the program.[24] Why so few, if rural hospitals are in such bad financial shape? "Closing the inpatient department is a big emotional thing for a hospital," says healthcare consultant Mike La Penna. "That means it's not really a hospital anymore. It's an urgent care center, or an urgent care center with a recovery area or an overnight stay area. And a lot of times, the EMS [Emergency Medical Service] system won't recognize it as a place where you can take patients [by ambulance]. They may not even realize there's a rural hospital out there. Or, even if they do, they know the patient isn't going to get the care they need."

Harold Miller, president and CEO of the Center for Healthcare Quality and Payment Reform, notes, "For some hospitals that have very few inpatients, it doesn't make sense to have an inpatient unit. But many critical access hospitals admit hundreds of patients every year. And for some of these patients, that's critical. An elderly woman with heart failure, for instance, gets pneumonia and needs to be admitted for a few days. It makes no sense to send her 50 miles away to an urban hospital, rather than being taken care of in the community."

Westfall, who recently retired from his post as a professor of family medicine at the University of Colorado School of Medicine, agrees. The Rural Emergency Hospital Program "is not an adequate policy, because there are so many people who don't want to leave the rural community," he points out. Moreover, the common belief that mortality rates are higher in small rural hospitals is false, he says. Based on his research, he notes, younger, healthier heart attack patients get transferred to urban hospitals far more often than older patients with the same condition. This skews the mortality rates and makes the rural facilities look worse.

It's also a myth that rural hospitals are losing money mainly because of their inpatient services, Miller says. "Most of them are losing money on their other service lines, like emergency care and their rural health clinics. And that comes back to commercial insurance payments."

In addition, he points out, "Rural hospitals that close their inpatient units are giving up their cost-based CAH payments. And what they are getting in return is the standard Medicare outpatient payment plus

5%, compared to the 7% extra they get as a sole community hospital." Since most of a rural hospital's services are outpatient, he notes, they're actually getting paid less if they become a rural emergency hospital. But he admits that must be weighed against the extra $3.3 million in facility payments.

More federal funding for rural hospitals is coming. When the One Big Beautiful Bill (OBBB) was being debated, experts warned that its nearly $1 trillion in Medicaid cuts would particularly hurt rural hospitals in districts where many Republican voters live. To mitigate the impact, Congress added the Rural Health Transformation Program to the measure. To be dispensed over five years, the Rural Health Transformation funds total $50 billion.

However, observers say the program won't benefit the highest-need hospitals and won't be nearly sufficient to counterbalance the Medicaid and Medicare cuts under the new tax law. While some of the new money will go to keeping rural hospitals open, much of it will be spent on partly related goals such as boosting clinical recruitment and training programs.[25]

Moreover, the states will control only half of the spending; HHS will determine where the rest of the money goes. Michael Cannon, a healthcare expert at the conservative Cato Institute, has called the program "a government slush fund where politics decide where the money goes."[26]

Survival Techniques

Rural hospitals have adopted a variety of strategies to survive the dismal environment in which they find themselves. Among these approaches are merging with a bigger healthcare system, cooperating with an urban health system in a hub-and-spoke arrangement, and forming clinically integrated networks (CINs) with other rural hospitals.

From 2010-2018, one study found, 7% of money-losing rural hospitals closed and 17% of them merged with other hospitals — most of them outside their markets. Merging with another hospital or health system increases market power and can lead to higher prices. Moreover, the study said, "aggregating volume into fewer, larger facilities can help hospitals leverage economies of scale and improve quality in situations in which higher volume is associated with better outcomes."[27] On the other hand, notes La Penna, rural hospitals may be shut down or stripped of some services after mergers with outside health systems.

Isolated hospitals, the study observed, were less likely than facilities with competitors to merge with other hospitals, and CAHs experienced out-of-market mergers at a lower rate than other hospitals did. Small-market hospitals were also less likely to close than large-market hospitals. These findings point to the community need for these hospitals and their reluctance to give up the CAH designation. It's also notable that 77% of the unprofitable hospitals survived during the study period. The researchers speculated that these hospitals "may have had other financial resources to draw from, outside of short-term profits." These resources may have included grants and community tax funds.

Hub-and-Spoke Model

Another way to alleviate the rural health crisis is to adopt a "hub-and-spoke" strategy. In this model, independent rural "spoke" hospitals partner with large "hub" health systems to access resources they can't obtain on their own. Regional or national hospital chains can extend their technology, staffing, medication discounts and other assets to rural hospitals to boost revenue and expand specialty care. This strategy empowers rural hospitals to survive without surrendering their independence.[28]

An important part of the hub-and-spoke model is telehealth services that, where available, enable rural hospitals to access specialty care services while reducing costs. Chat-based platforms, e-consults with providers and virtual triage can be used where residents have access to broadband Internet.[29]

Rural broadband is still missing in many rural areas. While 72% of rural people had broadband access in 2021, compared to 77% of urban dwellers and 79% of suburbanites, 35% of rural areas had no broadband access at all. Some residents in those areas had dial-up Internet access.[30]

What does a metropolitan health system get out of forming a hub-and-spoke network with rural hospitals? Major hospitals need referrals from rural facilities, La Penna observes, "So when the rural hospitals close, there's a secondary impact."

Moreover, he points out, these urban hospitals are competing with other health systems, often in different cities, for the rural business. As a result, some specialists visit rural hospitals on a regular basis to provide care and pave the way for referrals. When people need heart surgery, for example, they're more likely to use the tertiary-care hospital where the cardiologist they have seen in their local hospital is on staff. "They follow their doctor."

Westfall has observed the same phenomenon. "Historically, the large hospitals have sponsored specialists to come to rural hospitals as part of a balance of doing something good and as a loss leader, or case finding. They'd send a cardiologist out to Yuma to see patients one day a month, and they'd capture the heart procedures. And the gastroenterologist would capture GI procedures."

Clinically Integrated Networks

Rural hospitals have created an increasing number of clinically integrated networks (CINs) in recent years. Decades ago, CINs usually consisted of independent physician practices that formed them to get around the FTC ban on competitors bargaining with insurers on price. Today, rural hospitals are building these networks partly for the same reason. In addition, CINs can provide these facilities with data infrastructure, shared equipment and service contracts, and the ability to get value-based-care contracts from health plans.[31]

For example, 10 rural hospitals in Wisconsin with a combined net revenue of $880 million formed a CIN in 2025. Similar networks have emerged in Montana, Ohio, Minnesota, North Dakota, Nebraska, and West Virginia.[32-33]

Harold Miller says that the CIN approach is superior to merging with a health system. "For one thing, the hospitals have much greater negotiating power with commercial health plans because the plan can't say, 'We have a contract with this other hospital down the road.' Now you have all these hospitals across a broad area. More important, they can also share services."

Noting that physicians are often involved in these CINs, La Penna likens them to the physician-hospital organizations (PHOs) that emerged in the first wave of managed care. "It's like the old PHO model, where the hospital, the PCPs and the specialists all are somehow related economically and structurally. That has existed in some form for a long time. Some of the current CINs are huge and are private equity connected."

PHYSICIAN SHORTAGES AND RURAL CLINICS

As noted earlier, rural areas have a chronic physician shortage. Eighty percent of them are medically underserved. In rural areas, there are 39.8 physicians per 100,000 people, versus 53.3 physicians per 100,000 in urban areas.[34]

In many rural ERs, there are no attending physicians onsite, and physician assistants or nurse practitioners provide care. According to one study, in 2022, 7.4% of ERs across the United States didn't have an attending doctor; more than 90% of these ERs were in low-volume or critical access hospitals. In North and South Dakota and Montana, about half of the ERs lacked attending physicians.[35]

Some healthcare observers say NPs or PAs can oversee ERs, and that requiring a physician to be present might force some rural hospitals to close. But it's not just ERs. Some rural hospitals don't have any doctors onsite at all or much of the time, although physicians may oversee the care of midlevel practitioners.

Michael Tuggy, MD, a family physician in rural Washington, explains the nuances of this situation. "In a lot of the hospitals in our area, we have an NP there during the day while the doctors are in clinic," he says. "And they'll come in in the morning and round on the patients with the nurse and create care plans together. Then they hand off to the NP to handle the cases during the day. The NPs will take care of the paperwork and early stabilization, but they often need physicians to oversee that work."

In some cases, he adds, NPs and PAs staff the ER, and the hospital brings in locum tenens physicians for at least one shift per week. "But they're often not from the community and don't know the system very well."

Tuggy notes that, although every community wants to have its own hospital, that's not realistic in many cases. "They just don't have enough volume to maintain a hospital. They don't want to drive 10 miles to the next town, but if you combined their hospital with the one 10 miles away, they'd have enough capacity to keep the hospital going.

"That's what happened with our obstetric program: we had one delivery per week at two hospitals, and eight deliveries at the other one, so we combined them, and now we have 10. And that paid for the OB nurses and so on. It was more realistic to combine them."

Heterogenous Care System

As mentioned previously, there are rural counties without hospitals. In many of those areas, the main sources of healthcare are federally qualified health clinics (FQHCs). "Typically, FQHCs exist in small towns with under 2,000 people," Tuggy points out. "A significant proportion of those towns don't have a hospital within 10 or 20 miles. In the town I live in, we have an FQHC 10 miles away, and we're 50 miles from the nearest [full-service] hospital."

FQHCs are also found in medium-sized communities of 10,000-20,000 people or more, he adds. Even if those towns have hospitals, they're usually very small, so FQHCs are essential. In his very large county, which has about 30,000 people, there are several FQHCs, and most people live within 10-20 miles of one.

Besides clinicians, support staff, and ancillary services such as lab and X-ray units, he notes, FQHCs have social workers and, in some cases, behavioral health therapists. An FQHC without a hospital nearby functions partly as an urgent care center, he says. If someone needs a higher level of care, the clinic staff stabilizes the patient and sends him or her to the nearest hospital with an ED. If that is insufficient, they will be sent to the major urban hospital in the area.

Tuggy, who is now transitioning out of practice, works for a bigger clinic that is part of an urban health system and has a satellite clinic in his area. The group also includes specialists who are available to the critical access hospitals. Most of the primary care doctors work for either the group or one of the FQHCs in the area.

"There are very few independent rural practices that are doing pretty well," he notes. "They're usually attached to the hospital, so they get pulled into the hospital structure, and they get cost-plus reimbursement to cover their costs."

Westfall's hospital employs its PCPs, who work both in an affiliated rural health clinic and the ED. Six doctors, including him, share 24/7 ED coverage, he says. Not all of them live in Yuma — he himself lives in Denver — but they each spend two or three days a week in the hospital and the clinic.

The nearest FQHC, he adds, is about an hour's drive away. "We're the only medical team in town. There's no other clinic, but there's a pharmacy and a dentist."

Not every town is like Yuma, he adds. Nearby Sterling, Colorado, for example, has a small hospital that employs ED specialists and hospitalists. There are four primary care clinics in Sterling that are independent of the hospital. One of them is part of the University of Colorado, and another is a private practice with an FP who does obstetrics, including C-sections.

FQHCs: The Workhorses of Rural Healthcare

One in five rural residents was served by a federal qualified health center in 2024, according to the Health Resources and Services Administration (HRSA). FQHCs that receive HRSA grants are required to "provide a set of comprehensive, high-quality primary care and preventive services regardless of patients' ability to pay." They're also supposed to "deliver care coordination and other enabling services that facilitate access to care."[36]

Also known as community health centers, FQHCs serve as the primary care home for 10 million rural patients. Of these patients, 84% have low incomes. They include 2.6 million children, 1.6 million seniors, 215,000 veterans, and 235,000 homeless people. Nearly three quarters of the clinics provide treatment for opioid use disorder, and some have mobile units that travel to remote areas.

FQHCs contributed $13.3 billion in spending to rural communities in 2023. They provided 130,000 jobs, including those of 20,000 physicians, NPs, PAs, and nurses, 11,000 behavioral health professionals, 7,000 dental services staff, and 42,000 other staff members.[37]

Like CAHs, FQHCs receive cost-based reimbursement from Medicare. But, by shutting off access to federal grant funding early in 2025, the Trump Administration endangered the viability of FQHCs in both rural and urban areas.[38] Despite court orders to release the appropriated funds, the money continued to trickle in slowly, and recent HRSA staff cuts have further constricted the flow of federal funds to rural health clinics.[39]

Instead of cutting off grants to FQHCs, the federal government should ensure they are adequately funded. Congress should also provide money to expand the FQHC network to areas where they are sorely needed.

Alleviating the Physician Shortage

There are various reasons why primary care physicians prefer to work and live in metropolitan, rather than rural areas, but money is not one of them. Rural PCPs earn roughly the same as their urban counterparts do, although the income range is wide. In 2024, one survey found, median compensation for a rural family physician who didn't do obstetrics was about $260,000, with earnings ranging from $179,500-$420,000.[40] The national average salary for FPs, by comparison, was $242,000.[41]

Tuggy notes that private practice physicians can earn significantly more than that in rural areas, but they have to work very hard and long to do it. In contrast, he says, FQHCs pay modest salaries to primary care doctors, resulting in high turnover rates.

Many suggestions have been made about how to alleviate the primary care shortage in rural areas. Some of them apply to underserved urban areas as well. For example, the National Health Service Corps (NHSC) tries to attract physicians to underserved areas by paying back part of their student loans or by providing scholarships in return for a commitment to practice in an underserved community for two years.[42]

Currently, over half of NHSC members work in community health centers, and a third of NHSC and Nurse Corps members work in rural communities where patients have difficulty accessing care. But this approach has filled only a small portion of the primary care gap.[43]

Many international medical graduates (IMGs) do their residency or fellowship training under a J-1 visa. Upon completion of their training, U.S. immigration law gives them two options: they can return to their home country for at least two years before applying for a visa to re-enter the United States, or they can obtain a J-1 visa waiver that eliminates the home country return requirement if they are willing to practice in a medically underserved area. State health departments can each request J-1 visa waivers for up to 30 IMG doctors per year, and the program recruits about 800-1,000 IMGs annually.[44] But again, this meets only a small portion of the need — and it's likely to diminish in importance as the Trump Administration limits immigration to the United States.

Nurse practitioners are increasingly being used as primary care providers across the United States, and they are more likely than primary care physicians to practice in underserved areas. They treat a high proportion of uninsured patients and other vulnerable populations. However, nurses are in short supply, too. More than a million nurses are expected to retire by 2030, and a shortfall of 328,000 RNs, 42,000 LPNs, and 33,800 NPs is expected by 2032.[45]

It's often said that physicians who train in rural residency programs are more likely to stay in those areas and practice medicine there. But rural residencies are not numerous and may not be all they're cracked up to be, says La Penna. Noting that an effort by Michigan State University (MSU) to place resident doctors at rural hospitals has "fallen aside," he suggests that the motivation of young physicians to practice where they want to live and in their desired specialty usually trumps other considerations.

"People are desperate to go to medical school, so maybe they'll end up going to MSU. At the end of the [rural residency] program, they'll subspecialize in dermatology or cardiology. Their program never showed it was able to get doctors to stay in the rural areas. Instead of converting a rural residency into a primary care practice in the same town, the physicians left as soon as they could and went into a specialty fellowship program [at an academic medical center]."

VALUE-BASED CARE IN RURAL AREAS

It might seem that rural healthcare providers are too small and underfunded to participate in value-based-care arrangements. That is not the case, however, in some regions. For example, we earlier encountered the Rio Grande Valley Health Alliance, which has done quite well in the Medicare Shared Savings Program (MSSP).

Aledade, a company that finances and manages small ACOs, has also had success in the MSSP with ACOs in underserved areas. In 2023, all eight Aledade ACOs made up exclusively of community health centers earned MSSP shared savings. Of the 300 FQHCs with which Aledade partners, nearly two-thirds are in healthcare shortage areas.[46] But most ACOs are concentrated in urban areas, and many rural regions lack a significant ACO presence.

In some respects, FQHCs — both rural and urban — are well positioned to move into value-based care. They already offer more comprehensive care than most other primary care practices do. They also provide coordinated care, as shown by the fact that three quarters of them have been recognized as a patient-centered medical home (PCMH). In addition, they understand the importance of social determinants of health (see Chapter 12).

According to HRSA, "The PCMH model of care enables health centers to have strong patient outcomes at lower costs despite treating a sicker and poorer population in comparison with other health care settings." In one study, the HRSA report found, "Health centers had 24% lower spending compared to non-health center patients across all services provided."[47]

State VBC Experiments

Private insurers take financial risk from most state Medicaid programs. More than half of the states require these Medicaid managed care organizations (MCOs) to use alternative payment models (APMs) for a specific percentage of provider payments. For most of these states, the requirements for APMs range from 25%-50% of the payments.[48] Some states contract directly with community health centers, including FQHCs and rural health clinics, using APMs such as upside-only shared savings and two-sided risk contracts.[49]

Some states have designed population-based payments (PBP) specifically for FQHCs. California, Oregon, and Washington have such models.[50]

In Washington, Medicaid MCOs contract with providers using the state's FQHC-specific approach. In Oregon, safety-net providers in the PBP model are paid by regional care coordination organizations (CCOs), which are part of the Oregon Health Plan. In both states, FQHCs receive capitated payments for each Medicaid beneficiary plus care management fees.[51]

Some FQHC networks accept prepayment for all or part of the care provided to Medicaid patients. Yakima Valley Farm Workers Clinic, which has 42 clinics in Oregon and Washington, takes downside risk for spending on specialty care, pharmacy and hospital care. In addition, Yakima also has an ACO that belongs to the MSSP. According to a Commonwealth Fund brief, "The investment [in APMs] has paid off: in a given year, Yakima's additional revenue from quality incentives and shared savings can be upward of $10 million — a substantial segment of Yakima's $250 million operating budget."

Mosaic Medical, which has 15 FQHCs in Oregon, has also taken some downside financial risk for its Medicaid patients, the report points out. The population-based payment has allowed the clinics' providers to deliver care between visits in a variety of locations. Clinical pharmacists also play a key role in helping patients manage their chronic diseases. Community health workers screen patients for social needs and track their progress in finding community resources to meet those needs.[52]

FQHC patients in these and other states are benefiting from state-led VBC models. For example, health centers participating in Oregon's Alternative Payment and Advanced Care model can offer nontraditional services such as home visits, telemedicine and telephone visits, clinical follow-up and transitions, dental care coordination, transportation assistance, case management, and health education.[53]

A NEW VISION OF RURAL CARE

The key innovation in my health reform model — splitting financing between basic care and major medical services — can be retained in rural healthcare, but with one important difference: Instead of the two halves of the financing being divided on the basis of what *type* of care is being delivered, the separation will depend mainly on *where* the care is delivered.

If a patient is treated in a rural area, and the cost is below a certain level, the case is part of basic care, whether or not a hospital stay is involved. If the rural patient is treated in an urban facility, his or her stay is covered by major medical insurance. (Urban specialists also receive insurance payments for rural patients.) As in the other part of my model, basic care is covered by a subscription, and major medical services, by health insurance.

The reason why rural hospital care is considered part of basic care is that it's part of the continuum of local healthcare that ranges from FQHCs, rural health clinics and private practices to critical access hospitals and other small facilities. Providers must work closely together because they constitute the sole healthcare resources in the community. Since providers are in such short supply, there is no competition among them; they must cooperate to survive.

In the mainstream model, large primary groups charge subscription fees, which collectively form their budget. But in the rural areas, there are only small practices, and most primary care doctors are employed by either hospitals or FQHCs. So they are not in a position to take financial responsibility for care.

Rural hospitals can be budgeted, and as discussed below, they have been in Maryland and Pennsylvania. In this model, however, the budget would cover all healthcare in a community. Every kind of provider, whether it be an FQHC, an independent practice, or a visiting specialist or locum tenens physician, would be covered under the same budget as the hospital. The funds would come from subscription fees paid by all residents living within a certain radius of the hospital or clinic that serves as the local healthcare hub. As in the urban model, those fees would be subsidized by employers and the government.

Another major difference between this model and the mainstream approach is that the subscription fees would be determined through negotiations with the state. The local providers can't be allowed to set the fees, because they have no competition. So, the state would work out the amount with the local providers. Perhaps those providers could form a bargaining unit like the physician-hospital association (PHO) discussed earlier. Using data gathered from their combined financial records, they could establish and propose a budget sufficient to cover their combined expenses for the following year.

In an area with one or more FQHCs, part of the budget could be used to fund a population health management infrastructure along the lines of the West Coast initiatives described above. If there is a hospital in the area, it should be part of this organization, which would resemble an ACO in some ways.

The local healthcare systems would not be big enough to build and implement such an infrastructure by themselves. They would require support from a larger organization — one not tied to the state or to a private health system. I propose the creation of Rural Healthcare Cooperatives on a regional or statewide basis. These cooperatives would combine some of the functions of the current FQHC networks and rural hospitals' clinically integrated networks. They would purchase supplies at scale, provide health IT support, and process claims, as the health utilities would in more populated areas. These claims would come from visiting or remote specialists, locum tenens physicians, durable medical equipment suppliers, and other parties.

Boundary Issues

The boundaries of local healthcare communities would also have to be determined. In the vast expanses of rural America, particularly in the West, those are fluid and not always obvious. Depending on where they live, people may be more likely to go to a clinic or a hospital in one town than in another. For certain health conditions or emergencies, they might travel to a different location for care. Moreover, they can't be bound to one place; for example, they might need care in a rural specialty clinic that isn't part of the local healthcare system.

Another boundary issue is to define what a rural area is. To start with, there is a gradation between exurban, semi-rural and rural areas. Also, some medium-sized cities are surrounded by rural areas. Where does the market of that urban area end? Hospital service areas have been mapped out, and they provide a reliable guide to the catchment areas of individual hospitals. But states must figure out how those service areas overlap in rural regions.

Nevertheless, boundaries can be set between rural healthcare communities, based on where most people go for their care most of the time. And a budget can be constructed by using historical costs plus one other factor: the additional cost of maintaining hospital capacity, even when it's not needed. As mentioned earlier, this is a major reason why rural healthcare costs more than urban healthcare. A "standby capacity payment" — say, 10% extra — should be tacked onto the budget to provide the financial wherewithal to sustain that capacity.

Global budgeting of rural hospitals might create an incentive for them to transfer patients to urban hospitals, even if they could be treated in their communities. But there are at least two safeguards against that: First, interhospital transfers, especially to tertiary care hospitals, are declining because of ED overcrowding and rising hospital occupancy levels.[54] Second, rural patients often prefer to be treated at the nearest hospital rather than travel long distances, as we've seen.

History of Global Budgeting

In Chapter 5, I discussed the implications of Maryland's system of global budgeting of hospitals within an all-payer rate-setting system. Maryland prepared for the transition to global budgets by introducing the system in selected rural hospitals, beginning in 2010. A paper comparing the results in these facilities to a group of non-budgeted Maryland hospitals found that there were no significant changes in admissions, readmissions, ED visits, or hospital costs at the budgeted facilities during a three-year period.

This was a disappointment to policy analysts at the time. However, the rural hospital budgets did not include physician payments or other services provided outside the hospital — both of which are part of the MSSP's total cost of care model and would also be included in my rural hospital model. If physicians had an incentive to reduce costs, unnecessary hospital utilization might decline.

One other factor stands out in Maryland's experience: The hospitals didn't receive prospective payments to cover their costs. Instead, as explained earlier, they billed for services at the all-payer rate. Depending on whether they underspent or overspent relative to their budgets, they later lowered or increased their charges within narrow limits. For rural hospitals, the researchers regarded this approach, not as an asset, but as a liability:

> This payment structure might have limited hospitals' incentives to lower utilization, since price increases were generally limited to no more than 5 percent (Larger price adjustments were subject to the review and approval of state regulators.).[55]

Direct budgeting of rural hospitals has also been tried in Pennsylvania. The voluntary Pennsylvania Rural Health Model (PARHM), introduced in 2017, provided participating rural hospitals with prospective, multi-payer global budgets rather than traditional fee-for-service payments to improve financial stability.

A comparison of 17 PARHM hospitals with 40 non-participating hospitals found mixed results. Among the hospitals that joined the program in 2019, the mean operating margin improved (from a substantial loss to near breakeven), whereas operating margins among the comparison hospitals declined in 2019 and 2020. After adjustment for several variables, however, the changes in operating income were deemed nonsignificant.[56]

Again, it should be emphasized, these global budgets did not cover local physicians. Where physicians have an incentive to improve population health and keep people out of the hospital — whether they are in urban or rural areas — it is likely that they will do so. Rural providers' experience with value-based care, especially among FQHCs, shows that they can use the VBC approach to improve quality and lower costs.

Primary Care Versus Hospitals

Global budgeting didn't seem to harm the finances of rural hospitals in either Maryland or Pennsylvania, so it shouldn't in this model, either. That still leaves two questions about this financing approach: Would it enable more rural hospitals to survive, and, if so, should all of those facilities continue to exist?

Better population health should lower costs at every level of the healthcare system, including rural hospitals. Moreover, designing budgets to include standby capacity payments would be a real boon for those hospitals. However, that doesn't mean that all hospitals should be kept in business.

Tom Campanella, a rural health policy expert who used to be a rural hospital administrator, acknowledges the importance of rural hospitals to their communities. However, to save rural healthcare, he says, more emphasis must be placed on increasing the supply of primary care.

"What we need is a ground-up approach, which starts with the residents' needs in rural communities, instead of a narrow focus on the hospitals," he wrote in an August 2025 blog post. "Obviously, hospitals play a significant role in residents' health and well-being, but to have a long-term impact on rural America, addressing primary care shortages may be more of a priority."[57]

La Penna agrees with this view. "Various studies have shown that primary care has a higher yield of value to a patient population than a hospital bed does," he says.

Miller takes the opposite position. "If you say we should have primary care in a community, and let's give them a lab and an imaging center, and they're going to be open 24/7, sure. But if you have primary care in a community and no hospital, where do people go for an emergency? Where do they get their labs done for diabetes management? Primary care isn't going to do all that."

Based on my conversations with rural physicians, it appears that in areas where no hospitals exist, FQHCs do a reasonably good job of providing care. In cases where a higher level of care is needed, they can send patients to nearby or urban hospitals. And, for a lot of purposes, such as surgical follow-ups and certain kinds of specialty care, telehealth will do just fine. Congress just has to place a greater priority on making broadband Internet available in rural areas.

This is not to say that there aren't failing rural hospitals that we need to keep in place. That is absolutely true, and perhaps a community-wide budget can help do that. But where hospitals no longer fill enough beds to justify their existence, it may be time for them to close their doors and make way for a new kind of rural healthcare.

Getting More Rural Doctors

A nationwide commitment is required to ameliorate the rural physician shortage. We need an "all-of-the-above" approach to address this glaring problem. Perhaps we could start by making medical school free to any student who pledges to become a family physician and serve in an underserved area for at least two years. If they choose to become an internist — and thus have the option to later subspecialize — maybe 50% of their tuition could be paid. We should also make it easy — not hard — for international medical graduates who want to practice in rural areas to become legal U.S. residents, so they don't have to worry about being sent home later. And states should be able to take as many IMGs as they can find who want to practice medicine in their rural areas.

Finally, incentives could be provided to academic medical centers to start rural residency programs. These don't have to be outposts of little-known medical schools in the heartland. Of course, there are a limited number of graduates of Harvard Medical School or Johns Hopkins who would want to undertake such missions. But I believe in the fundamental idealism of young doctors — especially if they don't have to pay off medical school loans.

Ultimately, rural healthcare will never be as good overall as the care that people can obtain in urban centers. But it can be a lot better and much more affordable than it is today. This form of health inequity should not exist — and it doesn't have to, if we're willing to try something new.

CHAPTER 12.

Addressing Health-Related Social Needs

HOW TO MEET PATIENTS WHERE THEY ARE

Jeremy Seals was once the kind of person known in the healthcare business as a "frequent flyer." In a single year, he visited the emergency department at Oregon Health & Science University in Portland 15 times and was admitted to the hospital 11 times, according to a report by Oregon Public Broadcasting. At the age of 40, his health was poor: he had had a heart attack when he was 35; he had congestive heart failure and terrible nerve pain in his legs.

What made his situation worse was that, because of his ill health, he was no longer able to hold a job. Then he became homeless and started living in his car.

"I basically lived at the emergency department," he told Oregon Public Broadcasting. "Ever since I'd had a heart attack, anytime my chest hurt, I'd either call the ambulance or go up to the hospital, and I think it was also out of desperation to just get out of my car and off the street."

Because of his frequent ED visits, Seals came to the attention of one of Oregon's coordinated care organizations (CCOs), which the state had created with federal funding to lower its Medicaid costs. The care manager assigned to work with Seals helped him schedule doctor appointments, get dialysis and take his medications correctly. But that wasn't all. She also got him new boots (his old ones had holes in them) and a sleeping bag. She made sure he had passes for a local community center so he could shower. Eventually, she helped him land a spot in adult foster care, so he had a place to live.

As a result of these and other interventions, Seals had only four ED visits and four hospitalizations the year after he entered the CCO program. Just averting a single hospitalization more than paid for the time his care manager had spent with him.[1]

Seals' case shows how addressing the "social determinants of health" can make a big difference in patient outcomes and health costs. Social determinants of health (SDOH) include a broad range of factors, such as socioeconomic status, race, environment, housing stability, food security, transportation, interpersonal violence, and alcohol and drug abuse, that influence a person's health.

Health care accounts for only 10%-25% of the variance in individual health over time, according to the World Health Organization. A much greater influence is exerted by genetic factors (up to 30%), health behaviors (30%-40%), social and economic factors (15%-40%), and physical environmental factors (5%-10%).[2]

Health behaviors are strongly affected by the other non-medical factors, so they are viewed as part of SDOH. And, as we'll see, mental health — which has an important influence on physical health — can be affected by social determinants such as poverty and violence. So all these factors need to be considered together in devising a strategy to address SDOH as part of population health management.

Widespread Social Issues

Social determinants of health don't affect only the poor. Fifty-three percent of consumers who responded to a McKinsey & Co. survey said they were impacted by social determinants such as food, transportation, safety, housing and social support. Those reporting higher ED and hospitalization rates were more likely to have unmet social needs.[3]

The impact of SDOH — and of increasing inequality — can also be seen in life expectancy. Better educated, more affluent Americans have a rising life expectancy, while the opposite is true for the poor and uneducated. In the 1970s, a 60-year-old man in the top half of the income distribution could expect to live 1.2 years longer than a man in the bottom half. By the turn of century, such an individual could expect to live 5.8 years longer than a less well-off man.[4]

A frequently cited 2002 article about social determinants found that about 60% of early deaths could be attributed to factors other than poor medical care and genetic predispositions. It is clear that SDOH interventions can lead to better health, the coauthors said. However, they added, "The cost-effectiveness of various interventions to improve population health is less clear."[5]

What has made SDOH interventions more cost-effective today, observers agree, is the growth of value-based care. Melinda Abrams, executive vice president for programs at the Commonwealth Fund, says that the gradual shift to value-based payments has already changed the conversation about integrating healthcare with social services to address the needs of very sick patients. However, with the healthcare system still largely reliant on fee-for-service payments, investing in social services remains a question mark for most providers.

Universal Coverage and SDOH

Seals was uninsured, which was one reason why he didn't have a regular source of care and was a frequent visitor to the ED. He wound up in that state partly because of his health problems and partly because he was poor and lacked a primary care doctor. His care cost a fortune that he didn't have, and the rest of us ended up paying for it.

Under my reform model, this would never happen. Seals would have the same subscription to basic care that everyone else had, and he'd be assigned a primary care doctor if he didn't choose one. His physician would be part of a basic care group that managed the health of its entire population, including individuals like Seals who now fall through the cracks. Specialists would be more likely to accept him as a patient than they are today, since his care would be as well reimbursed as that for any other patient.

Of course, universal coverage would remedy only one of his social determinants — poor access to care. But that is a powerful asset for someone who has chronic conditions. It could affect everything else in his or her life.

Another facet of the model that would help address SDOH is population health management. The basic care groups would have a strong incentive, as mentioned earlier, to keep everyone healthy or prevent their conditions from worsening. Part of that would be screening them for health-related social needs (HRSNs) and referring them to community-based organizations (CBOs) like social services agencies, housing bureaus and food banks. Much more could be done by the care teams within each group, as I'll explain later in this chapter.

Ultimately, of course, it is society's responsibility to address social determinants such as food insecurity, lack of affordable housing, and environmental factors. The best way to do that would be to integrate healthcare and social services, as other countries do. However, the United States has not been inclined to go in that direction. "In the United States, for every $1 spent on health care, about 90 cents is spent on social services, while other advanced countries spend $2 on social services for every $1 spent on healthcare," said a 2019 report from the National Academies of Sciences, Engineering and Medicine (NASEM).

According to the report, the time has come for the nation to develop a program to make SDOH an intrinsic part of health care. The report said that SDOH data needs to be better integrated into healthcare delivery and that providers should make organizational commitments to addressing social factors.[6]

PROVIDER SDOH PROGRAMS

Other than community health centers, most healthcare providers have not viewed social services as part of their remit until recently. But, partly due to the spread of value-based care, some of them are now grappling with the effects of SDOH.

To lower health costs, the majority of organizations that take financial responsibility for care deliver certain kinds of social support to high-risk patients or, more commonly, refer them to community resources.

A wide range of such activities are undertaken by integrated delivery systems, ACOs and other at-risk entities.

Fee-for-service healthcare systems, on the other hand, have been reluctant to get involved in SDOH. Although major systems such as Dignity, Trinity and Northwell have launched significant SDOH initiatives, most healthcare organizations are still just nibbling at the edges.

For example, a survey of Michigan emergency departments found that SDOH screening of super-utilizer patients is rare. There are several barriers to implementation of screening, including lack of financial support for programs that address social needs, the authors said.[7]

Another reason why many health systems don't pay much attention to SDOH is that better population health can actually cost them money. For example, Nemours Children's Health System in Jacksonville, Florida, started a home visit program to identify triggers of asthma. This program reduced ED visits and readmissions of children with asthma, but it hurt the healthcare system financially because fewer kids used hospital services.[8]

Most healthcare systems that intervene to help patients who lack adequate food, housing, and/or transportation, have some type of financial exposure to the cost of care, says David Nash. "As the care delivery systems take on more risk on the road to value, they'll be more stimulated to participate in this process," he predicts.

Montefiore Shows It Can be Done

One provider that has long been involved in meeting health-related social needs is the Montefiore Health System, which takes care of an underserved population in Bronx, New York. Montefiore, which has a global budget as part of a New York State Medicaid project, has built up three decades of experience with value-based payments and has an advanced population health management infrastructure. Having a fixed annual budget gives Montefiore an unusual degree of flexibility to innovate and invest in care delivery and PHM without volume-driven pressures. One of the system's main areas of focus is social determinants of health.[9]

Back in 2017, Montefiore had about 600 care managers, including nurses, social workers and health educators, who addressed the chronic disease of high-cost patients and linked them with community resources.

In a *Medical Economics* article on SDOH, I quoted Asif Ansari, MD, medical director of the Montefiore Medical Group's Grand Concourse practice, as saying that the system's efforts to address patients' HRSNs helped their doctors care for them. Ansari said he and his colleagues know the socioeconomic cards are stacked against their poorer patients, many of whom have trouble paying for their medications, and lack transportation and access to healthy food.

"Our physicians understand that we need this collaboration, this support and these resources to impact our patients' lives and their health," he said, referring to the social workers and other non-medical professionals at Montefiore. "When I compare practicing here 10 years ago and now, the difference in what I can do for my patients is significant."[10]

Calculating Social ROI

Other health systems that take financial risk have also found SDOH programs worthwhile. For example, Kaiser Permanente, which combines a care delivery system with an insurance company, has a program that places community health workers in care teams to support patients who are likely to end up in the ED. According to Kaiser, this initiative has reduced the average length of stay for these patients by two days and has resulted in savings of $82 per member per month. Kaiser calculates that its return on investment has been about 2:1.[11]

For health systems that don't have risk contracts and are largely dependent on fee-for-service, it can be hard to justify SDOH interventions. Bon Secours Hospital in Baltimore, Maryland, for example, has invested in 800 units of affordable housing in 12 properties. The hospital — part of a larger health system — expected to reduce the number of uncompensated ED visits and planned to reinvest those savings in other community benefit programs. However, it proved difficult to show that this investment paid off.

The traditional ROI method for demonstrating value is ill suited for analyzing investments such as these, noted the authors of a study on Bon Secours' approach. But a program like this has social value, which can be quantified, in their view. They estimated that the Bon Secours program has generated between $1.30 and $1.92 of "social return in the community" for every dollar in yearly operating costs.[12]

Food is Medicine Programs

Programs to help people feed themselves have had a clearer, more quantifiable effect on health and health costs than have programs to meet other social needs. In fact, these initiatives have scored enough success to spark a Food Is Medicine movement.

One reason for the elevation of food above other SDOH factors is its easily discernible impact on outcomes. In a study of Medicare Advantage plan members with type 2 diabetes, for example, food insecurity was the health-related social need most consistently associated with higher acute care utilization, inpatient encounters, and avoidable hospitalizations. Other HRSNs such as housing insecurity, lack of transportation, and loneliness affected the ability of Medicare patients to adhere to their medications, but insufficient food was the marker most often correlated with a need for acute medical care.[13]

In a study of how SDOH influenced North Carolina's Medicaid spending, researchers looked at a state program that allowed Medicaid to fund nonmedical services such as healthy food boxes and housing navigation in three regions. Comparing people with HRSNs who were in the program to those who were not, the study showed increased spending on the former group at enrollment, followed by a lower spending trend. Eighty-five percent of the social services provided to the patients in the intervention group were related to food security.[14]

Federal food programs such as WIC and SNAP have lowered healthcare spending, according to studies. For instance, a 2018 study found 5.8% lower expenses among older adult SNAP participants who were hospitalized as compared to hospitalized older adults without SNAP. Similarly, WIC has been associated with improved maternal and child health outcomes, including reduced likelihood of preterm births, lower odds of mortality within the first year, and reductions in disparities in low birthweight and extended infant hospitalizations.[15]

The Food Farmacy program of Geisinger Healthcare, an integrated delivery system in Pennsylvania, has also been notably successful. For diabetic patients who received food "prescriptions" from their doctors, HbA1c values decreased by an average of 20%. Geisinger estimated that every percentage point decline in HbA1c saved $8,000 in long-term health costs, compared to the annual investment in the program of $1,000 per patient. But there was no comparison group in the study.[16]

Besides programs aimed at increasing food security in general, there are other programs that deliver medically tailored meals (MTMs) to people with certain conditions. Under a model based on the health effects of MTMs, researchers projected that this intervention would be cost saving in nearly all states, according to a 2025 paper. Assuming full uptake by all eligible patients, the researchers estimated that a one-year implementation would yield net savings of $32 billion, and savings would total $151 billion over five years. MTM initiatives are rapidly expanding, including in some state Medicaid programs, they noted.[17]

Food-is-medicine programs are catching on elsewhere, too. For example, Elevance, a major health insurer, is partnering with the National Association of Community Health Centers (NACHC) to boost its FIM initiatives. Elevance has also partnered with Tufts Medicine's Food Is Medicine Institute. In 2025, Tufts and Elevance joined with Kaiser Permanente to form a national network to share best FIM practices. Other founders of the network include Blue Cross Blue Shield of North Carolina, CVS Health, Devote Health, Geisinger and Highmark Health.[18]

Screening for HRSNs

The most common approach to tackling SDOH is to screen patients for health-related social needs and to refer those who have HRSNs to community-based organizations (CBOs), such as social service and housing agencies, food pantries and homeless shelters. There are many variations on this theme. For example, some practices, hospitals and ACOs refer people directly to CBOs, while others use outside teams or networks to make the handoffs to community resources.

Before patients can be referred to community services, they must be screened for unmet social needs. Most often, the screening is limited to high-risk patients, because helping these patients meet their HRSNs has the most immediate payoff, both clinically and financially. In a recent survey of ACOs, 47% of respondents screened only high-risk patients, 14% screened all patients, and 36% didn't screen but planned to.[19]

The prevalence of HRSN screening is still fairly low, despite government efforts to encourage it. While nearly half of the states require Medicaid managed care plans to ensure that their members are screened, a national survey in 2019 found that only 24% of hospitals and 16% of physician practices screened patients for at least five HRSNs, and 8% of hospitals and 33% of practices did not screen at all. Medicaid providers such as FQHCs and practices participating in Medicaid ACOs reported higher screening rates, but the percentages of those providers that screened for all five social determinants were only 30% and 22%, respectively.[20]

A more recent study of primary care clinics in a large urban health system found that 17% of visits included HRSN screening. Only 7.7% of office visits in small clinics included screening, compared with 21.9% of visits in mid-sized facilities and 17.4% in large facilities. Screening was more likely in zip codes with lots of uninsured residents.[21]

Why have physicians not paid more attention to screening patients for health-related social needs?

According to a national survey, most physicians believe unmet social needs lead to worse health and that patients' HRSNs can have as big an impact on their health as their medical conditions do. However, 80% of the respondents said they didn't know how to deal with their patients' social needs.[22]

In a fee-for-service environment, moreover, primary care doctors are not being paid for anything other than face-to-face office visits.

They try to do the best they can by advising patients to quit smoking or drinking or leave boyfriends who beat them up. But behavior change is difficult, and physician advice alone has a limited impact on compliance.

Referrals to Community Organizations

When a patient is screened and found to have an HRSN, his or her physician must then decide where to refer the patient. It helps to have ongoing relationships with CBOs, so that the clinician knows how to get help for the patient. In addition, it would be ideal to have a way to communicate electronically with the CBOs. At the least, providers should be able to find out whether the referred patient has applied for services.

None of this is simple. CBOs are not necessarily used to working with healthcare organizations. Moreover, they are historically underfunded, and they don't have the resources to handle a big increase in the number of clients.

In a *Health Affairs* paper describing ACOs' efforts to address SDOH, Robert Mechanic and Ashley Fitch noted the disparity between the demand and the supply of social services. "Although health system demand for social service referrals is growing, many communities lack sufficient capacity to accommodate the new demand," they said. Many CBOs, they observed, lack funding to handle increased requests from healthcare organizations.[23]

Most social services are provided by local governments, public health agencies and nonprofit agencies. None of these entities has been adequately funded in their work with the poor, and that situation has worsened in recent years.

Even if the capacity were there, the relationships are not, in many cases. A 2019 study of 22 ACOs engaged in SDOH interventions shows that efforts to integrate social services and health care were limited among this set of early adopters. Staff members were just starting to talk to CBOs about how many ACO members they should be serving and about documentation requirements. Contracts with these partners were rare, and the majority of ACOs had not yet determined how to formalize their relationships with CBOs.

There were three main factors that inhibited the implementation of SDOH plans in these ACOs. First, the ACOs had limited information on social needs to use in making decisions. Second, the partnerships with CBOs were often difficult to develop. And third, ACOs did not know how to approach the issue of return on investment, "given shorter funding cycles and longer time horizons to see returns on social determinants investments."[24]

Navigation of Patients to CBOs

ACOs are not the first providers to traverse the difficult terrain of SDOH. In a 2007 survey of community health centers, including FQHCs, more than 90% of them provided eligibility assistance for government programs (including Medicaid and WIC), health education, parenting education, delivered meals, and/or assistance in obtaining suitable shelter, and referred patients to food banks and other community resources. Slightly fewer CHCs made referrals for employment and education counseling and/or environmental health risk reduction programs.[25]

A more recent study found that most CHC interventions related to SDOH originate as a response to an issue or a problem brought to their attention by patients, staff or clinic leadership. CHCs endeavor to address these issues, but they lack the necessary resources and skills to do it alone. So, many CHCs create partnerships at the local, state and federal levels, often using time-limited grants.[26]

The Accountable Health Communities (AHC) model, which the Center for Medicare and Medicaid Innovation (CMMI) tested from 2017-2022, measured the effectiveness of SDOH screening, referral, and navigation aid. The goal was to find out whether connecting Medicare and Medicaid beneficiaries with CBOs could improve outcomes and lower costs by addressing HRSNs. More than two-thirds of eligible patients reported food insecurity, and about half needed help with housing and transportation.[27]

Among the key findings of the AHC demonstration is that while the acceptance of navigators' help was high, they had limited success in resolving the patients' HRSNs. Less than a fifth of beneficiaries completing 12 months of navigation had been linked with a CBO or had resolved any HRSNs. The AHC navigators attributed this to insufficient community resources for referrals, especially to address housing and transportation needs.[28]

How Many People Can be Helped?

Another challenge to addressing SDOH is that the focus of healthcare providers is different from that of public health departments. As at-risk physician groups and ACOs see it, population health management, including HRSNs, is mostly about healthcare for their defined population. While the groups that are more experienced with PHM increasingly emphasize SDOH, it's still secondary to the main task of improving health through care coordination, patient engagement, and better preventive and chronic care.

Organizations involved in PHM must decide how much emphasis to place on managing care for various population segments. Smaller organizations and those that are new to PHM tend to focus on high-risk and rising-risk individuals. But the overriding goal of PHM is to optimize the health of all patients to prevent them from getting sick or sicker.

The budgets that at-risk groups must manage within are designed to cover health care, not SDOH interventions. Those interventions, whether they be referrals to community resources or the delivery of certain services by the healthcare organization, may reduce health costs and help the at-risk entity succeed financially. But the cost of the infrastructure to execute on SDOH must also be considered, and there is a limit to how many people can receive HRSN services through the organization.

So one issue that confronts any group or ACO that takes on SDOH is how much of its patient population to include in its SDOH initiative. To some extent, that depends on whether the organization is mainly referring patients to housing agencies, food pantries, legal aid and the like, or whether it also delivers some services, such as free transportation or home visits to assess patient living conditions. But ultimately, the decision comes down to whether SDOH interventions can reduce health costs enough to guarantee the organization a return on investment.

Considered in that perspective, helping high-risk, high-cost patients with HRSNs is a no-brainer. But it's unclear how far down in the population risk hierarchy an organization should go. Should it also provide such services to rising-risk patients, who, along with the high-risk people, comprise about 20% of the population? Should a patient with diabetes and who is overweight with social needs, but who isn't an ED frequent flyer, also be included, for example?

"Probably, and that probably makes it difficult to afford it," says Melinda Abrams. "In addition to identifying those who have the greatest needs and are at greatest risk, you have to identify those who are amenable to change. Another way of doing it is to start with the highest-need, highest-cost patients, because that's where you're going to see the greatest savings. And with those savings, you can invest not just in the top 1% or 5% [of high-cost patients], but also in the top 10% or 15%."

HOW PAYERS VIEW SDOH

Private and public payers — including insurance firms, Medicare and Medicaid — view SDOH as a natural complement to their other efforts to reduce health costs. Like providers, they have limits on what they can do to address health-related social needs. But payers have been stepping up their SDOH efforts in recent years.

Among private insurers, Kaiser Permanente is in the forefront of this movement. In January 2019, the big national HMO announced it was investing more than $100 million in a multiyear initiative to address homelessness across eight states and the District of Columbia. The company also announced a new care network that allows Kaiser providers to connect patients with community resources that address social needs.[29]

Recently, as noted above, Kaiser helped found a network to share information with other insurers about best practices in fighting food insecurity, and it now uses community health workers in its efforts to meet patients' social needs.

CVS and Aetna, its health insurance subsidiary, have launched a social needs network similar to Kaiser's. In partnership with SDOH software developer Unite US, CVS is giving providers the ability to refer patients to community resources, starting with Aetna's Medicaid and dual-eligible patients. CVS has also invested $100 million in affordable housing for at-risk and underserved patients.[30]

UnitedHealthcare, the nation's largest private health insurer, is also taking on SDOH. Providers in United's Medicare Advantage plans made 560,000 referrals to social services in 2017 and 2018, the company said. Through a partnership with Mom's Meals, United also distributed over 2.5 million meals to its members in 2018.[31]

In 2021, United started using predictive analytics on claims data and over 100 other metrics to identify who was most likely to need support with SDOH, such as access to food and housing. United call center representatives use this information to help individuals in challenging circumstances. United has made over 1 million referrals to social services and contributed over $500 million to support affordable housing across the country.

Several years ago, the Blue Cross Blue Shield Association founded the BCBS Institute, which is focused on social determinants. The institute has partnered with Lyft, enabling Blues plans to offer transportation to members who need it to access health care. The organization has also worked with CVS and Walgreens to improve accessibility to pharmacy services.[32]

Horizon Blue Cross Blue Shield of New Jersey has teamed with RWJ Barnabas Health to address the social determinants of frequent ED visitors in Newark. Using community health workers, Horizon targeted 1,000 frequent flyers and enrolled 40% of them in the program. Horizon reported that care costs for this population dropped 25% as a result.[33]

Government Programs

In addition to providing financial support for FQHCs, the federal government has sought to address health-related social needs, including interventions related to housing services, home improvements, food access, non-emergency medical transportation, case management and social service connections, and community health workers.[34]

The Accountable Health Communities demonstration has already been discussed. In addition, Medicare Advantage plans have been allowed to offer certain kinds of non-clinical supplemental benefits, In 2022, the majority of MA plans offered benefits related to HRSNs, including meals (68%), transportation (39%), nutrition (30%) and in-home support services (11%).[35] Recently, however, MA insurers have been pulling back on their supplemental benefits as they seek to raise profitability.[36]

CMS has also given state Medicaid programs waivers to pursue programs designed to meet beneficiaries' social needs. As of 2021, 25 states had utilized these waivers to address HRSNs such as housing insecurity, nutrition needs, transportation, and interpersonal violence. Medi-Cal in California has also coupled clinical care with reimbursable nonmedical services, including housing supports, medical respite, personal care, and medically tailored meals.

The Affordable Care Act also authorized state-based Health Homes, which coordinate care across the spectrum of care for Medicaid beneficiaries who have chronic conditions.[37] As of 2021, there were 37 Health Home models across 21 states and the District of Columbia. All these models must include comprehensive case management, individual and family support, and referrals to community and social services. Medicaid programs in 37 states mandate that the private managed care organizations they contract with maintain relationships with social service providers and include HRSNs in care coordination.[38]

Some states have gone much further with their own SDOH programs. For example, SDOH was a key component of Oregon's 2012 plan to bolster its Medicaid program. Under this scheme, the federal government gave Oregon $2 billion, to be paid back in future savings from its Medicaid program.

The state used the money to create 15 coordinated care organizations (CCOs), which are locally governed networks of healthcare providers that deliver care to Medicaid recipients. The CCOs' goal is to save money by focusing on prevention, reducing ED visits and hospitalizations. Part of their approach, as we saw in the case of Jeremy Seals, is to address HRSNs for the sickest patients.[39] Through 2019, the program saved over $1 billion.[40]

In Vermont, 85% of primary care practices participate in the Vermont Blueprint for Health, a state program that has organized community health teams (CHTs) to help practices deal with HRSNs. These teams, which include nurse care managers, social workers, behavioral health counselors, dieticians and health educators, help physicians care for complex patients who have significant social issues. Private insurers, Medicare and Medicaid fund the Blueprint, including payments to CHTs and incentives for physicians to participate.[41]

Community Care of North Carolina (CCNC), a similar program, fields care managers who work closely with primary care physicians and a multidisciplinary team including physician assistants, psychiatrists, pharmacists and community health workers. CCNC focuses on complex patients, especially those with multiple chronic conditions.[42] Under the state's current Medicaid overhaul, all Medicaid recipients must be screened for HRSNs, and a free software platform is available to providers to refer patients to CBOs and follow up on them.[43]

RACIAL HEALTH DISPARITIES

Besides the social determinants of health that have been discussed so far, racially based health inequities are a key driver of poor health. Black and Hispanic people and Native Americans are particularly affected by racism and by the socioeconomic circumstances that often go with it.[44] These include unstable housing, homelessness, food insecurity, interpersonal violence, drug and alcohol addiction, stress-related mental illness, and lack of transportation. Moreover, environment factors such as air and water pollution, turned-off utilities, and mold in homes also affect the health of minorities.

Racial and ethnic disparities cannot be separated from the poverty in which so many minority people live, but it is not the whole story. As one study notes,

> Socioeconomic status is...one of the strongest known determinants of variations in health status globally...At the same time, race and socioeconomic status are two related but not interchangeable systems of social ordering that jointly contribute to health risks.[45]

Being Black makes it more likely that you will receive inferior health care, regardless of your socioeconomic status. A recent study of electronic health records underlines this reality. The researchers analyzed 13 million clinical notes for 1.5 million patients seen between 2016 and 2023. They discovered that clinical documentation undermining patient credibility disproportionately stigmatized Black people and favored Asian individuals. "As stigmatizing language in medical records has been shown to negatively influence clinician attitudes and decision making, these racial differences in documentation may influence patient care and outcomes and exacerbate health inequities," they concluded.[46]

Racial disparities also affect patient safety. One recent study found that Black patients had a higher rate of adverse safety events than did White patients when they were admitted to the same hospital, regardless of insurance coverage type or the percentage of hospitalized patients who were Black.[47]

Former Jefferson Health CEO Stephen Klasko, MD, commented on that study in his book as follows:

> Of everything we have discussed in this book and in my previous writings on what is right and wrong with American healthcare, this [finding] is among the hardest to explain. In my long career in medicine, I've met very few doctors, nurses, residents or students who expressed racist inclinations. Nevertheless, because of our segmentation of Medicaid and commercially insured

> patients, there is clearly an inherent bias that may subconsciously or unconsciously affect care.

Minority patients also tend to distrust White male physicians, he added, partly because of "past race- and gender-based biases and outright abuses in clinical trials and healthcare..."[48]

Worse Access Means Worse Health

Minority individuals have worse access to care than White people do, on average. In 2023, Native Americans and Hispanics under age 65 had the highest uninsured rates at 18.7% and 17.9%, respectively. Uninsured rates for Native Hawaiian or Pacific Islander people (12.8%) and Black people (9.7%) under age 65 were also higher than the rate for Whites (6.5%).[49] As most people can't afford any but the most basic healthcare on their own, the uninsured rate is a pretty good marker for access to care.

This unequal access, along with other social determinants, is reflected in the health status of different racial and ethnic groups. For brevity's sake, I'll just consider the contrast between Blacks and Whites. In 2017, 13.8% of Blacks reported being in fair or poor health, compared with 8.3% of Whites. Eighty percent of Black women were overweight or obese, compared to 64.8% of White women. The rate of Black children with asthma was 12.6%, compared with 7.7% of White children. Forty-two percent of Black adults over age 20 suffered from hypertension, compared with 28.7% of White adults.[50] Blacks were almost four times more likely than Whites to have kidney failure.[51]

Black people also have the highest mortality rate for all cancers combined, compared with any other racial or ethnic group. There are 11 infant deaths per 1,000 live births among Blacks, nearly twice the national average of 5.8 infant deaths per 1,000 live births.[52]

Impact of Universal Coverage

Earlier in this chapter, I noted that access to care is only one social determinant of health. But, in reference to minorities, instituting my model — or any other type of comprehensive, universal coverage — would make a huge difference in outcomes. By simply ensuring that every person has the same access to basic care, a large portion of health disparities could be eliminated.

What we're doing right now is not working. Despite all the public and private efforts to reduce health disparities, little progress has been made, said Margarita Alegria, chief of the Disparities Research Unit at Massachusetts General Hospital, at a *Health Affairs* event in 2024. In fact, she said, the quality of care for minority patients is often so poor that they drop out of treatment early.[53]

Meanwhile, the Trump Administration and the Republican-led Congress are busy knocking out the pillars of the social safety net. New Medicaid work requirements are expected to result in about 10 million people losing their health insurance, starting in early 2027.[54] And, as noted in this book's introduction, Congress' refusal to extend enhanced subsidies for Obamacare health plans is expected to result in 4 million people losing their coverage.[55] While these developments will affect many White people, they are also exacerbating racial health disparities.

ROLE OF VALUE-BASED CARE

As stated earlier, the growth of value-based care has increased the healthcare industry's interest in the social determinants of health. For any entity that takes financial risk, addressing SDOH is now part of the toolkit for lowering costs. Conversely, it has become clear that taking risk gives providers the flexibility to provide services that would be hard to justify in the fee-for-service world. From that viewpoint, VBC arrangements are creating the necessary conditions for a more robust response to health-related social needs.

A 2019 paper about screening for HRSNs acknowledges that identifying and addressing social needs have not historically been part of medical practice. "Despite these challenges, the movement toward value-based care has accelerated the focus of physicians and hospitals on population and whole-person health by incentivizing physicians and hospitals to address needs that may be outside of traditional clinical care yet are associated with health spending."[56]

Some at-risk ACOs and medical groups are tackling SDOH head-on. Rio Grande Valley Health Alliance, for example, has contracted with Uber and Lyft to ensure that patients can get to doctor appointments. In addition, the ACO directs food-insecure patients to food pantries, and in some cases, has even intervened to get their lights turned on. If an elderly or disabled patient can't afford a walker, the ACO will pay for that.[57]

The Heritage Provider Network in the Los Angeles area has long intervened to help patients with unmet social needs where necessary. "When we look back, the way Heritage became successful in some markets is by paying attention to some things just because the doctors, nurses and social workers who worked with the practices knew this patient was going to become sicker unless we got him some help on this thing that had nothing to do with his [insurance] benefits," says Mark Wagar, president of Heritage Medical Services.

Wagar has been very encouraged by payers' interest in SDOH. "Some payers, including Medicare Advantage plans, are starting to provide resources for this. If you do these things the right way, you'll get paid for it," he says. "We were doing some of that already, but now we can be more aggressive on it when we know there's some return."[58]

Enhanced Screening and Referrals

Clearly, the basic care groups in my model should embrace SDOH interventions. The big question, as noted earlier, is how many patients with HRSNs can they help without breaking their budgets?

One approach the groups can take is to establish a system that I call "enhanced screening and referrals." To see how this might work, let's go back to the PHM infrastructure I laid out earlier in this book. To recapitulate, this infrastructure includes not only software and data but also health IT experts, nurse care managers, disease educators, health coaches, nutritionists, pharmacists and behavioral health specialists.

While patients should be asked to fill out HRSN questionnaires, these care team members can augment the survey data with what they pick up from working with patients, especially in the home. Although behavioral health therapists can't break their confidentiality with patients by sharing what they learn with other clinicians, they can suggest certain kinds of referrals with their clients' consent.

The Role of Mental Health

Behavioral healthcare, which is part of the basic care package, can also play a key role in helping patients take better care of themselves. According to a seminal 2002 paper, 40% of early deaths are caused by behavioral patterns that could be modified by preventive interventions. "Behavior patterns represent the single most prominent domain of influence over health prospects in the United States. The daily choices we make with respect to diet, physical activity, and sex; the substance abuse and addictions to which we fall prey; our approach to safety; and our coping strategies in confronting stress are all important determinants of health."[59]

Stress is a prime factor in behavioral health, which encompasses mental health and drug and alcohol addiction. Behavioral health may also be impacted by the individual's environment and other social determinants of health. For these reasons, efforts to address social needs are often combined with an emphasis on behavioral healthcare.

Behavioral health conditions affect nearly 20% of Americans. Individuals with behavioral health or substance abuse conditions cost 2.5 to 3.5 times more to care for than do patients who have none of these issues. Depression leads the list of the five conditions that drive the largest share of health costs, followed by obesity, arthritis, back/neck pain and anxiety.[60]

For all these reasons, behavioral healthcare should be integrated with primary care in the basic care groups. Although few primary care practices do this today, it has a good experimental basis. For example, integrating depression treatment with medical care has been shown to be twice as effective as traditional depression care.[61]

Tackling the Referral Quandary

Community-based organizations will continue to have limited resources, making it difficult for them to provide aid to all the patients that basic care groups refer to them. Nevertheless, there are some things that can be done to facilitate the process.

A survey of healthcare organizations and CBOs involved in SDOH partnerships found some common themes:

1. Most partnerships have some kind of formal agreement in place.
2. Most commonly, partnerships provide services to impact immediate-term clinical needs, such as reducing hospital admissions or length of stay. Fewer partnerships are addressing HRSNs to improve long-term health.
3. Partnerships rely on an evolving variety of funding sources, including private foundations, healthcare systems, and government entities.
4. Nearly all organizations expanded skills and capacities through their partnerships.
5. Advancing the field will require partners and funders to work on building relationships, to engage a wide range of stakeholders, and to identify and fund the cost of partnership.[62]

The basic care groups should also find ways to communicate online with CBOs. While the computer systems of social services agencies are incompatible with the EHRs used by healthcare providers, there are several commercial platforms designed to connect providers and CBOs, including Unite US, Now Pow, Innovacer, and Zeomega.[63] The software developed by Unite US, for example, combines screening, decision support, electronic referral management, assessment and care plan management, and outcome tracking. Specifically, the platform includes a list of community-based organizations, along with contact information. Referring providers use Unite US to track their referrals and find out whether the patient contacted an agency and, if so, what the result was.

What Groups Can Do on Their Own

Because CBOs can't handle all the cases thrown at them, the basic care groups will have to figure out how to maximize their own impact on HRSNs.

To begin with, they should make a concerted effort to reduce racial health disparities. Some of this will be taken care of automatically by universal coverage, as noted earlier. But physicians and nurses must also acknowledge their own subconscious biases and work to remedy them. They could start by providing the same evidence-based care to everyone. In addition, they should pay close attention to the data on the care they provide and the outcomes of their patients of different races.

Wherever possible, the basic care groups should emulate FQHCs that have been addressing unmet social needs for decades. FQHCs help with parenting, obtaining long-term care or home care, food security, shelter, employment counseling, and environmental risk reductions.

While they often refer patients to CBOs, some FQHCs go further to help patients with HRSNs. For instance, an FQHC in Ridgewood, South Carolina, inspects the homes of elderly patients for safety and aids with fall prevention. To help eradicate soil-borne parasitic worms in children, the community health center created an environmental health team that built cluster wells and installed bathrooms in low-income residents' homes, using funds from the local United Way and federal grants.[64]

How can basic care groups duplicate this approach? In part, by training their care teams to address HRSNs in specified ways. In addition, those teams should include social workers or community health workers who can be sent out to check on what's going on with certain patients at home. These professionals can also play key roles in interfacing with CBOs.

This approach has much in common with a model for integrating medical, behavioral and social services in the treatment of very sick and frail elderly patients. In their paper on this model, experts at the Commonwealth Fund said, "Multidisciplinary teams of clinicians, case managers, and patients working together can better tailor treatment plans to address medical needs by managing behavioral health conditions such as severe depression and non-medical issues such as unstable housing."[65]

Melinda Abrams strongly supports this team approach. She also believes that non-physicians should carry most of the load, since doctors already have too much on their plates. In her view, physicians just need to have the right information about a patient's HRSNs served to them at the right time, so they can discuss it with patients and make the appropriate referrals.

"You don't need a ton of doctors; you need midlevel people, and you bring in doctors when necessary," she says.

Social determinants of health will always be with us and will always have a bigger impact on health than medical care does. So any serious effort to reform our healthcare system to improve health and lower costs must encompass SDOH. In the final chapters of this book, I'll explore another important facet of healthcare that is driving up health costs: the relentless advance of new medical technologies.

CHAPTER 13.

Technology and Health Spending

TECHNOLOGY'S EFFECT ON COSTS

In every advanced country, regardless of what kind of health system it has, the cost of healthcare has been relentlessly advancing for many years. The growth in global affluence accounts for much of this increased spending, but health costs are rising faster than wealth everywhere.

About 20 years ago, Princeton health economist Uwe Reinhardt told me that a 1% increase in per-capita GDP will push up health costs between 1.2% and 1.4%, depending on the nation. "In the U.S., that ratio has been about 1.4. So every time income rises 10%, health care spending rises 14%," he said. "That's the big cost driver."

A 2024 report by the Peterson-KFF Health Tracker System found that U.S. per-capita health spending has risen faster than per-capita GDP since 1970. From 1970-2019, the average difference per decade was nearly two percentage points. From 2020-2023, during the COVID-19 pandemic and the inflation that followed it, GDP grew faster than healthcare costs.[1] However, CMS expects national health expenditures to grow by 5.8% per year, on average, from 2024-2033, while GDP is expected to grow only 4.3% annually, for a difference of 1.5%.[2]

While the industry restructuring proposed in this book could slow and perhaps even reverse cost growth, the wild card in this effort is the evolution of new technology. "Technology" in this context refers to new drugs and medical devices, as well as new kinds of tests and procedures and the growth of AI. Health economists attribute about half of the rise in health spending to this factor, because new technology leads to increases in the volume and intensity of care.[3] The higher intensity level accounts for part of technology's impact on raising costs, and the rest comes from excess medical price growth.[4]

How new technology is used can drive up costs. For example, new technologies don't necessarily replace earlier ones. To use a couple of older examples, the introduction of MRI and CT scanners didn't put X-ray machines out of business, and coronary artery bypass grafts didn't go away after stents became commonplace.

In addition, there is a tendency for doctors to perform certain kinds of procedures more often when they're less invasive and patients are more willing to undergo them. When minimally invasive gall bladder operations came along in the late 1980s, for example, they were much less expensive and dangerous than open surgery; as a result, the number of procedures rose so much that the total cost increased.[5] Today, many other "laparoscopic" procedures are now being done, including hernia repairs, colon and rectal surgery, heart surgery, brain surgery, kidney removal, spine surgery, operations to remove adrenal glands and the spleen, endovascular surgery, neurosurgery, and urologic surgery.[6] All of these advances have driven up the volume of surgical procedures.

Joint Replacements Proliferate

Joint replacement provides another great example of how medical advances have raised costs. Not too many years ago, "undergoing a total hip or knee replacement and recovery was a grueling and often painful ordeal," according to a blog post by Brandon Bukowski, MD, an orthopedic surgeon at the Mayo Clinic. "While these are still major surgeries, new techniques and technologies are redefining them — and people's outcomes."[7]

For most patients, he pointed out, total hip replacement surgery is either a same-day surgery or involves a one-night hospital stay. Patients can walk right after surgery, and the majority of patients can follow a self-directed physical therapy plan at home. The same is true of total knee replacements, except that part of the recovery entails visits to a physical therapy facility.

Patients may receive robot-assisted hip replacements, which help surgeons tailor the hip implant to the individual patient. As part of this approach, 3D preoperative planning and modeling helps ensure there is no impingement or pinching of nerves or tissues, and the technology helps the surgeon insert the hip implant with an unprecedented level of precision. 3D printing also allows the designing and creation of custom implants to address challenging problems such as deformities and bone loss.

The advent of this robot-assisted technology, improved anesthesia techniques, and the spread of joint procedures from hospitals to ambulatory surgery centers have all helped drive up the number of total joint replacements.[8-9] From 2000-2019, one study found, the annual growth rate of total hip replacements for Medicare patients was 5.2% and that for total knee replacements was 4.4%. The number of hip replacements for traditional Medicare patients jumped from 94,846 in 2000 to 262,369 in 2019 — far faster than the growth in this population. For knee replacements, the number soared from 188,118 in 2000 to 480,958 in 2019.[10]

Without insurance, a hip replacement in a hospital can cost from $31,000-$45,000.[11] For Medicare beneficiaries, the average cost is $13,803 in a hospital outpatient department or $10,500 in an ambulatory surgery center.[12] Based on these prices, it can be seen that just this one procedure is consuming a large and growing chunk of national health spending because of technological advances.

What is the Cost to Society?

Social and economic forces will continue to spawn new technologies that will push up the cost of care. Besides joint replacements, we can also look at the rise of GLP-1 weight loss drugs (see Chapter 14), as well as the growing use of AI in disease diagnosis and prevention. The rapidly increasing cost of all this new technology gives rise to the questions of who can afford it today and who will be able to afford it in the future.

Some economists dismiss this problem as a matter of choices. Mark Pauly, an eminent economist of an earlier generation, pointed out that there is no "natural" limit to the share of GDP that health care can commandeer. "All that matters," he wrote, "is whether the value of medical spending at the margin is higher or lower than the other spending that it displaces."[13]

Medical advances will continue, regardless of their cost to society, noted Arthur Caplan, a bioethicist at the NYU Grossman School of Medicine. Speaking with me in the late 2000s, he explained that both the government and private companies have invested heavily in medical research, and entrepreneurial businesses will continue to capitalize on the results. The real challenge, he said, is that "we have lots of technology that doesn't do anything; it just costs money." He cited much end-of-life care and end-stage cancer care.[14]

The prevailing view among health policy experts, as noted earlier, is that we're going to have — or already have — a two-tiered system, in which some people have more access than others to the latest medical technologies. But, while that is happening, it's difficult to deny anyone access to a technology that may save his or her life ("the rule of rescue"). Meanwhile, giant aggregate costs for some new drugs, devices and other technologies could squeeze out funding for some of the basic care that average people need to live healthy, productive lives. And, if healthcare gets so expensive that only a minority of people can afford it, the benefits of medical advances will accrue only to the few.

MEDICAL DEVICES, TESTS AND PROCEDURES

In discussions of healthcare costs, medical devices get far less attention than prescription drugs do. Nevertheless, the device industry is very substantial. Worldwide, device sales totaled $810.4 billion in 2024 and were expected to grow to $1.3 trillion by the end of 2029.[15] While U.S. sales figures are elusive, total device revenues for the United States and Europe were $584 billion in 2024 and were expected to grow 5-6% in 2025.[16] So the U.S. device industry is roughly half the size of the drug business in this country.

Most medical devices receive FDA approval with limited or no clinical testing. If a manufacturer can show that a new device is similar to one already authorized by the FDA, it doesn't need to be clinically studied. Even for devices that do require clinical trials, the studies fall short of the standards required for testing new drugs. Many studies are either not randomized or don't use a control group. Moreover, the follow-up periods last an average of only six months, not long enough to capture most safety risks. Not surprisingly, some devices must be recalled after they're on the market and being used in patients.[17]

There were 157 urgent Class I recalls of heart devices — such as pacemakers, stents, and defibrillators — from 2013 to 2022, according to a recent study. Only a fifth of the recalled devices had been subjected to clinical testing — and some of those studies fell short. In a clinical trial of a Medtronic stent graft system, the patients were followed only for a month after surgery. In 2021, more than 33,000 units were recalled because some fractured or leaked in patients' bodies. Overall, more than a million patients have received high-risk heart devices that have been subject to a Class I recall.[18]

Cardiac devices are not the only culprits. Metal-on-metal hip replacements, for example, have four times the rate of revision surgery within five years, compared with other kinds of hip replacement prostheses. Yet some surgeons still use this FDA-approved device.[19]

Low-value Devices Drive up Costs

Because medical devices usually require surgical intervention, they incur large expenses but don't always provide value commensurate to their costs. According to a study of low-value device-based procedures, "Medical devices often receive FDA approval with limited or no clinical testing and are key drivers of low-value care. The sharply higher reimbursement of procedures compared to medical therapy can create incentives to perform procedures when medical treatment would be at least as effective."

In this study, the Louisiana Medicaid program distributed evidence-based guidelines on the use of four low-value medical devices to clinicians and the leaders of Medicaid managed-care plans. At the end of the study, there was no significant decrease in utilization for any of the procedures that used one of these devices. Evidently, the profit motive or personal beliefs trumped the scientific evidence in the view of some surgeons.[20]

To establish the cost-effectiveness of devices, it is first necessary to know whether they are effective. The best way to do this is with a randomized controlled trial (RCT). A review of 96,000 U.S. clinical trials, however, found that fewer than a third of device and procedure studies were RCTs. Thus, most clinical evidence for devices comes from observational studies and registries.[21]

There are good reasons why RCTs are less common for devices and procedures than for drugs. Some experts question the ethics of sham procedures and random allocations in medical device trials, and doctors and patients tend to agree with them.

Robotic surgery offers a perfect example, notes Joel Selby, the former director of the federal Patient-Centered Outcomes Research Institute. "Some people just believed robotic surgery was better, and some doctors had been trained in robotic surgery. So, they and their patients didn't want to be in a randomized trial, even if that was the best way to answer the question."[22]

Even fewer studies than those focused on effectiveness have been done to establish the cost-effectiveness of new medical devices. Nevertheless, some studies on this topic have been published. One of them was recently done on a left-ventricular assist device (LVAD), which may be implanted in a person awaiting a heart transplant or who is ineligible for a transplant.

While thresholds for cost effectiveness vary from one country to another, a standard guideline is that a device or drug is considered cost-effective if it can save a "quality-adjusted life year" (QALY) for less than $100,000. (QALYs are further explained in Chapter 14.)

In the LVAD study, it was found that the LVAD cost per QALY gained was $79,446 for patients dependent on the heart drug inotrope and $130,445 for those not dependent on the drug. The conclusion was that LVAD is "marginally cost effective" for inotrope-dependent patients.[23] But that doesn't mean that physicians won't insert LVADs in patients who need them. Currently, there are more than 4,000 Americans waiting for a heart transplant.[24]

Skin Substitutes Invite Fraud

Fraud, waste and abuse don't always involve lawbreaking. Sometimes, a new technology comes along, and it takes a while for CMS to recognize that private actors are taking advantage of a loophole in its regulations. Until late in 2025, this was the case with a new class of skin substitutes made from biological or synthetic materials.

These skin substitutes are valuable for healing hard-to-treat wounds such as diabetic foot ulcers and venous stasis ulcers.[25] But, because of how traditional Medicare reimbursed the use of these substances, many other patients with other kinds of wounds have been treated at an astonishing cost. From 2019-2024, Medicare outlays for skin substitutes exploded from $250 million to more than $10 billion.[26]

For payment purposes, CMS classified these wound-care products as prescription biologics and reimbursed them under Medicare Part B. The allowed payment rate was 106% of the average sales price, which created a tremendous incentive for suppliers to raise their prices. It also induced some physicians to profit on the "spread" between what they paid the suppliers for skin substitutes and what they charged patients for them.

The results were predictable. There was a large increase in the number of Medicare enrollees with skin substitute claims and the amount of product billed for each enrollee, especially in home care. As prices rose, providers tended to shift to more expensive products that were more profitable. Some fraud schemes allowed bad actors to quickly get paid millions of dollars when billing for a small number of Medicare beneficiaries.

Just between 2022 and 2024, the amount paid for skin substitutes tripled from $40,015 to $121,501 per case. From the first quarter of 2023 to the third quarter of 2024, the number of Part B enrollees with a skin substitute claim climbed by 53%; the total number of skin substitute units increased by 83%; and the average payment per unit increased by 153%. While some brands were priced at $125 per square centimeter or less, other products cost as much as $4,700 per square centimeter. Total spending was expected to rise to $15 billion in 2025.[27]

Finally, CMS got wise. In October 2025, the agency announced it would reclassify skin substitutes as "incident-to supplies" and pay a flat rate of $127 per sq. cm. for them, starting January 1, 2026.[28]

AI-assisted Devices

A whole new category of AI-assisted devices is moving into the mainstream of medicine. For example, a small number of cardiologists and radiologists are offering AI analyses of CT angiograms that can pinpoint the location and volume of plaque in coronary arteries.[29] The Mayo Clinic is using AI and genetic data to detect early signs of a rare, often fatal heart condition.[30]

In the past decade, the FDA has approved nearly 1,000 AI-enabled and machine learning-enabled medical devices. Clinical applications include diagnostic workups, patient risk assessments, and clinical decision support.[31]

Many hospitals and physicians receive payments from device firms in return for trying these devices and algorithms.[32] Some doctors charge patients out of pocket for AI analyses. For example, one cardiologist who uses AI to detect coronary artery plaque charges $850 per test.[33] Medicare recently agreed to pay over $1,000 for such analyses, and private insurers are also beginning to cover this type of test.[34]

AI applications of this kind don't cost a fortune at the individual level, but they are part of an entirely new area that will increase national health spending. Is it cost effective to pinpoint plaque at an early stage, when we can do the same later with CT scans? The value of these tests remains unproven, but we're all going to pay for them.

CT, MRI and PET scans

These high-technology diagnostic tests have proved their value over the years, but they're not always used appropriately. When hospitals and outpatient providers invest in the pricey machines used for these tests, they have an incentive to run as many tests as they can medically justify. Moreover, physicians have another reason to order some tests: to protect themselves against malpractice suits stemming from missed diagnoses.

The availability of CT and PET scanners and MRI units has increased rapidly in most advanced countries over the past few decades. According to a 2023 survey by the Organisation for Economic Cooperation and Development (OECD), Japan had the highest number of CT scanners and MRI units per capita, and the third highest number of PET scanners per capita among OECD countries. The United States had the second highest number of MRI units and PET scanners. The usage of these machines was highest in the United States, Luxembourg, Korea, France and Austria, all of which had a combined total of over 360 exams per 1,000 people in 2021.[35]

"Clinical guidelines exist in several OECD countries to promote more rational use of MRI and CT exams," the OECD said. Through the Choosing Wisely campaign, an international effort to reduce the use of low-value care (see Chapter 8), some medical societies have identified cases where an MRI or a CT exam is not necessary — for example, in patients with low back pain or migraine headaches. Other studies have found that many lumbar spine MRIs[36] and MRIs related to total knee arthroplasty[37] are inappropriate.

It's not only high-end imaging equipment that is overused. A systematic review of mostly U.S. studies also found many instances of inappropriate use of lab tests, electrocardiograms, chest X-rays, and pulmonary function tests in low-risk patients having low-risk surgery; baseline lab and bone mineral density tests for the same kind of patients; preoperative baseline lab tests, and echocardiography or exercise stress tests.[38]

While it's impossible for the average patient to discern which of the tests or procedures he or she receives are unnecessary, physicians might also disagree on how to diagnose or treat a particular case. That is why clinical guidelines have been developed. However, the guidelines themselves may diverge, and some doctors don't always follow widely accepted, evidence-based protocols. Consequently, the basic care groups in each region must agree on which guidelines to follow, and their performance scores should include measures of how well they follow these protocols. Of course, exceptions must be allowed in individual cases; but, to the extent that doctors subscribe to guidelines that avoid low-value care, patients benefit and costs are lower.

PRESCRIPTION DRUGS

The percentage of U.S. healthcare spending represented by prescription drugs has not changed much in the past 15 years: it's still 10-11%.[39-40] But brand name drugs, which account for 15% of prescriptions but nearly 90% of drug spending,[41] have increased rapidly in price.

Brand-name drugs covered under Medicare Part D have nearly doubled in price, and the prices of 25 of them — including many commonly prescribed medications — have risen 98% since they went on the market, according to an AARP Policy Institute analysis. The average period from the drug's launch date to the 2022 analysis was 11 years.[42]

From 2020-2023, drug spending rose faster than outlays on hospital or physician services. In 2023, drug costs jumped 8.6%, partly because of the popularity of GLP-1 weight-loss drugs.[43] But other new products also drove costs higher. The median annual list price of newly approved drugs was more than $300,000 — roughly $80,000 higher than the median price of $222,000 in 2022. For one-time gene therapy treatments, list prices in 2023 were even higher, ranging from $2.2 million to $3.2 million.[44] Drug makers raised prices on 250 brand name drugs in 2025 and nearly 1,000 prescription products in 2024.[45]

Compared to other advanced countries, the United States pays a disproportionate amount for prescription drugs. Overall, the prices of prescription drugs (including generics) in the U.S. were 2.78 times as high as the prices in 33 other OECD countries in 2022. Prices for brand-name drugs were 422% higher than prices in comparison countries, although U.S. generic drug prices were a bit lower.[46]

The value of the U.S. market to drug makers is enormous. The United States made up about 60% of drug sales revenues and 24% of unit volume among OECD member countries. And the gap is rapidly increasing. Total U.S. drug sales grew from $582 billion in 2017 to $716 billion in 2022 — a 23% increase. During the same period, the other OECD countries saw a 2% sales increase.[47]

For the top 50 drugs, ranked by U.S. sales revenue, the U.S. market comprised 75% of worldwide sales revenues and 21% of unit volume. Prices for these drugs also increased much faster here than in other nations.[48]

WHY ARE DRUG PRICES SO HIGH?

So why are U.S. prescription drug prices so high that almost nobody can afford many of the latest medications without insurance?

To begin with, other advanced countries have national health insurance, and their governments are authorized to negotiate drug prices. The United States never did that until recently. In fact, the 2003 law that created a Medicare drug benefit specifically prohibited the agency from bargaining with drug companies on price. The Inflation Reduction Act (IRA) of 2022, however, enabled CMS to negotiate prices on some drugs, as explained below.

Another major reason for high drug prices is that U.S. patent policies allow drug companies to extend their patents on brand-name drugs to prevent generic competition. Entitled to 20 years of exclusive marketing rights under their initial patents, drug companies may file multiple, overlapping applications to obtain new patents on existing brand name drugs. If the initial patent for a blockbuster drug was to expire in 2016, for example, the drug maker might have obtained several dozen new patents, allowing it to extend its monopoly to 2034.[49]

"Pay for delay" is another time-honored tactic to delay generic competition. Drug companies strike deals under which they agree to pay generic drug makers to postpone the introduction of their products on the U.S. market. Estimates are that pay-for-delay settlements drive up drug costs by nearly $12 billion per year. Of that, a quarter comes directly out of patients' pockets.[50]

Drug prices fall with an increasing number of generic competitors. Compared with brand name drug costs, generic prices decline by an average of 20% in markets with three competitors. They decline by 70-80% from the pre-generic level in markets with 10 or more competitors three years after the first generic entry, one study found.[51]

However, there is also growing concern about the rapid rise in costs of certain generic drugs. In some cases, these price increases have occurred with generic drugs that have only one or two competitors. And brand name manufacturers sometimes manage to maintain their drugs' prices despite generic competition. This happened in the case of the cholesterol-lowering drug Lipitor, which remained at the same price even after generic competitors appeared.[52]

Drug Marketing Strategies

Pharma firms generate the bulk of their profits from blockbuster drugs. These may be "one-and-done," very-high-priced biologic drugs or lower-priced medications that can be prescribed to hundreds of thousands or millions of people.

The drug makers' ideal is a high-priced medication that can be prescribed to a large portion of the population. One example is Aduhelm (aducanumab), which was designed to delay the full onset of Alzheimer's disease. Aduhelm was set to go on the U.S. market at $56,000 per year, but it was withdrawn before full Medicare approval amid a controversy over its efficacy and side effects. Biogen, its manufacturer, estimated the size of the U.S market for the drug at 6 million people.[53-54] If all those people had taken Aduhelm, it would have cost the country $336 billion annually.

So far, the blockbuster drugs on the market are not in that territory, but they still rack up very large sales. For example, Keytruda had 2024 sales of $29.5 billion in the United States; Eliquis netted $20.7 billion; and Skyrizi earned $11.7 billion.[55] Keytruda, a cancer drug with multiple indications, has a list price of $12,000 when given every three weeks or $24,000 at six-week intervals. That works out to $207,600 a year per patient.[56]

The most important feature of a blockbuster drug is that it must be taken regularly, in some cases daily. That's why drug makers are less interested in developing vaccines or medications for acute conditions — once a patient is cured, they stop taking the drug. The ideal customer for a pharma company is someone with a serious chronic condition who will have to take its drug forever.

Direct-to-Consumer TV ads

In 1997, drug makers received a great gift that keeps on giving to advance their blockbuster strategy. That was the year when the United States became one of only two nations (New Zealand is the other) that allowed direct-to consumer (DTC) drug advertising on television.[57]

Today, U.S. drug manufacturers spend more than $1 billion per month on these ads.[58] Most of the TV spots promote bestselling drugs or those that the drug makers are trying to turn into blockbusters. The results are what you would expect: Consumers see these drugs advertised in the context of happy, dancing people whose lives were apparently saved or whose health problems were mitigated after they began using the medications. Then, if they have the condition that that drug is intended for, they are likely to go to their doctors and ask for a prescription.

There is no doubt that DTC ads help drive prescription drug sales. In fact, about half of what Medicare spent on drugs from 2016-2018 was for DTC-advertised medications.[59] Meanwhile, the market for prescription drugs has greatly expanded. According to one study, 59% of U.S. adults used prescription drugs in 2011-2012 — a significant increase from the 51% who used them in 1999-2000, just after the ban on DTC ads ended.[60] In 2021, the percentage was 65%![61]

Some observers believe this situation stinks. "Pharma ads, designed to manipulate and persuade viewers into requesting medications they may not need, should not purposely drive a psychological desire in the viewer," Hal Rosenbluth, CEO of a company that sells a mental health coaching app, recently wrote in *STAT News*. "They exploit our fears of being sick, coercing us to take more prescriptions, leading to side effects that need to be addressed by more prescriptions. It's a costly cycle (both physically and fiscally) for the individual as well as the entire health ecosystem."[62]

Experts on the other side of this debate maintain that the harms of drug advertising have been greatly overblown. Abby Alpert and Neeraj Sood, a pair of academics who apparently have no connection to drug companies, argue in a recent *JAMA* commentary that studies showing that DTC ads mislead consumers are subjective and that evidence of patient harm is limited. The TV ads can have positive effects, including increased initiation of clinically beneficial medications, improved medication adherence, and reduced work absenteeism, they say.[63]

As for wasteful spending, although DTC advertising "may lead to some overuse," they state, there are "multiple layers of gatekeepers in the healthcare system (e.g., physicians and insurers) who can potentially limit inappropriate use." The key word here is "potentially": Physicians tend to prescribe what their patients want, and insurers have only indirect tools like tiered coverage to restrain overutilization of drugs that don't require prior authorization.

The experts also point out that the FDA requires drug ads to present a balanced view of a medication's benefits and risks, based on scientific evidence. However, it's often difficult to read the tiny print about a drug's side effects and contraindications at the bottom of the TV screen. Even if potential side effects are announced in the ad, they are downplayed. According to a recent *Washington Post* op-ed by Steven Woloshin and Baruch Fischhoff, "DTC ads don't communicate what consumers most need to know: how a drug works, in terms of how effective it is and what the possible harms are."[64]

Lately, there has been a bipartisan push to rescind the FDA's permission for DTC drug ads. Both HHS Secretary Robert F. Kennedy and President Trump have come out against them, and Senators Bernie Sanders (I-VT) and Angus King (I-ME) have introduced a bill to ban the ads.[65] This is an excellent idea that would reduce waste and lower the amount spent on drugs; but, considering the industry's lobbying muscle, it is doubtful that the legislation will pass.

Instead of having Congress prohibit drug ads, Woloshin and Fischhoff suggest, the FDA should more vigorously police them. Among other things, they write, the FDA could have focus groups of consumers view ads before they're released to find out whether they understand the drug's benefits and risks. However, TV viewers are not necessarily interested in being shown scientific information about a drug to help them decide whether to ask their doctor about it.

Drug Makers Defend Their Prices

Pharmaceutical companies claim that their outrageously high U.S. prices for brand-name drugs are justified because of the high cost of drug development. According to a study based on data from smaller pharma firms, the mean "capitalized" R&D cost for bringing a drug to market from 2009-2018 was $1.56 billion, counting expenditures on failed trials. (Capitalization is the opportunity cost of not investing the money elsewhere.) Confidential estimates from large drug companies range up to $2.8 billion per FDA-approved drug.[66]

Another study based on data from public and proprietary sources found that the mean cost of developing a new drug from 2000-2018 was $172.7 million (2018 dollars). When the cost of failures was included, the cost increased to $515.8 million, and it ballooned to $879.3 million when capital costs were included.[67]

Nevertheless, operating profits of the drug industry have increased steadily over the past 40 years, growing 3.5 times above 1979 levels, according to one study. In 2018, publicly traded pharma firms in the United States had operating profits of 23.4% of sales. Other studies found the average profitability of large drug companies was far above that of companies in other sectors (13.8% vs. 7.7%).[68]

It's also worth noting that the portion of sales that go to blockbuster drugs has accelerated over the past 15 years. In March 2022, specialty medicines — high-cost drugs that are often biologics — accounted for 55% of net drug spending, up from 28% in 2011. The increase was driven by growth in the autoimmune and oncology sectors. At the same time, the market share of traditional drugs and generics continues to decline.[69]

Net medicine spending in the United States increased by $50 billion, or 11.4%, from 2023 to 2024. Most of this growth was driven by just 31 blockbuster products. Sales of each of these drugs increased by more than $500 million in that year.[70]

FIGHTING HIGH DRUG PRICES

With government price negotiations still limited, the main mechanism for controlling the cost of drugs in the United States is the deeply flawed system of pharmacy benefit managers (PBMs). Three insurer-related PBMs — Express Scripts, CVS Caremark, and Optum — are the middlemen for 80% of U.S. drug prescriptions.[71]

What do PBMs do? According to the Kaiser Family Foundation, "PBMs negotiate with drug manufacturers and pharmacies to set prices, determine patients' access to different medications, and contract with pharmacies to participate in networks. Insurers pay fees to PBMs for performing these functions. PBMs also derive revenue in other ways: for example, they receive a share of the drug rebates they negotiate with pharmaceutical companies; they collect the difference between what insurers are reimbursed and the amount that pharmacies are paid (the 'spread'); and they steer business to their affiliated pharmacies."[72]

While PBMs are supposed to obtain lower drug prices, they have financial incentives that may contribute to higher prices, higher out-of-pocket costs for patients, and the closing of independent pharmacies. For example, they tend to include more expensive brand-name drugs in their formularies because that increases how much they receive from their share of drug rebates. This leads to higher drug copays for consumers. So does the exclusion of pharmacy discounts and manufacturer rebates in determining coinsurance amounts.

PBMs often charge insurers more than what they reimburse pharmacies for the drugs they buy at wholesale prices, profiting from the "spread."[73] And they steer patients to the retail pharmacies that their parent companies own (in the case of CVS) or the mail-order outfits that the PBMs own, while under-reimbursing independent pharmacies. This might be one of the reasons why 700 pharmacies closed in the United States from 2021-2023.[74-75]

After several failed attempts to pass legislation to rein in PBMs, in February 2026, Congress passed and President Trump signed a package of reforms as part of a large federal spending bill. The measure prohibits PBMs from linking rebates to the list prices of drugs and requires them to pass through 100% of rebates to health plans and corporate sponsors.[76]

Medicare Price Negotiations

Under the Inflation Reduction Act of 2022, CMS has the authority to negotiate prices with pharmaceutical companies on a relatively small number of drugs. Negotiated prices on the first 10 medications went into effect in 2026. Lower negotiated prices will be charged for 15 more drugs in 2027, 15 in 2028, and 20 per year after that.[77]

The drugs chosen by CMS for negotiation are brand-name drugs that have no generic or biosimilar equivalents and that generate some of the largest expenditures for Medicare Part D. The drugs are either costly, widely used or both.[78] To be included in the bargaining, a non-biologic drug must have been on the market for at least seven years; a biologic therapy, for 11 years. Low-volume and orphan drugs for rare diseases are off the table.[79]

The negotiated prices of the first 10 drugs — which went into effect on January 1, 2026 — were substantially reduced from their list prices. For example, the price of Januvia, a type 2 diabetes drug, dropped 79% from $527 to $113 for a 30-day supply. The prices of the other drugs declined from 50-70%. They included such brand names as NovoLog, Farxiga, Enbrel, Jardiance, Stelara, Xarelto, Eliquis, Entresto, and Imbruvica.[80]

The initial drugs subject to bargaining already enjoyed significant discounts to Medicare, so their negotiated prices represent only a modest savings, according to Laura Tollen, a senior editor of *Health Affairs*. It was unclear whether the price reductions would have much impact on patient access to these drugs, she wrote.[81]

In November 2025, the Trump Administration announced it had negotiated lower prices for the second group of 15 drugs. This tranche includes widely used inhalers and treatments for cancer, diabetes and depression. It also encompasses Novo Nordisk's blockbuster GLP-1 drug, sold as Ozempic (injectable) and Rybelsus (pill form) for type 2 diabetes and as Wegovy for obesity.

The negotiated prices are up to 85% lower than their list prices, but it isn't clear how much less they are than the discounted prices that Medicare currently pays. If the new prices had been in effect in 2024, the administration said, Medicare would have saved $12 billion, which would have reduced its spending on these drugs by 44% as a whole.[82-83]

In any case, this shows the power that the federal government has in negotiating drug prices. The big price drops in the first two rounds were only for Medicare. Imagine how much could be saved if the government bargained for prices across the board on behalf of everyone.

"Most-Favored-Nation" Pricing

The Trump Administration's other strategy for decreasing drug prices was to demand that pharmaceutical companies sell their products in the United States at the lowest price they sell them for in other wealthy countries.[84] Under this "most-favored-nation" (MFN) approach, in effect, the U.S. would piggyback on the prices negotiated by other advanced nations.

President Trump announced his new policy in an executive order in May 2025. For several months, there was no response from pharmaceutical companies. But in September 2025, after the President threatened to impose high tariffs on drug imports, Pfizer agreed to lower prices on some of its U.S. medications to the levels charged in other countries in return for avoiding tariffs for three years.[85]

Most of Pfizer's promised price cuts are only for state Medicaid programs, which already have extracted deep discounts from drug makers. And, although Pfizer also agreed to list discounted drugs on the Trump Rx website for direct sales to uninsured consumers, the industry was already doing something similar. By one estimate, Pfizer's deal with the Trump Administration would cost it up to $723 million a year — only a bit more than 1% of its total revenues in 2024.[86]

By the end of 2025, most major pharmaceutical firms had struck similar deals with the U.S. government, presumably to avoid regulatory actions that could sharply lower their profits. Many of the drugs that these companies pledged to list on Trump Rx either have cheaper generic alternatives or are nearing the end of their patent periods and will soon be facing generic competition. Some discounted drugs on the website, like the hepatitis C therapy Epclusa, will still be too pricey for most consumers. Moreover, the discounted drugs tend to be those usually prescribed by primary care doctors rather than more specialized, expensive treatments for cancer and other life-threatening conditions.[87-88]

While lower prices for some drugs will benefit state Medicaid programs, these deals don't apply to Medicare or private insurers. So, though some consumers will pay less because of TrumpRx, the MFN arrangements won't have much impact on overall drug prices in the United States.

The pharmaceutical companies have always argued that they need to charge high prices in the U.S. to fund innovative research on new cures. One of the implicit assumptions in the Trump MFN program is that, if drug prices drop in this country, they'll rise in other affluent nations to finance this research. But policy experts noted in a recent *JAMA* article that this is unlikely to happen. Other countries have lower drug costs because their governments negotiate prices or allow multiple payers to negotiate them as a group, they pointed out.

"Instead of importing prices from other countries, we should import the process that these countries use to negotiate fair prices," the authors asserted.[89] This would include cost-effectiveness analysis, which CMS has eschewed in Medicare coverage determinations (see Chapter 14).

Value-Based Payment

There is no way of knowing how much financially at-risk organizations like basic care groups might reduce drug spending, for one simple reason: drug costs are not included in most value-based payment arrangements. Currently, PBMs negotiate drug prices, and employers, insurers and consumers cover the costs. Most healthcare organizations that take risk for the cost of care from private payers are not on the hook for drug spending.

The same is true for value-based payment (VBP) contracts under Medicare and Medicaid, including those involving Medicare Advantage and Medicaid plans. Medicare Part D plans for traditional Medicare beneficiaries complicate the ability of Medicare to include prescription drugs and care in VBP models, according to an analysis by the Commonwealth Fund. State Medicaid programs do not delegate drug coverage to Medicaid managed care organizations.[90]

There are some other challenges to the inclusion of drug costs in VBP arrangements, the report said. For one thing, clinicians lack information about patient out-of-pocket costs for different drugs, as well as their comparative effectiveness and prices. There are also relatively few quality measures that assess the appropriate uses of pharmaceuticals.

TAKING RESPONSIBILITY FOR DRUG COSTS

Despite these challenges, my basic care groups would take financial responsibility for outpatient drugs below a specified annual cost level. Major medical insurance would cover more expensive medications, as well as those used in hospitals, ambulatory surgery centers, cancer centers, nursing homes, and other institutions. However, the insurers would delegate drug risk to globally budgeted hospitals for inpatient and post-acute care.

The federal government would negotiate drug prices on behalf of all U.S. residents. As a result, drugs would be priced much more fairly than they are today, and there would be no need for PBMs. Without these middlemen getting in the way, without Medicare Part D drug plans, and without a role for Medicaid programs in drug prices, there would be no structural impediments to basic care groups taking drug risk.

As for information about the comparative prices and comparative effectiveness of drugs, all this data would be available online to clinicians and patients alike. A new government organization would also do cost-effectiveness research on new drugs, like that now done in European countries. This would not only weed out many low-value medications but would also provide some of the basis for evidence-based guidelines that could be used to measure the appropriateness of drug utilization.

Both the basic care groups and the specialists they referred patients to would have incentives to manage drug utilization to stay within basic care budgets. Thus, they'd have a reason to favor generics over brand-name drugs and more-effective drugs over less-effective ones. At-risk healthcare providers would weigh the benefits of a long-term maintenance drug against its risks and would consider prescribing lifestyle interventions when they could provide as much or greater benefit than taking a drug forever.

How about the impact of all this on biomedical innovation? If the U.S. government negotiated all drug prices, and if the cost-effectiveness of new drugs became a factor in their approval, there is little doubt that pharmaceutical companies would develop fewer drugs at a slower pace. Health policy expert James D. Robinson suggests that this impact could be mitigated if the government provided grants for new product commercialization, similar to those for COVID-19 vaccines under Operation Warp Speed. In addition, he writes in *Health Affairs*, expanded R&D tax credits and advance purchase commitments for innovative products would encourage R&D investment by drug makers.[91]

Those policy changes might help maintain the pipeline for innovative drugs. But it's also important to remember that the federal government already supports most basic drug research through NIH grants. There is also a strong case to be made that innovation should not proceed more quickly and expensively than society can afford to pay for it.

The primary consideration should not be whether pharmaceutical companies are richly rewarded enough to invent these wonder drugs. We need to bear in mind that healthcare resources are limited, and that we need to use them wisely. The next chapter proposes a way to do that in relation to new technologies.

CHAPTER 14.

What We Owe Each Other

In healthcare, as in life, everybody can't have everything they want. To guarantee affordable access to high-quality care, we must distribute healthcare resources judiciously, in ways that benefit the whole population. Nevertheless, this doesn't mean that the needs of sick individuals should be ignored. I'm not proposing a utilitarian system in which "the greatest good for the greatest number" dictates all distributional decisions. Instead, as explained below, I favor a democratic system of healthcare choices, based on the relationship between health spending and outcomes.

This is not a radical concept. Countries with universal healthcare systems must make these kinds of choices, and so would our government if it adopted Medicare for All. Comprehensive healthcare should be guaranteed to everyone in the United States, just as it is in other advanced nations. But, to make that a reality, we might have to restrict access to some potentially beneficial technologies. That could occur if unlimited access were so expensive that it might impair the ability of many people to obtain basic care.

In Chapter 13, I mentioned Aduhelm, the withdrawn Alzheimer's drug of questionable efficacy. That medication would have cost hundreds of billions of dollars a year if it had been prescribed to most of the people who were in the early stages of the disease. Because its net benefit was small, its value for patients was low in relation to its cost.

On the other hand, there are much less expensive therapies that have high efficacy, can save many lives, and promise to lower long-term health costs. One example of this are the relatively new biologic treatments for hepatitis C, which now cost a modest amount for a single, curative cost of therapy that averts liver cirrhosis and reduces mortality. While the initial prices for the drug were very high, contributing to a significant rise in U.S. drug costs, they have dropped to a total net cost of $11,500 to $17,000 for a course of treatment.[1] Even at that price, they could add substantial cost because of the number of people with hepatitis C (2.7 million-3.9 million), many of whom are unaware they have it. Nevertheless, public health officials maintain that we should increase the reach of these drugs.[2]

GLP-1 weight-loss drugs, which are also less expensive than they were initially, also offer solid health benefits, and there is an expectation that they will lower health costs in the long run. However, GLP-1 drugs like Wegovy and Zepbound are different from hepatitis C therapies and other recent innovations in a key respect: Because of the huge number of people who could benefit from these medications, they pose a significant threat to the financial stability of our healthcare system. The next section delves into the pros and cons of GLP-1 drugs.

THE GREAT GLP-1 CONTROVERSY

Glucagon-like peptide 1 (GLP-1) receptor agonists were originally approved by the FDA for diabetes treatment. The agency approved semaglutide (Wegovy) for chronic weight management in June 2021 and tirzepatide (Zepbound) for the same indication in November 2023.[3] Both drugs are GLP-1s, but Zepbound includes another agent as well. The two medications are identical to the diabetes drugs Ozempic and Mounjaro, respectively.

Besides helping people lose weight, Wegovy also been shown to reduce the risk of cardiovascular events in patients with heart disease.[4] The FDA has approved its use to decrease the risk of heart attacks, stroke, and cardiovascular mortality in adults with heart disease who are obese or overweight.[5] In 2025, the FDA expanded Ozempic's label to allow use of the drug for treating worsening kidney disease and kidney failure.[6]

Studies have found that GLP-1s can decrease risks for alcoholism, cannabis disorders, opioid use disorders, suicide attempts, bulimia, schizophrenia and seizures. In addition, they may lower risk for bacterial infections, clotting disorders, pulmonary hypertension, acute pulmonary embolism, deep vein thrombosis, and chronic phlebitis.[7]

The most common side effects of the drugs are nausea, vomiting, diarrhea and constipation. A few patients have dangerous stomach complications. According to a Canadian study, people taking GLP-1s have an elevated risk of pancreatitis, bowel obstruction and gastroparesis. The risks of these side effects are all about 1% or less per year of GLP-1 use.[8] In addition, rapid weight loss leads to loss of lean muscle mass unless it is accompanied by an exercise regimen.

GLP-1s are effective at lowering weight, although studies differ on how much weight patients lose on the drugs. A systematic review found that, compared with placebo, tirzepatide resulted in a weight loss of up to 17.8%, and that semaglutide decreased weight by up to 13.9%.[9] But in the study that established GLP-1s' cardiovascular benefits, the average weight loss of the patients who took the drugs was about 10%.[10]

Potential Costs Are Off the Scale

There are about 122 million people with obesity in the United States.[11] So, as the costs of GLP-1 medications drop, they are likely to create a tidal wave of spending that we have only begun to experience.

According to a 2024 report from the Senate Committee on Health, Education, Labor and Pensions, if half of all Americans with obesity took these weight-loss drugs, it would cost the healthcare system $411 billion annually. If half of all Medicare and Medicaid enrollees with obesity took weight-loss drugs, it would cost the government $166 billion every year. In the long run, the report warned, weight-loss drugs could raise total annual prescription drug spending by up to $1 trillion a year.[12]

On the other hand, weight loss can reduce health costs for other conditions, including diabetes, heart disease, and musculoskeletal and pulmonary conditions. In a modeling study of privately insured adults and Medicare beneficiaries with a body-mass index (BMI) of 25 or higher, people on GLP-1 drugs who lost 5% of their weight were estimated to spend a mean of $670 (8%) less on healthcare per year, and those who lost 25% of their weight had average lower spending of $2,849 (34%). Among those with one or more comorbid conditions, a 5% weight loss translated into reduced health spending of $1,262 (7%), and a 25% weight loss decreased healthcare spending by a mean of $5,442 (31%).[13]

These estimates drew some skepticism from Peter Neumann, PhD, director of the center for the evaluation of value in risk and health at the Institute for Clinical Research and Health Policy Studies at Tufts Medical Center. "The problem with those kinds of projections is that, first, a lot of people don't stay on the drugs," he said in a recent interview. "There's also a lot of uncertainty about long-term effects, including side effects.

"Also, a recent Yale study showed that, after two years, people on these [GLP-1] drugs cost more money," Neumann continued. "And one reason why they may cost more money is they're more plugged into the system. They may go to the doctor more, which may not be a bad thing. But the idea that you're going to save money quickly is probably not right. And whether or not you save money in the long term, people living longer use more healthcare, which costs money."

The Institute for Clinical and Economic Review (ICER), a private U.S. research firm that assesses the value of new health technologies, recently analyzed the cost-effectiveness of GLP-1s. Using the quality-adjusted life year (QALY) methodology, which calculates how much a drug costs in relation to how many quality-adjusted years of life are gained, ICER assumed net prices of $6,830 per year for injectable or oral semaglutide and $7,973 for injectable tirzepatide. It concluded that all these drugs were cost effective because they fell well below the threshold of $100,000 per QALY that is commonly used in the United States.[14] "Despite these therapies being highly cost-effective, their potential budget impact is huge," the ICER report added. "This raises serious concerns about affordability."

Coverage Varies as Costs Drop

During the initial period of GLP-1 drugs' use for weight loss, their list prices topped $12,000 per year. From 2018-2023, U.S. sales of GLP-1s jumped by more than five times, from $13.7 billion to $71.7 billion.[15]

In 2024, the drugs' prices started coming down. By the following year, the net price of GLP-1s for large employers was $550-$650 a month, and the uninsured could buy the drugs directly from the manufacturers for $349-$499 a month.[16]

In November 2025, the Trump Administration announced deals with Novo Nordisk and Eli Lilly to cut the prices on Wegovy and Zepbound, respectively. By summer 2026, the drugs will be priced at $245 per month, plus a $50 copay, for Medicare and Medicaid beneficiaries. Orally taken GLP-1s, one of which has been approved by the FDA, will cost as little as $150 per month for the lowest dose. People without insurance will be able to buy the injectable drugs directly for an average of $350 per month, depending on the dose.

The drug companies agreed to cut their prices in exchange for tariff relief and CMS' promise to broaden coverage for Medicare patients. Initially, CMS said it still wouldn't cover GLP-1 drugs for weight loss alone. The agency planned to cover it for people with obesity accompanied by diabetes, prediabetes, kidney disease, heart failure, or established cardiovascular disease.[17] Just weeks later, however, CMS Administrator Mehmet Oz announced a new demonstration project called the Better Approaches to Lifestyle and Nutrition for Comprehensive Health (BALANCE) model. Scheduled to begin in 2026 and to conclude in 2031, BALANCE will allow Medicare and Medicaid to cover GLP-1 drugs for beneficiaries who are obese but have no comorbid conditions.[18] The floodgates are now officially open.

A 2024 study estimated that if CMS covered GLP-1 weight-loss drugs for 5% of Medicare Part D enrollees with obesity or overweight and one or more relevant comorbidities, Medicare costs would rise by $3.1 billion annually, or $6.1 billion if 10% were covered.[19] By that logic, annual Medicare costs would rise $30.5 billion if half of eligible beneficiaries were covered. And that's only a small fraction of what these drugs might cost if all obese Americans — with or without comorbidities — had insurance for GLP-1s.

At the 2026 price of $300 per month (Medicare cost plus patient copay), the annual cost of GLP-1s would be $3600 per prescription. If half of the U.S. population with obesity — about 61 million people[20] — were covered for GLP-1s, were prescribed the drugs, and filled their prescriptions, the total annual cost at that price would amount to $219.6 billion. The ultimate cost would be lower than that, because 60% of people on GLP-1s quit them within the first year.[21] But it's still a staggering bill — and one that wouldn't be partially offset by cost savings in healthcare for a long period of time.

Payers Slow-walk GLP-1 Drugs

Unsurprisingly, payers have been reluctant to pull the trigger on these weight-loss drugs. As earlier mentioned, Medicare currently covers GLP-1 drugs only for diabetes and some other comorbidities of obesity. Just 13 states cover GLP-1s for weight loss under their Medicaid programs, and some of them are pulling back.[22] Although two-thirds of large employers cover GLP-1s for weight loss, these medications have raised their drug costs by up to 50%. So, many businesses have passed that expense onto employees by increasing their premium charges.[23] Eleven of 18 commercial insurers cover GLP-1s for weight loss, but those that do have made it difficult to get prescriptions for the drugs.[24] Independence Blue Cross in Pennsylvania ended coverage of GLP-1s for weight loss in 2025 after spending $500 million on them in 2024.[25]

At Blue Cross Blue Shield of Massachusetts, 49,000 members, or just 3.6% of its policyholders, were taking GLP-1 medications as of January 2025, Chief Medical Officer Sandhya Rao, MD, told *Modern Healthcare.* Yet the health insurer and its employer clients spent more than $300 million on these drugs in 2024.

"If we stay on the current trajectory, we forecast that we'd spend close to a billion dollars on just these drugs in 2026, which would mean significantly higher premiums for everyone, whether they use these medications or not," Rao said. "There has never been a greater urgency to address the rising cost of healthcare for our members and customers."[26]

COST-EFFECTIVENESS ANALYSIS

The lesson to be learned from the GLP-1 saga is that, in some cases, lines must be drawn around innovative technologies to prevent them from breaking the bank. It is hard to determine where those limits should be imposed, however. That depends not only on healthcare resources, but also on the value that society attaches to particular medical advances. In addition, we must come to grips with the central question of which is more important, the benefit of a technology to an individual who needs it, or the value to society of being able to provide good healthcare to all within a budget. If they're both important, how do we help the individual without make healthcare unaffordable for everyone else?

Before we get to that issue, it is imperative to consider how to prevent the widespread dissemination of low-value drugs and other low-value technologies and procedures that add substantial cost to healthcare without providing a commensurate benefit to the population. GLP-1 drugs are clearly not in this category; but many other innovations, as well as older technologies and techniques, aren't worth their cost.

We visited some of these tests and treatments in Chapter 13. Others include PSA tests for men over 70 years old;[27] imaging for uncomplicated low-back pain within the first six weeks after onset;[28] placing vena cava filters in all patients who have blood clots, instead of prescribing a blood thinner if they can tolerate it and don't have certain other indications;[29] and whole-body CT scans to detect cancer in people with average cancer risk.[30]

When it comes to drugs, cost-effectiveness analysis (CEA) can help establish which medications are worth the cost and should be included in a standard benefit package. As mentioned earlier, CMS is prohibited from using cost in its coverage decisions. While the private Institute for Clinical and Economic Review (ICER) does these kinds of analyses, its decisions aren't binding on payers.

Types of Technology Assessment

CEA is one branch of health technology assessment (HTA), which also includes comparative effectiveness research (CER). CEA depends on CER, but health technology assessment doesn't necessarily include CEA. For example, the Patient-Centered Outcomes Research Institute (PCORI), which was established by the Affordable Care Act, compares the effectiveness of tests and treatments but is prohibited from doing CEA.

At the other end of the HTA spectrum is the United Kingdom's National Institute for Health and Care Excellence (NICE). NICE is a governmental organization that tells the National Health Service (NHS) which new drugs and other technologies to cover. Its recommendations, based on a combination of CEA and CER, are legally binding.

Many countries with national health insurance have adopted CEA because it helps them select the new technologies that will provide the greatest health benefit within a budget. CEA is rarely applied to coverage decisions in the United States, however. During the run-up to Obamacare, the debate over whether to consider CEA in coverage decisions "raised the specter of rationing and government interference in patient care," noted Alan Garber and Harold Sox in a 2010 article.[31]

According to Garber and Sox, cost-effectiveness analysis "is a method designed to assess the comparative impacts of expenditures on different health interventions....It is based on the premise that for any given level of resources available, society...wishes to maximize the total aggregate health benefits conferred....Cost-effectiveness compares the health effects that result from alternative uses of a given amount of health resources."[32]

Opportunity Costs for Society

NICE goes further than that by estimating the "opportunity costs" created by the adoption of a new technology. These opportunity costs result when the technology absorbs resources that might otherwise be devoted to other healthcare services or even to the non-healthcare needs of a country, such as education or defense. Because the United Kingdom has a fixed healthcare budget, NICE has repeatedly stated that it considers an appropriate threshold for product approval to be the "opportunity cost of programs displaced by new, more costly technologies."[33]

The cost-effectiveness thresholds used in CEA, as earlier noted, are expressed in "quality-adjusted life years" (QALYs). A QALY combines the additional years of life that can be gained through the use of the technology with the expected quality of those years. The QALY scale is based on such health states as "completely healthy," "blind," "immobilized," and "dead." There are multiple health states for each condition, adding up to thousands of these categories.[34]

Joe Selby, MD, the former director of PCORI, views the quality-of-life aspect as the Achilles' heel of CEA. A healthy person and a sick person, for example, might have different evaluations of what their quality of life would be if they were on dialysis, he points out.

Peter Neumann of Tufts, in contrast, says it's wrong to look at CEA from the perspective of individual patients who have a disease. "We should think about what the insurance would cover before we know we have the disease. Through insurance, you're buying a package of benefits that would be covered in case you have the illness. So how much would you be willing to pay to add some new technology to that package on the very small chance you'll need it? It's a hard calculation to do. But that's how we should think about it."

Defining C/E Thresholds

The span of cost-effectiveness thresholds in various countries is huge, ranging from about $25,000 to $200,000 per QALY gained. Moreover, HTA bodies build flexibility into their thresholds. Even NICE, which did not increase its 2001 threshold range of 20,000-30,000 British pounds ($26,400-$39,000) until recently, makes exceptions for treatments of "very rare diseases" and the later stages of terminal diseases.[35]

Near the end of 2025, the United Kingdom agreed to raise its threshold for cost-effectiveness and to pay more for certain drugs as President Trump threatened to impose tariffs on imported pharmaceuticals. Britain will allow the National Health Service to pay 25% more for new medications than it does now. NICE has also set a new CEA threshold of 25,000-35,000 pounds ($33,000-$46,200) per QALY gained.[36]

ICER uses a threshold range of $100,000-$150,000 per QALY gained — a gamut that some experts consider reasonable for the United States. The lower end of this range comes mainly from what the World Health Organization has calculated that our country can afford to pay, based on its GDP per capita, says David Whitrap, former vice president of communications and outreach for ICER.

Cost-effectiveness thresholds also can be based on the amount that patients would be willing to pay for an additional year of life, he notes. Many surveyed patients say that they'd give about two years of their income to live an extra year.

NICE uses a third CEA approach tied to opportunity costs, as mentioned earlier. Its experts compare "the incremental cost-effectiveness of a new technology with the cost-effectiveness threshold. This indicates whether or not the health expected to be gained from its use exceeds the health expected to be lost elsewhere as other health-care activities are displaced."[37]

There is no evidentiary basis for the cost-effectiveness threshold used by NICE, one report noted.[38] The same is true for HTA bodies in other nations. A systematic review published in 2018 found that 17 countries had formal cost-effectiveness thresholds, of which 13 were based on willingness to pay. Most of the thresholds fell within the WHO range of one to three times GDP per capita. But the authors concluded, "Presently, there is no commonly agreed-upon value or method for determining C/E thresholds."[39]

Nevertheless, CEA is important for two reasons, says Amitabh Chandra, a professor of public policy and business administration at the Harvard Kennedy School. First, in the absence of CEA, we end up paying for a raft of new technologies that cost more in insurance premiums and taxes than their incremental benefit to patients. Second, he says, not subjecting new products to CEA sends a signal to manufacturers that they should create more of these "dubious new technologies," because we'll pay for them. "So, the lack of cost-effectiveness analysis creates strong incentives to bring less cost-effective drugs and devices to markets."

INTERNATIONAL COMPARISONS

The U.K. single-payer system imposes more rigorous government control over technology than any other healthcare system in the world. So, it's not surprising that NICE also takes a more rigorous approach to CEA than other countries do. While NICE recommends that the NHS cover most things that it deems to be clinically effective, it draws the line at some expensive, low-value technologies.

This approach sometimes leads to clashes with public opinion. One example involved NICE's rejection of coverage for five drugs because their cost far exceeded its cost-effectiveness threshold. According to one report, "this decision resulted in patients suffering from chronic lymphocytic leukemia and mantle cell lymphoma not having access to medication that could improve their quality of life."[40]

In another case, NICE declined to approve Pfizer's crizotinib for advanced lung cancer. While this drug targeted only a small subset of lung cancer patients with a specific genetic mutation, Pfizer priced at it at 7,800 pounds ($10,000) per month, which translated to 195,000 pounds ($250,000) per QALY. After the company offered to reduce the price, the drug still would have cost over 100,000 pounds ($129,000) per QALY, and NICE decided it was not cost-effective.[41]

Chandra takes a dim view of NICE's low C/E threshold range. "British taxpayers routinely forgo medical treatments that are cost-effective but are deemed cost-ineffective by NICE," he says. "Folks in the U.K. might love that and say, 'look how little we spend on healthcare.' But if you were to ask a sick child or the parents of a child who has cystic fibrosis in the U.K., 'where would you rather live, in America or the U.K.,' the answer would be America. So the U.K. has erred too much on one side of the tradeoff. I don't think what they've done is responsible. It's an irresponsible country in the way they treat the sick."

Canadian Approach

Canada has national health insurance, but it doesn't cover outpatient drugs. Hence, Canadians have to pay for medications out of pocket or buy private drug insurance. The government sets drug prices using an international reference price system; however, while costs are far below those of the United States, Canada has the second-highest drug prices in the world.[42]

In response to public protests, the Canadian government in 2019 announced new policies to reduce drug prices and allow the government to consider cost-effectiveness in coverage decisions.[43]

The Canadian Agency for Drugs and Technologies in Health (CADTH), an independent, not-for-profit organization created by the government, already does this on an advisory basis.[44] CADTH performs health technology assessments, including CER and CEA. It uses a cost-effectiveness threshold of just under $100,000 per QALY gained for new drugs.[45] When a new medication exceeds that threshold, CADTH sometimes recommends it only for particular types of patients or in particular situations.

For example, the agency has recommended that lanadelumab be reimbursed for routine prevention of attacks of hereditary angioedema (HAE) only if the patient is at least 12 years old, the diagnosis is made by a specialist in the condition, and the patient has experienced at least three HAE attacks within any four-week period before initiating lanadelumab therapy. It also has recommended that the drug's price, currently $534,000 a year, be reduced by at least 59%. At the lower price, CADTH concluded, the incremental cost-effectiveness ratio of lanadelumab would be $50,000 per QALY compared with Cinryze, another therapy for HAE.[46]

The German Solution

Germany doesn't use an explicit C/E threshold to determine the value of new drugs. Instead, the government allows a new drug approved by the European Medicines Agency (EMA) to go on the market at whatever list price its manufacturer sets for the first year. During that year, the country's Institute for Quality and Efficiency in Health Care (IQWiG) evaluates the drug's comparative effectiveness based on clinical evidence, including the studies that the manufacturer submitted to the EMA. The IQWiG sends its report to a government committee, which, after public hearings, decides whether the medication offers major, moderate, minor, or no incremental benefit compared to existing treatments.

If a drug offers more benefit than its comparators do, the German "sickness funds" association negotiates a price with the drug company based on comparative effectiveness and other factors. If the medicine offers no added benefit, the insurers will pay no more for it than they pay for the alternatives in its therapeutic class. If the sickness funds and the drug maker can't reach an agreement, an arbitration panel sets the price or the company withdraws the drug.[47]

Coverage with Evidence Determination

Although CMS doesn't consider cost in its coverage decisions, the United States has a back door to delaying or preventing widespread use of expensive new technologies: Medicare's coverage with evidence development program (CED). Under this program, CMS conditionally covers a new technology while collecting additional evidence on the technology's effectiveness. The patients who receive the drug, device, or procedure must be in a clinical trial.[48]

Current examples of these technologies include cochlear implantation, transcatheter aortic valve replacement, percutaneous image-guided lumbar decompression for lumbar spinal stenosis, and vagus nerve stimulation for treatment-resistant depression. About two dozen technologies currently are covered under CED, although others have been covered, as well, in the two decades since CMS launched the program.[49]

In some cases, CMS's efforts to control the introduction of these technologies have failed. In February 2019, for example, CMS announced it would provide CED for CAR T-cell cancer therapies.[50] These personalized biologic drugs cost \$373,000-\$475,000, and the supportive care they require can double those prices.[51] According to Neumann, CMS tried to negotiate an agreement to cover the drugs only if short-term outcomes were positive, but the deal fell apart. In late 2019, CMS announced a national coverage determination for CAR-T therapies.[52]

History of U.S. Technology Assessment

Besides the information CMS derives from the CED program, the Medicare Evidence Development and Coverage Advisory Committee (MEDCAC) advises CMS on specific clinical topics. According to the agency, MEDCAC "reviews and evaluates medical literature, reviews technology assessments, public testimony and examines data and information on the benefits, harms, and appropriateness of medical items and services that are covered under Medicare or that may be eligible for coverage under Medicare." But it doesn't look at costs.[53]

Another technology assessment body, the Agency for Healthcare Research and Quality (AHRQ), does health services and patient safety research; at one time, it also housed the most extensive library of clinical guidelines in the United States. AHRQ's predecessor, the Agency for Health Care Policy and Research (AHCPR), went further than that, establishing Patient Outcomes Research Teams that looked at practice variations, measured patient outcomes, and disseminated the results to clinicians. AHCPR ran into a snag in 1995 when it recommended against spinal fusion surgery and was assailed by spine surgeons with pull on Capitol Hill.[54] The agency survived but morphed into AHRQ, which carried on its mission without doing outcomes research. In 2018, the first Trump Administration closed AHRQ's clinical guidelines database,[55] and in spring 2025, the federal government partly defunded AHRQ and laid off much of its workforce.[56]

Technology assessment in the private sector has also mostly faded out, except for cursory reviews that outside firms do for insurance companies. The Blue Cross Blue Shield Association (BCBSA) used to have a Technology Evaluation Center (TEC) that assessed the value of new technologies on behalf of its member companies and, in some cases, did "special reports" on cost-effectiveness. TEC also worked closely with Kaiser Permanente, which factored the center's findings into its own coverage decisions.[57] Neither TEC nor Kaiser ever explicitly used CEA in their technology assessments. However, ICER reports do, and their conclusions are increasingly taken into account by health plans.[58-59]

NEW DIRECTIONS FOR TECHNOLOGY ASSESSMENT

The introduction of new technologies must be controlled in some manner to constrain the growth in health spending. In addition, the comparative effectiveness of existing technologies must be studied to find out which ones really contribute to health and which ones don't.

To restate what was said in Chapter 13, the federal government should negotiate prices with pharmaceutical companies on behalf of the whole country as part of any effective program to reduce drug prices. But, instead of whacking drug spending across the board, the government should consider CEA, where appropriate, to determine how best to allocate healthcare resources.

To provide the requisite data to the government, we should establish a U.S. health technology assessment body along the lines of ICER or the United Kingdom's NICE. Although this entity would be under the government's control, it need not be an official agency. Much of the government's work is done by outside contractors, and perhaps HHS could contract with a private organization like ICER. Considering that ICER has been doing this work for 20 years and has accumulated a great deal of expertise, that might be the best way to go to ramp up this essential work quickly.

Strong political opposition to this move can be expected. One line of that opposition is likely to be that CEA is too rigid to accommodate new research and changes in scientific thinking. The legislation establishing the health technology assessment entity could deflect this attack by requiring the entity to be flexible in its determinations. For example, if a technology were shown to be effective for a wider range of indications than what the FDA approved it for or if its price dropped significantly, the HTA body could revisit its original decision on whether to recommend the technology or what to use it for.

Another inevitable source of criticism would be that individual patients might be condemned to avoidable deaths or needlessly painful lives if the technology assessment body were to consider cost in its coverage decisions. As explained earlier, healthcare resources are not infinite, and some limitations must be placed on coverage of very expensive technologies to spare resources for basic care and other lifesaving treatments. But still, these decisions involve human values that cannot be blithely dismissed. How can these values be applied to technology assessments and who should do that?

HOW PATIENTS CAN BE INVOLVED

Here we can take another lesson from the U.K. Starting in 2002 and continuing through at least 2016, NICE had a citizens council that provided the U.K. agency "with a public perspective on overarching moral and ethical issues that NICE should take into account when producing guidance [on NHS coverage]. Made up of members of the public…the Council operates through a 'citizens jury' style meeting, to explore and respond to a question set by NICE."[60]

NICE didn't ask the council to consider issues related to coverage of any new drug or technology by the National Health Service. Instead, NICE asked the citizens council to opine on more general areas such as "what are the social values that need to be considered when making decisions about trade-offs between equity and efficiency?" As a result, U.K. patient advocacy groups described the citizens' council as a "toothless tiger" when it was initially convened. One critic said that patients should be involved in decisions on drugs at every step in NICE's process. Michael Rawlins, the chairman of NICE, responded by saying that the citizens council was not qualified to do that, "because so many of the appraisals require scientific judgements."[61]

While the citizens council is no more, NICE has established independent advisory committees that include patients as well as clinicians and experts in health and social care. There are a limited number of paid slots on these committees, with terms lasting from several months to three years. For example, "lay members" recently served for nine months on a committee addressing "heart valve disease presenting in adults: investigation and management." NICE sought people who had had a transcatheter aortic valve implantation to treat aortic stenosis. Another qualification was "a good understanding of the issues important to patients and their families or unpaid carers."[62-63]

In this country, ICER also has patients review its reports. These patients are involved right from the start of the research. When ICER begins reviewing a new drug — usually about eight months before the FDA is expected to approve it — the organization reaches out to patient communities and starts getting their input on the burden of the disease and what outcomes matter most to them. This dialogue continues throughout the assessment process and public hearings that also involve experts and manufacturers, says David Whitrap.

U.S. Consumer Council

Based on these examples, it is possible to envision a U.S. citizens council that would be empowered to make recommendations on the moral and financial issues that the introduction of an expensive new therapy or test entail. In fact, because so many new technologies involve human values and economic tradeoffs, it is imperative that citizens — who are also patients — be allowed to weigh in on these consequential decisions.

David Eddy, MD, an expert on health technology analysis and clinical guidelines, came up with such a proposal in the 1990s. His idea of a "consumer council" has many advantages, although it would not be easy to assemble such a body and make it work properly. Specifically, Eddy proposed that the government assemble a nationally representative group of people, present them with information on the benefits and harms of a medical intervention, tell them what it would cost, "and observe their choices."[64]

In an interview I did with Eddy about 20 years ago, he elaborated on this idea, suggesting that the consultative body should consist of several thousand people who would represent a broad cross-section of the population by age, gender, race, geography and income. Since they would have to be able to understand basic concepts of medicine and mathematical probability, he added, they'd have to be of above-average intelligence — a requirement that could be met by picking only people who'd had at least some college education.

Eddy also felt strongly that consumer "judges" should be required to buy their own insurance, with the premiums adjusted according to income and net worth so that everyone would feel the same economic pain when premium costs increased. That way, he explained, they'd know how the cost of whatever new technologies were adopted would affect them.

This suggestion makes sense, except that it is unnecessary to have a special insurance system for the consumer judges. The insurance costs they pay should be what people encounter today in the real world, where most working-age people have employer-provided insurance. The council members would be sensitive to the additional cost of, say, unrestricted access to GLP-1s for weight loss both in their share of insurance premiums and in the Medicare taxes they paid. Under my reform plan, they'd feel it directly in their share of basic care subscription fees and premiums for major medical insurance.

The situation would be different, however, for the poor, whose insurance would be entirely subsidized by the government, and for the wealthy, who would not feel the pinch of additional health costs. So perhaps participation in the consumer council should be limited to people of moderate means, who would notice if coverage of a very expensive drug or test increased their insurance costs.

The Internet has made it much easier to construct a consumer council than it would have been when Eddy first set forth his proposal. Several thousand consumer judges could easily be recruited, vetted, educated, and polled through a website. The more active members of the council, which would include committees looking at specific products, could also have virtual video meetings to discuss their ideas.

The council members would have to be paid for their time, of course, and their terms should probably be limited to a year or two to minimize burnout and attrition. Above all, their identities would have to be guarded to protect them from political and commercial pressures, as well as pleas from patients and their advocates.

Dividing the Wheat from the Chaff

The consumer council should be asked to evaluate only particular kinds of technologies and procedures. Among these would be interventions that are high-cost and low-benefit; those that would generate tricky conflicts among different patient values; and those that would be so expensive that they'd limit access to other important technologies or even basic services. Following are a few examples where human values play an important role.

I've already discussed the cost implications of Aduhelm. Another Alzheimer's disease treatment, lecanemab (Leqembi), has been approved by the FDA and is covered by Medicare and Medicaid. Leqembi can delay disease progression for up to 36 months, and it enables patients in the early stage of the disease to perform activities of daily living for 10 months.[65] A third Alzheimer's therapy, donanemab (Kisunla), enables diagnosed patients to take care of themselves for 13 months, on average.[66] The costs of the latter two drugs are $26,500 and $32,000 per year, respectively, not counting the cost of diagnostic and tracking tests. With 7.2 million Americans currently diagnosed with Alzheimer's,[67] these are pricey therapies that don't cure the disease and that slow its progression for a relatively short time. But how much is an extra year of being able to function as a sentient human being worth?

To cite a more obscure example, the FDA recently approved a therapy called brensocatib for non-cystic fibrosis bronchiectasis, a chronic lung disease that affects breathing and coughing. The disease affects more people than cystic fibrosis — about 350,000-500,000 at any given time. Exacerbations occur when symptoms worsen, requiring antibiotics and sometimes hospitalizations.

ICER did a report on brensocatib and concluded that it had a minimal cost benefit. While clinical trials showed that it reduced exacerbations of bronchiectasis, it had little effect on the deterioration of lung function. At an annual net price of $61,600, ICER concluded, brensocatib would not meet commonly used cost-effectiveness thresholds. Moreover, only 4% of the 461,208 potentially eligible patients could be treated without crossing the ICER budget impact threshold of $880 million.[68] So, to be affordable, the drug's price would have to come down. But, for someone with this condition, brensocatib might make living worthwhile.

The GLP-1 Conundrum Revisited

GLP-1s would present a much bigger quandary for a consumer council. Although these drugs are considered cost-effective, they could ruin healthcare economics if everyone who was obese or overweight could get them. To recapitulate, the upper boundary of annual costs for GLP-1s in that case might be $1 trillion — about 20% of current annual health spending in the United States.

So, the members of the consumer council would have to weigh the human considerations against the cost to society of allowing unrestricted access to these drugs. Let's say that one option was to follow Medicare's lead and limit coverage to people with a comorbid condition that a GLP-1 prescription might alleviate (which, as noted earlier, might be expanded). That would still be very expensive, but it might be affordable for the country as a whole. On the other hand, obese people without comorbidities like diabetes or heart disease might develop them later because they didn't have access to GLP-1s. In addition, as the TV ads for these drugs make clear, there is a social dimension of weight loss that is very important to people with obesity.

For a moment, imagine that you are on the consumer council. You have received training in how to evaluate new technologies, as well as extensive educational material about obesity and GLP-1s. You've also been told how much your basic care subscription fees and major medical premiums are likely to increase if you decide to make GLP-1s available to everyone, rather than only to people with certain comorbid conditions. How do you process this information?

If your family income is modest, as suggested above, a significant increase in your health insurance/subscription costs would have a noticeable impact on your ability to afford healthcare or to buy other things. Unless you yourself are obese, you're going to make your decision based on the tradeoff between your own economic well-being and the possibility that someone who you don't know might get sick or sicker if they can't take the drug.

One other factor might be brought to your attention: the opportunity cost of investing so much in one new drug category, which we encountered earlier in our discussion of NICE. If we spent hundreds of billions a year on GLP-1 drugs, would we be able to fund prenatal care? Would we have enough money to spend on mental healthcare or dental care? And if an effective treatment for Alzheimer's disease were finally developed, would we be able to afford it at all?

These are questions that, by and large, are being ignored outside of policy circles. Yet they are fundamental to the kind of healthcare we'll have in the future and the kind of society we'll live in. No matter what we do to reform healthcare and to ensure a more equitable division of resources, the march of medical technology will rob us of the care we need unless we learn how to control it.

AFTERWORD.

A New Deal for Healthcare

Too many people, institutions, and corporations make too much money from U.S. healthcare. It's a classic case of capitalism gone wild. Healthcare should be about health, not profits.

That said, we do live in a capitalist country. But, unlike the people in other advanced capitalist societies, Americans are not overly concerned about social solidarity. Our individualism makes it difficult for some people to understand why everyone deserves healthcare. The ideal of individual freedom — so inculcated in American culture — also makes it difficult to accept the need to restrict access to some new technologies because they consume resources needed for other kinds of healthcare.

At the beginning of this book, I explained why our current healthcare system is unsustainable. Neither of our major political parties has a practical plan to save healthcare, but public pressure is growing for them to come up with a solution. The likelihood is that politicians will continue to embrace incremental steps — which, after all, is the safest position. Unfortunately, however, the time for half-measures is over. Unless our system is radically changed, it will collapse, and most people will have less access to worse healthcare.

Having pondered this dilemma for 30 years, I'm convinced that we can build on the system we have, preserving enough of it to satisfy the healthcare players while providing high quality, comprehensive, affordable care for all. Is this a compromise? Of course it is. But, rather than continuing to pursue the mirage of Medicare for All, progressive reformers would have a better chance of rescuing healthcare if they could figure out how to work within the parameters of our current, profit-driven system.

I believe that the model proposed in this book could do that. Although it involves a complete restructuring of healthcare delivery and financing, insurance companies and hospitals would do well under this model, and pharmaceutical companies would do no worse than they would if the United States kept enlarging drug price negotiations. Also, the major players would be much better served under this arrangement than they would be if the system fell apart.

As for physicians, my model would give them much more control over the health system than they have now. Primary care physicians would effectively run most ambulatory care, which would not only lead to big improvements in health but would also give them the opportunity to earn more than they do today. While we'd still have a shortage of primary care physicians, the additional money and the new respect they'd receive would induce more young doctors to enter the field.

Specialists would have the hardest time adjusting to the new model. Their compensation would likely shrink unless they were in rare specialties. And they'd have to deliver value to the basic care groups if they wanted to receive a steady stream of referrals. But those who provided high-quality care at a reasonable price would get not only referrals, but also the opportunity to work with primary care teams to enhance chronic disease management. And, with every patient covered by the same level of insurance, specialists could be assured that they would be reimbursed for every covered service they provided.

Bifurcated healthcare financing might seem like an eccentric idea, because it's never been done before. The current U.S. healthcare system, however, is also unprecedented and unique in many ways. Employment-based insurance, for example, is largely an historical accident that grew out of the labor shortage during World War II. To lure scarce workers, companies offered them health benefits. Due to the government's decision to exempt those benefits from taxation, along with the rise of labor unions that bargained with employers for health insurance, it became our de facto method of financing healthcare.

So, let's stipulate that, just because something has never been done, that doesn't mean it can't work. Perhaps the way to get the ball rolling is with a proof of concept in one state. Since Maryland already has a global budgeting system for hospitals, maybe we could start in that state (with its consent, of course). Let Maryland use its corporate practice of medicine law to liberate PCPs from hospital and corporate ownership. Give these doctors incentives to form basic care groups that charge subscription fees, ban other insurance for basic care, and let insurers form major medical plans. Try it out for a while and measure the results. If it succeeds in Maryland, it can work elsewhere.

The biggest obstacle to the implementation of my model is time. We have a limited amount of time left before care becomes unaffordable for most Americans. And, as I noted in Chapter 6, it would take at least five years to transform the system in the ways I propose. So, there's no time to waste. Starting in 2029, when the next Democratic Administration takes office, we should try this or something else that can accomplish the same goals.

Whatever it turns out to be, a healthcare reform plan must be all-encompassing. Half-measures won't do; they will fail. Congress must devise and pass far-reaching legislation on a par with, but better than the Affordable Care Act. We can hope that the two parties, at long last, will come together for the good of the American people. They have to, because we're all in this together.

References

Introduction

1. Cox C. ACA insurers are raising premiums by an estimated 26%, but most enrollees could see sharper increases in what they pay. Kaiser Family Foundation Quick Take. October 28, 2025. Accessed January 26, 2026. https://www.kff.org/quick-take/aca-insurers-are-raising-premiums-by-an-estimated-26-but-most-enrollees-could-see-sharper-increases-in-what-they-pay/
2. Setting the Record Straight on Premium Tax Credit Enhancements. Center on Budget and Policy Priorities. January 12, 2026. Accessed January 26, 2026. https://www.cbpp.org/blog/setting-the-record-straight-on-premium-tax-credit-enhancements
3. Appleby J. Trump team offers its answer to rising premium costs: catastrophic coverage. Miami Herald. Feb. 15, 2026. Accessed Jan. 26, 2026. https://www.yahoo.com/news/articles/trump-team-offers-answer-rising-175420945.html
4. Fiedler M. The outlook for US health spending growth: a blast from the past? Health Affairs Forefront. June 17, 2024. doi:10.1377/forefront.20240614.517072
5. Glied SA and Lui B. Slowdown: Decomposing the Moderation in Health Spending Growth, 2009-19. Health Affairs Vol. 45, No. 1. January 2026. https://doi.org/10.1377/hlthaff.2025.00472
6. Emanuel EJ. Why haven't health care cost increases exceeded inflation? There's a very good reason. STAT. December 21, 2023. Accessed January 26, 2026. https://www.statnews.com/2023/12/21/health-care-costs-inflation-affordable-care-act/
7. Keehan SP, Madison AJ, Poisal JA, *et al.* National health expenditure projections, 2024-33: despite insurance coverage declines, health to grow as share of GDP. Health Aff. 2025;44(7):776-787. doi:10.1377/htlhaff.2025.00545
8. de Vise D. Why Americans pay so much more for health care in 2024. USA Today. December 28, 2024. Accessed January 26, 2026. https://www.usatoday.com/story/money/2024/12/28/why-american-health-care-costs-more/77264782007/
9. Hartman M, Martin AB, Lassman D, Catlin A, *et al.* National Health Care Spending Increased 7.2 Percent in 2024 As Utilization Remained Elevated. Health Affairs 45, No. 2 (2026). https://doi.org/10.1377/hlthaff.2025.01683.
10. Claxton G, Rae M, Damico A, Winger A, Wager E. Health benefits in 2025: family premiums rise 6 percent, large employers increase coverage of GLP-1s for weight loss. Health Aff. 2025;44(11):1359-1368. doi:10.1377/hlthaff.2025.01106
11. Kanimian S, Ho V. Why does the cost of employer-sponsored coverage keep rising? Health Aff Sch. 2024;2(6):qxae078. doi:10.1093/haschl/qxae078

12. Hughes S, Gee E, Rapfogel N. Health insurance costs are squeezing workers and employers. Center for American Progress. November 29, 2022. Accessed January 26, 2026. https://www.americanprogress.org/article/health-insurance-costs-are-squeezing-workers-and-employers/
13. Lopes L, Montero A, Presiado M, Hamel L. Americans' challenges with health care costs. KFF Issue Brief. March 1, 2024. Accessed January 26, 2026. https://www.kff.org/health-costs/issue-brief/americans-challenges-with-health-care-costs/
14. Lopes L, Montero A, Presiado M, Hamel L. Americans' challenges with health care costs. KFF Issue Brief. March 1, 2024. Accessed January 26, 2026. https://www.kff.org/health-costs/issue-brief/americans-challenges-with-health-care-costs/
15. Carter J. Federal court reverses federal medical debt protections. Medicare Rights Center. July 31, 2025. Accessed January 26, 2026. https://www.medicarerights.org/medicare-watch/2025/07/31/federal-court-reverses-federal-medical-debt-protections
16. Claxton G, Rae M, Damico A, Winger A, Wager E. Health benefits in 2025: family premiums rise 6 percent, large employers increase coverage of GLP-1s for weight loss. Health Aff. 2025;44(11):1359-1368. doi:10.1377/hlthaff.2025.01106
17. Percentage of small employers offering health benefits in decline; nearly all large employers offer coverage. Employee Benefit Research Institute. December 5, 2024. Accessed January 26, 2026. https://www.ebri.org/publications/research-publications/fast-facts/content/percentage-of-small-employers-offering-health-benefits-in-decline--nearly-all-large-employers-offer-coverage
18. Collins SR, Gupta A. The state of health insurance coverage in the U.S. Commonwealth Fund. November 21, 2024. Accessed January 26, 2026. https://www.commonwealthfund.org/publications/surveys/2024/nov/state-health-insurance-coverage-us-2024-biennial-survey
19. National uninsured rate at 8.2 percent in the first quarter of 2024. ASPE Office of Health Policy. August 2024. Accessed January 26, 2026. https://aspe.hhs.gov/sites/default/files/documents/ee0475e44e27daef00155e95a24fd023/nhis-q1-2024-datapoint.pdf
20. Oberlander J. Progress lost—the unraveling of Medicaid and the Affordable Care Act. N Engl J Med. 2025;393(7):628-629. doi:10.1056/NEJMp2509768
21. Blumenthal D, Gumas ED, Shah A, Gunja MZ, Williams RD II. Mirror, mirror 2024: a portrait of the failing U.S. health system. Commonwealth Fund. September 19, 2024. Accessed January 26, 2026. https://www.commonwealthfund.org/publications/fund-reports/2024/sep/mirror-mirror-2024
22. Blumenthal D, Gumas ED, Shah A, Gunja MZ, Williams RD II. Mirror, mirror 2024: a portrait of the failing U.S. health system. Commonwealth Fund.

September 19, 2024. Accessed January 26, 2026. https://www.commonwealthfund.org/publications/fund-reports/2024/sep/mirror-mirror-2024

23. Rosenthal E. The shrinking number of primary care physicians is reaching a tipping point. KFF Health News. September 8, 2023. Accessed January 26, 2026. https://kffhealthnews.org/news/article/lack-of-primary-care-tipping-point/
24. Taylor M. NP workforce grows 8% in 1 year. Becker's Clinical Leadership. November 13, 2023. Accessed January 26, 2026. https://www.beckershospitalreview.com/nursing/nurse-practitioners-grow-8-in-1-year.html
25. AMN Healthcare survey: physician appointment wait times up 8% from 2017, up 24% from 2004. AMN Healthcare. September 12, 2022. Accessed January 26, 2026. https://ir.amnhealthcare.com/news-releases/news-release-details/amn-healthcare-survey-physician-appointment-wait-times-8-2017-24
26. Dennison B. Interview with author. Date not specified.
27. PBGH publishes purchaser policy priorities for the new Congress and administration. Pacific Business Group on Health. January 31, 2025. Accessed January 26, 2026. https://www.pbgh.org/pbgh-publishes-purchaser-policy-priorities-for-the-new-congress-and-administration/
28. Claxton G, Levitt L, Gremminger S, Kramer B, Rae M. How corporate executives view rising health care cost and the role of government. KFF. April 29, 2021. Accessed January 26, 2026. https://www.kff.org/report-section/how-corporate-executives-view-rising-health-care-cost-and-the-role-of-government-findings/
29. Schubel J. The big Republican cost-shift: massive cuts to Medicaid and the ACA will increase costs for older adults and Medicare. Health Affairs Forefront. May 30, 2025. Accessed January 26, 2026. https://www.healthaffairs.org/content/forefront/big-republican-cost-shift-massive-cuts-medicaid-and-aca-increase-costs-older-adults-and
30. Report to the Congress: Medicare payment policy. Medicare Payment Advisory Commission (MedPAC). March 2024. Accessed January 26, 2026. https://www.medpac.gov/wp-content/uploads/2024/03/Mar24_MedPAC_Report_To_Congress_SEC.pdf
31. Cubanski J, Neuman T. FAQs on Medicare financing and trust fund solvency. Kaiser Family Foundation. May 29, 2024. Accessed January 26, 2026. https://www.kff.org/medicare/issue-brief/faqs-on-medicare-financing-and-trust-fund-solvency/
32. Mallory H. Private insurers pay 240% of what Medicare pays for hospital services. Healthcare Finance. September 18, 2020. Accessed January 26, 2026. https://www.healthcarefinancenews.com/news/private-insurers-pay-240-what-medicare-pays-hospital-services
33. Potts M, Burton C, Fuong H, Brown A. Americans are unhappy with the state of health care and insurance. ABC News. December 16, 2024. Accessed January

26, 2026. https://abcnews.go.com/538/americans-unhappy-state-health-care-insurance/story?id=116775693

34. Fiore K. Social media unleashes cruel responses to UnitedHealthcare CEO's murder. Medpage Today. December 5, 2024. Accessed January 26, 2026. https://www.medpagetoday.com/special-reports/features/113243
35. Lagasse J. More than half of healthcare consumers not fully satisfied with their insurance. Healthcare Finance. August 18, 2023. Accessed January 26, 2026. https://www.healthcarefinancenews.com/news/more-half-healthcare-consumers-not-fully-satisfied-their-insurance
36. Murphy N, Rapfogel N, Thornton A. Trends and consequences in health insurer consolidation. Center for American Progress. December 4, 2024. Accessed January 26, 2026. https://www.americanprogress.org/article/trends-and-consequences-in-health-insurer-consolidation/
37. Kanimian S, Ho V. Why does the cost of employer-sponsored coverage keep rising? Health Aff Sch. 2024;2(6):qxae078. doi:10.1093/haschl/qxae078
38. Berwick DM, Batchlor E, Chokshi DA, *et al.* From laggard to leader: why health care in the United States is failing, and how to fix it. Health Aff. 2025;44(2):179-188. doi:10.1377/hlthaff.2024.01007

Chapter 1

1. Starr P. The Social Transformation of American Medicine. New York, NY: Basic Books; 1982:428.
2. Brown EF, Singh Y, Whaley CM, Perkins J. The rise of health care consolidation and what to do about it. Health Affairs Forefront. September 9, 2024. doi:10.1377/forefront.20240906.397095
3. Updated report: hospital and corporate acquisition of physician practices and physician employment 2019-2023. Avalere Health, prepared for Physicians Advocacy Institute. April 2024. Accessed January 26, 2026. https://www.physiciansadvocacyinstitute.org/Portals/0/assets/docs/PAI-Research/PAI-Avalere%20Physician%20Employment%20Trends%20Study%202019-2023%20Final.pdf
4. Berenbrok LA, Tang S, Gabriel N, *et al.* Access to community pharmacies: a nationwide geographic information systems cross-sectional analysis. J Am Pharm Assoc (2003). 2022;62(6):1816-1822.e2. doi:10.1016/j.japh.2022.07.003
5. Welch WP, Oliveira I, Blanco M, Sommers BD. Ownership of skilled nursing facilities: an analysis of newly-released federal data. HHS Assistant Secretary for Planning and Evaluation (ASPE) Office of Health Policy. December 15, 2022. Accessed January 26, 2026. https://aspe.hhs.gov/sites/default/files/documents/fd593ae970848e30aa5496c00ba43d5c/aspe-data-brief-ownership-snfs.pdf
6. Stewart E, Baker J. Private equity: the metastasizing disease threatening health care. Health Affairs Forefront. December 18, 2023. doi:10.1377/forefront.20231213.928665

7. U.S. pharmaceutical industry—statistics & facts. Statista. Accessed January 26, 2026. https://www.statista.com/topics/1719/pharmaceutical-industry/
8. Trends and consequences in health insurer consolidation. Center for American Progress. December 4, 2024. Accessed January 26, 2026. https://www.americanprogress.org/article/trends-and-consequences-in-health-insurer-consolidation/
9. Competition in health care research. American Medical Association. November 19, 2024. Accessed January 26, 2026. https://www.ama-assn.org/health-care-advocacy/access-care/competition-health-care-research
10. Trends and consequences in health insurer consolidation. Center for American Progress. December 4, 2024. Accessed January 26, 2026. https://www.americanprogress.org/article/trends-and-consequences-in-health-insurer-consolidation/
11. Trends and consequences in health insurer consolidation. Center for American Progress. December 4, 2024. Accessed January 26, 2026. https://www.americanprogress.org/article/trends-and-consequences-in-health-insurer-consolidation/
12. Morse S. PwC: hospital mergers not yielding IT, clinical or operational efficiencies. Healthcare IT News. March 29, 2016. Accessed January 26, 2026. https://www.healthcareitnews.com/news/pwc-hospital-mergers-not-yielding-operational-efficiencies
13. Gaynor M, Mostashari F, Ginsburg P. Health care's crushing lack of competition. Forbes. June 28, 2017. Accessed January 26, 2026. https://www.forbes.com/sites/realspin/2017/06/28/health-cares-crushing-lack-of-competition/
14. Beaulieu ND, Dafny LS, Landon BE, *et al.* Changes in quality of care after hospital mergers and acquisitions. N Engl J Med. 2020;382(1):51-59. doi:10.1056/NEJMsa1901383
15. Condon A. 14 academic health systems acquiring hospitals. Becker's Hospital Review. December 4, 2024. Accessed January 26, 2026. https://www.beckershospitalreview.com/hospital-transactions-and-valuation/academic-systems-acquiring-hospitals-left-and-right.html
16. Kacik A. Beth Israel Deaconess and Lahey Health complete merger. Modern Healthcare. March 1, 2019. Accessed January 26, 2026. https://www.modernhealthcare.com/mergers-acquisitions/beth-israel-deaconess-and-lahey-health-complete-merger
17. Kacik A. Catholic Health Initiatives, Dignity Health combine to form CommonSpirit Health. Modern Healthcare. February 1, 2019. Accessed January 26, 2026. https://www.modernhealthcare.com/article/20190201/NEWS/190209994
18. Minemyer P. Advocate Aurora Health, Atrium Health close megamerger, forming the nation's 5th largest nonprofit system. Fierce Healthcare. December 2, 2022. Accessed January 26, 2026. https://www.fiercehealthcare.com/providers

/advocate-aurora-health-atrium-health-close-mega-merger-forming-nations-5th-largest-non

19. Kaiser Permanente and Geisinger come together to launch Risant Health and expand access to value-based care. Geisinger Health. April 26, 2023. Accessed January 26, 2026. https://www.geisinger.org/about-geisinger/news-and-media/news-releases/2023/04/26/15/46/kaiser-permanente-and-geisinger-come-together-to-launch-risant-health
20. Condon A. Kaiser's Risant Health to become $35B system in 5 years: 14 things to know. Becker's Hospital CFO Report. December 5, 2024. Accessed January 26, 2026. https://www.beckershospitalreview.com/finance/kaisers-risant-health-to-become-35b-system-in-5-years-14-things-to-know.html
21. Kaiser Permanente and Geisinger come together to launch Risant Health and expand access to value-based care. Geisinger Health. April 26, 2023. Accessed January 26, 2026. https://www.geisinger.org/about-geisinger/news-and-media/news-releases/2023/04/26/15/46/kaiser-permanente-and-geisinger-come-together-to-launch-risant-health
22. Melnick GA, Fonkych K. Hospital prices increase in California, especially among hospitals in the largest multi-hospital systems. Inquiry. 2016;53:0046958016651555. doi:10.1177/0046958016651555
23. White C, Whaley C. Prices paid to hospitals by private health plans are high relative to Medicare and vary widely. RAND Health Research Report. 2019. Accessed January 26, 2026. https://www.rand.org/pubs/research_reports/RR3033.html
24. The prices that commercial health insurers and Medicare pay for hospitals' and physicians' services. Congressional Budget Office. January 2022. Accessed January 26, 2026. https://www.cbo.gov/system/files/2022-01/57422-medical-prices.pdf
25. 37% of hospitals still losing money. Becker's Hospital Review. February 27, 2025. Accessed January 26, 2026. https://www.beckershospitalreview.com/finance/37-of-hospitals-still-losing-money/
26. National hospital flash report, December 2024 metrics. Kaufman Hall. Accessed January 26, 2026. https://www.kaufmanhall.com/sites/default/files/2025-02/KH-NHFR_Report-December-2024-Metrics.pdf
27. Chang JY, Martin K. Commercial inpatient hospital price growth driven by system affiliation and nonprofit-status hospitals. Health Aff Sch. 2024;2(11):qxae140. doi:10.1093/haschl/qxae140
28. Gaynor M, Mostashari F, Ginsburg P. Health care's crushing lack of competition. Forbes. June 28, 2017. Accessed January 26, 2026. https://www.forbes.com/sites/realspin/2017/06/28/health-cares-crushing-lack-of-competition/
29. Schencker S. FTC challenges NorthShore, Advocate mega-merger in Illinois. Modern Healthcare. December 18, 2015. Accessed January 26, 2026. http://www.modernhealthcare.com/article/20151218/NEWS/151219865

30. Brot-Goldberg Z, Cooper Z, Craig S, Klarnet L. Is there too little antitrust enforcement in the US hospital sector? Am Econ Rev. 2024;114(12):3941-3991. doi:10.1257/aer.20221475
31. Kole K, Poklop J. Determining the true value of primary care practices. ECG Management Consultants. Accessed January 26, 2026. https://www.ecgmc.com/insights/article/2596/determining-the-true-value-of-primary-care-practices
32. Optum now has 90,000 physicians. Becker's Hospital Review. November 29, 2023. Accessed January 26, 2026. https://www.beckershospitalreview.com/legal-regulatory-issues/optum-added-nearly-20-000-physicians-in-2023.html
33. Updated report: hospital and corporate acquisition of physician practices and physician employment 2019-2023. Physicians Advocacy Institute/Avalere Health. April 2024. Accessed January 26, 2026. https://www.physiciansadvocacyinstitute.org/Portals/0/assets/docs/PAI-Research/PAI-Avalere%20Physician%20Employment%20Trends%20Study%202019-2023%20Final.pdf
34. Newitt P. Physician practice consolidation skyrocketing: 10 GAO findings. Becker's ASC Review. September 25, 2025. Accessed January 26, 2026. https://www.beckersasc.com/asc-transactions-and-valuation-issues/physician-practice-consolidation-skyrocketing-10-gao-findings/
35. Over 77% of physicians are employed. Here's how that's shaping healthcare. The Advisory Group. May 30, 2024. Accessed January 26, 2026. https://www.advisory.com/daily-briefing/2024/04/16/pai-avalere-ec
36. Terry K. Hospitals continue to acquire more physician practices. Medscape Medical News. February 22, 2019. Accessed January 26, 2026. https://www.medscape.com/viewarticle/909411
37. Kane CF. Updated data on physician practice arrangements: for the first time, fewer physicians are owners than employees. AMA Policy Research Perspectives. May 2019. Accessed January 26, 2026. https://www.ama-assn.org/system/files/2019-05/prp-fewer-owners-benchmark-survey-2018.pdf
38. Garvey G. Smaller share of doctors in private practice than ever before. AMA News Wire. June 24, 2025. Accessed January 26, 2026. https://www.ama-assn.org/practice-management/private-practices/smaller-share-doctors-private-practice-ever
39. Singleton T, Miller P. The physician employment trend: what you need to know. Fam Pract Manag. 2015;22(4):11-15.
40. Terry K. One in 5 residents doubt career choice, despite ample job offers. Medscape Medical News. May 16, 2019. Accessed January 26, 2026. https://www.medscape.com/viewarticle/913082
41. Hancock J. When the hospital is boss, that's where doctors' patients go. Kaiser Health News. September 9, 2015. Accessed January 26, 2026. http://khn.org/news/when-the-hospital-is-boss-thats-where-doctors-patients-go

42. Terry K. Site-neutral payments are less than meets the eye, experts say. Medscape Medical News. December 6, 2018. Accessed January 26, 2026. https://www.medscape.com/viewarticle/906146
43. Terry K. Site-neutral payments are less than meets the eye, experts say. Medscape Medical News. December 6, 2018. Accessed January 26, 2026. https://www.medscape.com/viewarticle/906146
44. Levinson Z, Neuman T, Hulver S. Five things to know about Medicare site-neutral payment reforms. Kaiser Family Foundation. June 14, 2024. Accessed January 26, 2026. https://www.kff.org/medicare/issue-brief/five-things-to-know-about-medicare-site-neutral-payment-reforms/
45. Haelle T. Physician-hospital integration tied to higher prices. Medscape Medical News. October 20, 2015. Accessed January 26, 2026. http://www.medscape.com/viewarticle/852900
46. Evans M. Hospitals hire more doctors, outpatient prices increase. Modern Healthcare. October 19, 2015. Accessed January 26, 2026. http://www.modernhealthcare.com/article/20151019/BLOG/151019915
47. Kacik A. Rapid rise in hospital-employed physicians increases costs. Modern Healthcare. March 16, 2018. Accessed January 26, 2026. https://www.modernhealthcare.com/article/20180316/TRANSFORMATION02/180319913
48. Medical loss ratio. Centers for Medicare & Medicaid Services. Accessed January 26, 2026. https://www.cms.gov/marketplace/private-health-insurance/medical-loss-ratio
49. Newitt P. Optum physicians are paid 17% more than peers: study. Becker's ASC Review. November 7, 2025. Accessed January 26, 2026. https://www.beckersasc.com/asc-transactions-and-valuation-issues/optum-physicians-are-paid-17-more-than-peers-study/
50. Bannow T. FTC approves UnitedHealth-DaVita deal with conditions. Modern Healthcare. June 19, 2019. Accessed January 26, 2026. https://www.modernhealthcare.com/mergers-acquisitions/ftc-approves-unitedhealth-davita-deal-conditions
51. Condon A. Optum spending spree continues, adding to 70K+ physicians. Becker's Hospital CFO Report. April 11, 2023. Accessed January 26, 2026. https://www.beckershospitalreview.com/finance/optum-spending-spree-continues-adding-to-70k-physicians.html
52. Emerson J. Health systems take over Optum urgent care clinics. Becker's Hospital Review. October 18, 2024. Accessed January 26, 2026. https://www.beckershospitalreview.com/hospital-transactions-and-valuation/health-systems-take-over-optum-urgent-care-clinics.html
53. Pifer R. UnitedHealth closes $5.4B buy of home health business LHC. Healthcare Dive. February 22, 2023. Accessed January 26, 2026. https://www.healthcaredive.com/news/unitedhealth-lhc-group-closes-buy-home-health/643200/

54. Minemyer P. Humana opens 250th primary care center as it continues to focus on growth. Fierce Healthcare. June 6, 2023. Accessed January 26, 2026. https://www.fiercehealthcare.com/payers/humana-opens-250th-primary-care-center-it-continues-focus-growth

55. Elevance Health and Clayton, Dubilier & Rice sign agreement to launch strategic partnership to advance primary care delivery. Elevance Health. April 15, 2024. Accessed January 26, 2026. https://www.elevancehealth.com/newsroom/elevance-health-clayton-dubilier-rice-sign-agreement-launch-strategic-partnership-advance-primary-care-delivery

56. Global healthcare private equity report 2025. Bain & Company. Accessed January 26, 2026. https://www.bain.com/insights/topics/global-healthcare-private-equity-report/

57. Brown EF, Singh Y, Whaley CM, Perkins J. The rise of health care consolidation and what to do about it. Health Affairs Forefront. September 9, 2024. doi:10.1377/forefront.20240906.397095

58. Kacik A. Private equity infuses healthcare with $63B investment. Modern Healthcare. April 18, 2019. Accessed January 26, 2026. https://www.modernhealthcare.com/finance/private-equity-infuses-healthcare-63b-investment

59. Scheffler RM, Alexander L, Fulton BD, Arnold DR, Abdelhadi OA. Monetizing medicine: private equity and competition in physician practice markets. American Antitrust Institute. July 10, 2023. Accessed January 26, 2026. https://www.antitrustinstitute.org/wp-content/uploads/2023/07/AAI-UCB-EG_Private-Equity-I-Physician-Practice-Report_FINAL.pdf

60. Abdelhadi O, Fulton BD, Alexander L, Scheffler RM. Private equity-acquired physician practices and market penetration increased substantially, 2012-21. Health Aff. 2024;43(3):354-362. doi:10.1377/hlthaff.2023.00152

61. Singh Y, Song Z, Polsky D, Zhu JM. Increases in physician professional fees in private equity-owned gastroenterology practices. Health Aff. 2025;44(2):189-197. doi:10.1377/hlthaff.2024.00190

62. Singh Y, Song Z, Polsky D, Bruch JD, Zhu JM. Association of private equity acquisition of physician practices with changes in health care spending and utilization. JAMA Health Forum. 2022;3(9):e222886. doi:10.1001/jamahealthforum.2022.2886

63. Gondi S, Song Z. Potential implications of private equity investments in health care delivery. JAMA. 2019;321(11):1047-1048. doi:10.1001/jama.2019.1077

64. Global healthcare private equity report 2025. Bain & Company. Accessed January 26, 2026. https://www.bain.com/insights/topics/global-healthcare-private-equity-report/

65. What is a retail clinic? CVS MinuteClinic. Accessed January 26, 2026. https://www.cvs.com/minuteclinic/why-choose-us/retail-clinic

66. Minemyer P. CVS is expanding its MinuteClinics into primary care. Here's why. Fierce Healthcare. October 30, 2024. Accessed January 26, 2026. https://www.fiercehealthcare.com/retail/cvs-expanding-its-minuteclinics-primary-care-heres-why

67. Walgreens Boots Alliance makes $5.2 billion investment in VillageMD. VillageMD. October 14, 2021. Accessed January 26, 2026. https://www.villagemd.com/press-releases/walgreens-boots-alliance-makes-5.2-billion-investment-in-villagemd-to-deliver-value-based-primary-care-to-communities-across-america

68. Hudson C. What to expect from big retailers providing healthcare in 2025. Modern Healthcare. December 18, 2024. Accessed January 26, 2026. https://www.modernhealthcare.com/providers/cvs-health-walgreens-amazon-healthcare-services-2025

69. Hoff T. Why retail health clinics failed. Harv Bus Rev. October 10, 2024. Accessed January 26, 2026. https://hbr.org/2024/10/why-retail-health-clinics-failed

70. Hudson C. What to expect from big retailers providing healthcare in 2025. Modern Healthcare. December 18, 2024. Accessed January 26, 2026. https://www.modernhealthcare.com/providers/cvs-health-walgreens-amazon-healthcare-services-2025

71. Amazon and One Medical sign an agreement for Amazon to acquire One Medical. Amazon. July 21, 2022. Accessed January 26, 2026. https://press.aboutamazon.com/2022/7/amazon-and-one-medical-sign-an-agreement-for-amazon-to-acquire-one-medical

72. Healthcare just got less painful. Amazon One Medical. Accessed January 26, 2026. https://www.onemedical.com

73. Hagen J. Amazon's One Medical announces three new partnerships. Mobihealthnews. November 15, 2023. Accessed January 26, 2026. https://www.mobihealthnews.com/news/amazons-one-medical-announces-three-new-partnerships

74. Newitt P. The 15 largest independent physician groups. Becker's Physician Leadership. August 16, 2023. Accessed January 26, 2026. https://www.beckersphysicianleadership.com/leadership/the-15-largest-independent-physician-groups.html

75. Zhu JM, Shah D, Brown EF. Independent physician associations—a bulwark against corporate control? N Engl J Med. 2024;391(24):2283-2285. doi:10.1056/NEJMp2406792

76. Grover A, Orgera K, Pincus L, Senn S, Redford G. Why market power matters for patients, insurers and hospitals. AAMC Research and Action Institute. May 1, 2024. Accessed January 26, 2026. https://www.aamcresearchinstitute.org/our-work/data-snapshot/why-market-power-matters

77. Brown EF, Singh Y, Whaley CM, Perkins J. The rise of health care consolidation and what to do about it. Health Affairs Forefront. September 9, 2024. doi:10.1377/forefront.20240906.397095
78. Shrank WH, Rogstad TL, Parekh N. Waste in the US health care system: estimated costs and potential for savings. JAMA. 2019;322(15):1501-1509. doi:10.1001/jama.2019.13978
79. Abou-Atme Z, Alterman R, *et al.* Investing in the new era of value-based care. McKinsey & Company. December 16, 2022. Accessed January 26, 2026. https://www.mckinsey.com/industries/healthcare/our-insights/investing-in-the-new-era-of-value-based-care
80. Blumenthal D, Gumas ED, Shah A, Gunja MZ, Williams RD II. Mirror, mirror 2024: a portrait of the failing U.S. health system. Commonwealth Fund. September 19, 2024. Accessed January 26, 2026. https://www.commonwealthfund.org/publications/fund-reports/2024/sep/mirror-mirror-2024
81. Blumenthal D, Gumas E, Shah A. The failing U.S. health system. N Engl J Med. 2024;391(17):1566-1568. doi:10.1056/NEJMp2410855
82. McWilliams JM, Dusetzina SB. Affordability of health care in the United States—old problems awaiting a new administration. N Engl J Med. 2024;391(15):1372-1374. doi:10.1056/NEJMp2410638
83. Berwick DM, Batchlor E, Chokshi DA, *et al.* From laggard to leader: why health care in the United States is failing, and how to fix it. Health Aff. 2025;44(2):179-188. doi:10.1377/hlthaff.2024.01007
84. Johnson DW, Kusserow P. The revolutionary cure for U.S. healthcare. 4Sight-Health. March 25, 2025. Accessed January 26, 2026. https://mcusercontent.com/8a4bf5d1617f86a90e5a909f0/files/1bd6e6ef-fadb-bba5-6383-0086b3eecef6/4sightHealth.Johnson_Kusserow_Revolutionary_Cure_for_US_Healthcare.3_25_25.pdf

Chapter 2

1. Condon A. Physicians are doing more—but being paid less. Becker's Physician Leadership. Feb. 10, 2026. https://www.beckersphysicianleadership.com/compensation/the-physician-work-pay-gap-widens/?origin=PhysicianE&utm_source=PhysicianE&utm_medium=email&utm_content=newsletter&oly_enc_id=1405B9453478D7V
2. Habig C. Health care's hidden problem: hospital primary care losses. KevinMD. December 5, 2023. Accessed January 26, 2026. https://www.kevinmd.com/2023/12/health-cares-hidden-problem-hospital-primary-care-losses.html
3. Stanger K. Paying hospital-employed physicians for services performed by others. Holland & Hart Health Law Blog. July 9, 2018. Accessed January 26, 2026. https://hhhealthlawblog.com/paying-hospital-employed-physicians-for-services-performed-by-others/

4. Ianni KM, Sinaiko AD, Curto VE, *et al.* Quality-of-care outcomes in vertical relationships between physicians and health systems. JAMA Health Forum. 2024;5(8):e242173. doi:10.1001/jamahealthforum.2024.2173
5. Devereaux M. Physicians leaving private practice hurt patient care: survey. Modern Healthcare. December 5, 2023. Accessed January 26, 2026. https://www.modernhealthcare.com/providers/physicians-private-practice-physicians-advocacy-institute
6. Robertson R. Is healthcare consolidation fueling the physician burnout crisis? Medpage Today. September 19, 2024. Accessed January 26, 2026. https://www.medpagetoday.com/special-reports/features/112042
7. Newitt P. A private practice revival? Becker's ASC Review. March 11, 2025. Accessed January 26, 2026. https://www.beckersasc.com/leadership/a-private-practice-revival/
8. Glasser D. Primary Care Internal Medicine Is Dead. Medscape. July 17, 2024. https://www.medscape.com/s/viewarticle/primary-care-internal-medicine-dead-2024a1000ctb?ecd=wnl_infocu1_broad_broad_persoexpansion-algo_20240828_etid6783611&uac=302753BJ&impID=6783611
9. Ejnes YD. Deprofessionalization: An Emerging Threat to The Physician Workforce. Health Affairs Forefront, Sept. 5, 2025. 10.1377/forefront.20250904.611684
10. Eydis S. 5 trends shaping private practice. Becker's Physician Leadership. Feb. 13, 2026. https://www.beckersphysicianleadership.com/independent-practice/5-trends-shaping-private-practice/#:~:text=A%20Bain%20%26%20Co.,transition%20to%20physician%2Downed%20settings.
11. Galewitz P. Hospitals cash in on a private equity-based trend: concierge physician care. Fierce Healthcare. April 1, 2024. Accessed January 26, 2026. https://www.fiercehealthcare.com/providers/hospitals-cash-private-equity-backed-trend-concierge-physician-care
12. Dentzer S. Susan Dentzer: it is time to move past denying the perfect storm facing U.S. healthcare. HFMA Magazine. September 27, 2024. Accessed January 26, 2026. https://www.hfma.org/payment-reimbursement-and-managed-care/value-based-payment/susan-dentzer-it-is-time-to-move-past-denying-the-perfect-storm-facing-u-s-healthcare/
13. Clark C. Primary care doctors at Mass General Brigham want to unionize. Medpage Today. November 18, 2024. Accessed January 26, 2026. https://www.medpagetoday.com/special-reports/features/112982
14. Rooke-Ley H, Richman B, Bowling DS, *et al.* Unionization efforts by physicians between 2000 and 2024. JAMA. 2025;333(4):347-348. doi:10.1001/jama.2024.23721
15. Singh Y, Cardenas GB, Torabzadeh H, Borkar D, Whaley CM. Physician turnover increased in private equity-acquired physician practices. Health Aff. 2025;44(3):353-361. doi:10.1377/hlthaff.2024.00974

16. Ubel PA. Private equity acquisition of physician practices—looking for ethical guidance from professional societies. JAMA Health Forum. 2024;5(9):e242767. doi:10.1001/jamahealthforum.2024.2767
17. Singh Y, Radhakrishnan N, Adler L, *et al.* Growth of private equity and hospital consolidation in primary care and price implications. JAMA Health Forum. 2025;6(1):e244935. doi:10.1001/jamahealthforum.2024.4935
18. Singh Y, Song Z, Polsky D, Zhu JM. Increases in physician professional fees in private equity-owned gastroenterology practices. Health Aff. 2025;44(2):189-197. doi:10.1377/hlthaff.2024.00190
19. Kannan S, Bruch JD, Song Z. Changes in hospital adverse events and patient outcomes associated with private equity acquisition. JAMA. 2023;330(24):2365-2375. doi:10.1001/jama.2023.23147
20. AMN Healthcare survey: physician appointment wait times up 8% from 2017, up 24% from 2004. AMN Healthcare. September 12, 2022. Accessed January 26, 2026. https://ir.amnhealthcare.com/news-releases/news-release-details/amn-healthcare-survey-physician-appointment-wait-times-8-2017-24
21. Health at a Glance 2019. Organisation for Economic Co-operation and Development (OECD). 2019:173. Accessed January 26, 2026. https://www.oecd.org/content/dam/oecd/en/publications/reports/2019/11/health-at-a-glance-2019_f58fa178/4dd50c09-en.pdf
22. New AAMC report shows continuing projected physician shortage. American Association of Medical Colleges. March 21, 2024. Accessed January 26, 2026. https://www.aamc.org/news/press-releases/new-aamc-report-shows-continuing-projected-physician-shortage
23. Devereaux M. Why physician, nursing staffing shortages persist. Modern Healthcare. March 7, 2024. Accessed January 26, 2026. https://www.modernhealthcare.com/labor/healthcare-workforce-shortages-2024-physician-nurse-staffing-hrsa
24. New Medicare-supported GME residency positions expand health care access, physician workforce. American Association of Medical Colleges. November 21, 2024. Accessed January 26, 2026. https://www.aamc.org/news/press-releases/new-medicare-supported-gme-residency-positions-expand-health-care-access-physician-workforce
25. Reichlin-Melnick A. President Trump expands his travel ban: what you need to know. American Immigration Council. December 19, 2025. Accessed January 26, 2026. https://www.americanimmigrationcouncil.org/blog/president-trump-expands-his-travel-ban-what-you-need-to-know/
26. Price T. America is running out of doctors. Congress must step up. STAT. June 4, 2025. Accessed January 26, 2026. https://www.statnews.com/2025/06/04/us-medical-school-international-students-j-1-physician-visa-residency-shortage/
27. Whitford E. Trump's visa ban is barring new foreign doctors from entering U.S. Forbes. June 13, 2025. Accessed January 26, 2026. https://www.forbes.com/sites

/emmawhitford/2025/06/13/trumps-visa-ban-is-barring-new-foreign-doctors-from-entering-us/

28. Taylor M. More states eye removing requirements for foreign-trained physicians. Becker's Hospital Review. March 3, 2025. Accessed January 26, 2026. https://www.beckershospitalreview.com/hospital-physician-relationships/more-states-eye-removing-requirements-for-foreign-trained-physicians/
29. Jabbarpour Y, Jetty A, Byun H, *et al.* The health of US primary care: 2025 scorecard report—the cost of neglect. Milbank Memorial Fund/American Academy of Family Physicians. February 18, 2025. Accessed January 26, 2026. https://www.milbank.org/publications/the-health-of-us-primary-care-2025-scorecard-report-the-cost-of-neglect/
30. McCauley L, Phillips RL Jr, Meisnere M, Robinson SK, eds. Implementing High-Quality Primary Care: Rebuilding the Foundation of Health Care. Washington, DC: National Academies Press; 2021. Accessed January 26, 2026. https://nap.nationalacademies.org/catalog/25983/implementing-high-quality-primary-care-rebuilding-the-foundation-of-health
31. Hoffer EP. Primary care in the United States: past, present and future. Am J Med. 2024;137(8):702-705. doi:10.1016/j.amjmed.2024.03.009
32. Afable R, Connelly MD. The decimation of primary care. 4sight Health. Accessed January 26, 2026. https://mcusercontent.com/8a4bf5d1617f86a90e5a909f0/files/95705d82-d9f1-822d-c165-ae774599af46/4sightHealth.Connelly.Afable_Patient_Care_Part_2_1.23.24.pdf
33. Andrews M. Compensation is key to fixing primary care shortage. KFF Health News. November 16, 2023. Accessed January 26, 2026. https://kffhealthnews.org/news/article/compensation-pay-primary-care-shortage-solution/
34. Landon BE, Fazio SB, Cluett JL, *et al.* Death by a thousand cuts—the crushing weight of nonclinical demands in primary care. N Engl J Med. 2025;392(18):1771-1773. doi:10.1056/NEJMp2415431
35. Afable R, Connelly MD. The decimation of primary care. 4sight Health. Accessed January 26, 2026. https://mcusercontent.com/8a4bf5d1617f86a90e5a909f0/files/95705d82-d9f1-822d-c165-ae774599af46/4sightHealth.Connelly.Afable_Patient_Care_Part_2_1.23.24.pdf
36. Rosenthal E. The shrinking number of primary care physicians is reaching a tipping point. KFF Health News. September 8, 2023. Accessed January 26, 2026. https://kffhealthnews.org/news/article/lack-of-primary-care-tipping-point/
37. Koller CF, Betancourt JR, Miller ME. Out of balance: fixing our health system's neglect of primary care. Health Affairs Forefront. September 5, 2024. doi:10.1377/forefront.20240904.902880
38. Kasaure HS, Neely NB, Howard LE. Primary care use and 90-day mortality among older adults undergoing cancer surgery. JAMA Surg. 2024;159(10):1170-1176. doi:10.1001/jamasurg.2024.2598

39. Cooney E. 11 experts on why gains in cardiovascular disease are stalling and what we can do about it. STAT. October 15, 2024. Accessed January 26, 2026. https://www.statnews.com/2024/10/15/cardiovascular-disease-rising-experts-on-causes/

40. Cooney E. 11 experts on why gains in cardiovascular disease are stalling and what we can do about it. STAT. October 15, 2024. Accessed January 26, 2026. https://www.statnews.com/2024/10/15/cardiovascular-disease-rising-experts-on-causes/

41. Rosenbaum L. Is a long-simmering crisis boiling over? U.S. primary care today. N Engl J Med. 2025;393(17):1537-1541. doi:10.1056/NEJMms2510425

42. Garvey G. In 6 specialties, desire to step away or scale back is common. AMA News. July 23, 2024. Accessed January 26, 2026. https://www.ama-assn.org/practice-management/physician-health/6-specialties-desire-step-away-or-scale-back-common

43. Swan G, Condon MJ, Altman W, *et al*. Does higher spending on primary care lead to lower total health care spending? Health Affairs Forefront. October 8, 2024. doi:10.1377/forefront.20241007.439293

44. Berenson RA, Schartzer A, Pham HH. Beyond demonstrations: implementing a primary care hybrid payment model in Medicare. Health Aff Sch. 2023;1(2):1-6. doi:10.1093/haschl/qxad024

45. Berenson RA, Schartzer A, Pham HH. Beyond demonstrations: implementing a primary care hybrid payment model in Medicare. Health Aff Sch. 2023;1(2):1-6. doi:10.1093/haschl/qxad024

46. McCauley L, Phillips RL Jr, Meisnere M, Robinson SK, eds. Implementing High-Quality Primary Care: Rebuilding the Foundation of Health Care. Washington, DC: National Academies Press; 2021. Accessed January 26, 2026. https://nap.nationalacademies.org/catalog/25983/implementing-high-quality-primary-care-rebuilding-the-foundation-of-health

47. Phillips RS, Altman W, Friedman C, Song Z. A value-based primary care model that doubles primary care investment. Health Affairs Forefront. December 16, 2024. doi:10.1377/forefront.20241212.213721

48. Rosenthal E. The shrinking number of primary care physicians is reaching a tipping point. KFF Health News. September 8, 2023. Accessed January 26, 2026. https://kffhealthnews.org/news/article/lack-of-primary-care-tipping-point/

49. Shah S, Gondi S, Navathe AS. Paying more for primary care—a new approach by Medicare. JAMA. Published online December 12, 2024. doi:10.1001/jama.2024.23933

50. Phillips RS, Altman W, Friedman C, Song Z. A value-based primary care model that doubles primary care investment. Health Affairs Forefront. December 16, 2024. doi:10.1377/forefront.20241212.213721

51. CMS, "ACO PC Flex (ACO Primary Care Flex) Model. https://www.cms.gov/priorities/innovation/innovation-models/aco-primary-care-flex-model
52. Phillips RS, Altman W, Friedman C, Song Z. A value-based primary care model that doubles primary care investment. Health Affairs Forefront. December 16, 2024. doi:10.1377/forefront.20241212.213721
53. Betancourt J, Schneider E. The future of primary care, brought to you by AI. Modern Healthcare. August 11, 2025. Accessed January 26, 2026. https://www.modernhealthcare.com/opinion/mh-primary-care-future-ai-regulation/
54. The Starfield Signal: a shared vision and roadmap for AI in primary care. American Academy of Family Physicians and Rock Health. 2025. Accessed January 26, 2026. https://www.aafp.org/dam/AAFP/documents/practice_management/ai-road-map.pdf

Chapter 3

1. Berwick DM, Nolan TW, Whittington J. The triple aim: care, health and cost. Health Aff. 2008;27(3):759-769. doi:10.1377/hlthaff.27.3.759
2. Smith B. CMS innovation center at 10 years—progress and lessons learned. N Engl J Med. 2021;384(8):759-764. doi:10.1056/NEJMsb2031138
3. Medicare Shared Savings Program accountable care organizations—updated performance year 2024 financial and quality results. Centers for Medicare & Medicaid Services. September 29, 2025. Accessed January 26, 2026. https://www.cms.gov/files/document/fact-sheet-ssp-py24-financial-quality-results.pdf
4. Keehan SP, Madison AJ, Poisal JA, *et al.* National health expenditure projections, 2024-33: despite insurance coverage declines, health to grow as share of GDP. Health Aff. 2025;44(7):776-787. doi:10.1377/hlthaff.2025.00545
5. Terry K, Muhlestein D. Medicare Advantage for all? Not so fast. Health Affairs Forefront. March 11, 2021. doi:10.1377/forefront.20210309.302220
6. Keehan SP, Madison AJ, Poisal JA, *et al.* National health expenditure projections, 2024-33: despite insurance coverage declines, health to grow as share of GDP. Health Aff. 2025;44(7):776-787. doi:10.1377/hlthaff.2025.00545
7. Value-based care report. Humana. 2021. Accessed January 26, 2026. https://humana.gcs-web.com/static-files/39bb066e-bca5-45ff-aab2-827fe03c92c1
8. Markowski J, Wallace J, Schlesinger M. Alternative payment models and performance in federally qualified health centers. JAMA Intern Med. 2024;184(9):1065-1073. doi:10.1001/jamainternmed.2024.2754
9. McDonald T, Debbarma A, Whaley C, Reid R, Dowd B. Barriers primary care clinic leaders face to improving value in a consumer choice health plan design. Health Aff Sch. 2023;1(4):1-6. doi:10.1093/haschl/qxad065
10. Fowler E, Rawal P, Calloway R. The spillover effect of the CMS innovation center. NEJM Catalyst. January 21, 2025. doi:10.1056/CAT.24.0427

11. Emanuel EJ. Why haven't health care cost increases exceeded inflation? There's a very good reason. STAT. December 21, 2023. Accessed January 26, 2026. https://www.statnews.com/2023/12/21/health-care-costs-inflation-affordable-care-act/
12. Shrank WH, Rogstad TL, Parekh N. Waste in the US health care system: estimated costs and potential savings. JAMA. 2019;322(15):1501-1509. doi:10.1001/jama.2019.13978
13. Berwick DM, Hackbarth AD. Eliminating waste in healthcare. JAMA. 2012;307(14):1513-1516. doi:10.1001/jama.2012.362
14. Keehan SP, Madison AJ, Poisal JA, *et al.* National health expenditure projections, 2024-33: despite insurance coverage declines, health to grow as share of GDP. Health Aff. 2025;44(7):776-787. doi:10.1377/hlthaff.2025.00545
15. Terry K. Rx for Health Care Reform. Nashville, TN: Vanderbilt University Press; 2007:177.
16. Davis K, Guterman S, Bandeali F. The Affordable Care Act and Medicare. Commonwealth Fund Issues Brief. June 9, 2015. Accessed January 26, 2026. https://www.commonwealthfund.org/publications/fund-reports/2015/jun/affordable-care-act-and-medicare
17. Castellucci M. Drop in hospital-acquired conditions saves $7.7 billion. Modern Healthcare. January 29, 2019. Accessed January 26, 2026. https://www.modernhealthcare.com/article/20190129/NEWS/190129927
18. CMS hospital value-based purchasing program results for fiscal year 2019. Centers for Medicare & Medicaid Services. December 3, 2018. Accessed January 26, 2026. https://www.cms.gov/newsroom/fact-sheets/cms-hospital-value-based-purchasing-program-results-fiscal-year-2019
19. Robbins KJ, Zheng J, Waken RJ, *et al.* Medical and surgical episodes among hospital participants in the bundled payments for care improvement-advanced program. JAMA Netw Open. 2024;7(12):e2451792. doi:10.1001/jamanetworkopen.2024.51792
20. Liao JM, Emanuel EJ, Polsky DE, *et al.* National representativeness of hospitals and markets in Medicare's mandatory bundled payment program. Health Aff. 2019;38(1):44-53. doi:10.1377/hlthaff.2018.05177
21. Verma S. 2018 quality payment program (QPP) performance results. Centers for Medicare & Medicaid Services Blog. January 6, 2020. Accessed January 26, 2026. https://www.cms.gov/blog/2018-quality-payment-program-qpp-performance-results
22. Crosson FJ, Bloniarz K, Glass D, Mathews J. MedPAC's urgent recommendation: eliminate MIPS, take a different direction. Health Affairs Forefront. March 16, 2018. doi:10.1377/forefront.20180309.302220
23. Calendar year (CY) 2024 Medicare physician fee schedule (PFS) final rule fact sheet and policy comparison table. Centers for Medicare & Medicaid Services.

Accessed January 26, 2026. https://www.cms.gov/files/document/2024qpppoliciesfinalrulefactsheet.pdf

24. CMS moves closer to accountable care goals with 2025 ACO initiatives. Centers for Medicare & Medicaid Services. January 15, 2025. Accessed January 26, 2026. https://www.cms.gov/files/document/2024qpppoliciesfinalrulefactsheet.pdf
25. Everhart AO, Lyu PF, Maddox KEJ, Hockenberry JM, and Johnston KJ. Changes in Clinicians' Participation Across Medicare Value-Based Payment Models, 2017-2022. Health Affairs Vol. 44 No. 8. August 2025. https://doi.org/10.1377/hlthaff.2024.01551
26. Bond AM, Civelek Y, Schpero WL, *et al.* Long-term spending of accountable care organizations in the Medicare Shared Savings Program. JAMA. April 28, 2025. doi:10.1001/jama.2025.3870
27. Medicare Shared Savings Program accountable care organizations—updated performance year 2024 financial and quality results. Centers for Medicare & Medicaid Services. September 29, 2025. Accessed January 26, 2026. https://www.cms.gov/files/document/fact-sheet-ssp-py24-financial-quality-results.pdf
28. Medicare Shared Savings Program accountable care organizations—updated performance year 2024 financial and quality results. Centers for Medicare & Medicaid Services. September 29, 2025. Accessed January 26, 2026. https://www.cms.gov/files/document/fact-sheet-ssp-py24-financial-quality-results.pdf
29. Shared Savings Program fast facts—as of January 1, 2025. Centers for Medicare & Medicaid Services. Accessed January 26, 2026. https://www.cms.gov/files/document/2025-shared-savings-program-fast-facts.pdf
30. Morken I, Brown K, Bonesteel R, *et al.* Medicare accountable care organizations in 2023: large savings with increasing value-based programmatic competition. Health Affairs Forefront. January 15, 2025. doi:10.1377/forefront.20250113.365291
31. Shared Savings Program fast facts—as of January 1, 2025. Centers for Medicare & Medicaid Services. Accessed January 26, 2026. https://www.cms.gov/files/document/2025-shared-savings-program-fast-facts.pdf
32. Terry K. Evaluating value-based care part 1: an in-depth analysis of federal initiatives, outcomes, and promise for the future. Institute for Advancing Health Value. February 2022. Accessed January 26, 2026.
33. Calendar year (CY) 2023 Medicare physician fee schedule final rule—Medicare Shared Savings Program. Centers for Medicare & Medicaid Services. Accessed January 26, 2026. https://www.cms.gov/files/document/mssp-fact-sheet-cy-2023-pfs-final-rule.pdf
34. Morken I, Brown K, Zulueta M, Muhlestein D. Medicare accountable care organizations in 2023: large savings with increasing value-based programmatic competition. Health Affairs Forefront. January 15, 2025. doi:10.1377/forefront.20250113.859128

35. Terry K. Evaluating value-based care part 1: an in-depth analysis of federal initiatives, outcomes, and promise for the future. Institute for Advancing Health Value. February 2022. Accessed January 26, 2026.
36. Ouayogode MH, Colla CH. Reflecting on 2 decades of Medicare ACO experience. JAMA. April 28, 2025. doi:10.1001/jama.2025.6175
37. APM measurement: progress of alternative payment models. Health Care Payment Learning & Action Network. 2024. Accessed January 26, 2026. https://hcp-lan.org/wp-content/uploads/2024/11/2024-HCPLAN-Methodology-Report-11-13.pdf
38. Robeznieks A. Nearly 60% of doctors work for a practice that's part of an ACO. American Medical Association. Accessed January 26, 2026. https://www.ama-assn.org/practice-management/payment-delivery-models/nearly-60-doctors-work-practice-s-part-aco
39. Accelerating and aligning primary care payment models. Health Care Payment Learning & Action Network. 2017. Accessed January 26, 2026. https://hcp-lan.org/workproducts/pcpm-whitepaper-final.pdf
40. Priorities in advancing high quality value-based health & health care. National Academy of Medicine. May 2021. Accessed January 26, 2026. https://nam.edu/wp-content/uploads/2021/05/CMMI_Expert-Panel-Overview_2021_5.19-F.pdf
41. Terry K. Physician-Led Healthcare Reform. Washington, DC: American Association for Physician Leadership; 2020:103-104.
42. Terrell GE and Bobbitt JD, Jr., Value-Based Healthcare and Payment Models: Including Frontline Strategies For 20 Clinical Subspecialties. Washington, D.C.: American Association for Physician Leadership; 2019:50.
43. Terry K. Evaluating value-based care part 3: an in-depth examination of healthcare providers' efforts and results in value. Institute for Advancing Health Value. 2023:5. Accessed January 26, 2026. https://www.advancinghealthvalue.org/evaluating-value-based-care-part-3-an-in-depth-examination-of-healthcare-providers-efforts-and-results-in-value/
44. Huber K, Gonzalez-Smith J, Wang A. Engaging specialists in accountable care: tailoring payment models based on specialties and practice contexts. Health Affairs Forefront. December 21, 2023. doi:10.1377/forefront.20231219.115250
45. Fowler E, Fogler S, Schreiber C, *et al.* The CMS innovation center's strategy to support person-centered, value-based specialty care: 2024 update. Health Affairs Forefront. April 2, 2024. doi:10.1377/forefront.20240328.868596
46. APM measurement: progress of alternative payment models. Health Care Payment Learning & Action Network. 2024. Accessed January 26, 2026. https://hcp-lan.org/wp-content/uploads/2024/11/2024-HCPLAN-Methodology-Report-11-13.pdf
47. Terry K. Evaluating value-based care part 1: an in-depth analysis of federal initiatives, outcomes, and promise for the future. Institute for Advancing Health Value.

February 2022. Accessed January 26, 2026. https://www.advancinghealthvalue.org/evaluating-value-based-care-part-1-an-in-depth-analysis-of-federal-initiatives-outcomes-and-promise-for-the-future/

48. Humana's 11th value-based care report. Humana. Accessed January 26, 2026. https://assets.humana.com/is/content/humana/2088482_CM-2024-VBC_Report_11x8.5pdf-1
49. Herman B, Ross C, Lawrence L, Bannow T. Health care's colossus: UnitedHealth pays its own physician groups considerably more than others, driving up consumer costs and its profits. STAT. November 25, 2024. Accessed January 26, 2026. https://www.statnews.com/2024/11/25/unitedhealth-higher-payments-optum-providers-converts-expenses-to-profits/
50. Humana's 11th value-based care report. Humana. Accessed January 26, 2026. https://assets.humana.com/is/content/humana/2088482_CM-2024-VBC_Report_11x8.5pdf-1
51. Cohen K, Vabson B, Podulka J, *et al.* Health outcomes under full-risk Medicare Advantage vs. traditional Medicare. Am J Manag Care. 2025;31(10):2. Accessed January 26, 2026. https://file-us.clickdimensions.com/capgorg-aedlw/files/apgdataprojectajmcstudyhealthoutcomesunderfull-riskmedicareadvantagevstraditionalmedicare5.9.25.pdf
52. Gilfillan R, Berwick DM. Medicare Advantage, direct contracting, and the Medicare "money machine," part I: the risk-score game. Health Affairs Forefront. September 29, 2021. doi:10.1377/forefront.20210927.623971
53. The Medicare Advantage program: status report. Medicare Payment Advisory Commission. March 2025:320. Accessed January 26, 2026. https://www.medpac.gov/wp-content/uploads/2025/03/Mar25_Ch11_MedPAC_Report_To_Congress_SEC.pdf
54. Terry K, Muhlestein D. Medicare Advantage for all? Not so fast. Health Affairs Forefront. March 11, 2021. doi:10.1377/forefront.20210309.302220
55. Performance year financial and quality results. Centers for Medicare & Medicaid Services. 2023. Accessed January 26, 2026. https://data.cms.gov/medicare-shared-savings-program/performance-year-financial-and-quality-results
56. Tepper N. These are the health insurers that quit Medicare Advantage. Modern Healthcare. October 6, 2025. Accessed January 26, 2026. https://www.modernhealthcare.com/insurance/mh-medicare-advantage-market-exits-2026/
57. Adams K. Why shared savings still isn't a viable business model for hospitals. MedCity News. November 16, 2025. Accessed January 26, 2026. https://medcitynews.com/2025/11/value-based-care-health-medicare-hospital/

Chapter 4

1. Blumberg Y. 70% of Americans now support Medicare-for-all—here's how single-payer could affect you. CNBC Money. August 28, 2018. Accessed January

26, 2026. https://www.cnbc.com/2018/08/28/most-americans-now-support-medicare-for-all-and-free-college-tuition.html

2. Brenan M. Majority in U.S. still say gov't should ensure healthcare. Gallup. January 23, 2023. Accessed January 26, 2026. https://news.gallup.com/poll/468401/majority-say-gov-ensure-healthcare.aspx
3. Medicare for All Act, S 1506, 119th Congress. Accessed January 26, 2026. https://www.congress.gov/bill/119th-congress/senate-bill/1506
4. Medicare for All Act, HR 3069, 119th Congress. Accessed January 26, 2026. https://www.congress.gov/bill/119th-congress/house-bill/3069
5. Jayapal, Sanders, Dingell, hundreds of health care workers introduce Medicare for All. Rep. Pramila Jayapal. April 29, 2025. Accessed January 26, 2026. https://jayapal.house.gov/2025/04/29/jayapal-sanders-dingell-hundreds-of-health-care-workers-introduce-medicare-for-all/
6. S. 1506: Medicare for All Act. Govtrack.US. Accessed January 26, 2026. https://www.govtrack.us/congress/bills/119/s1506
7. Terry K. Physician-Led Healthcare Reform: A New Approach to Medicare For All. Washington, DC: American Association for Physician Leadership; 2020:6.
8. Berwick DM, Hackbarth AD. Eliminating waste in healthcare. JAMA. 2012;307(14):1513-1516. doi:10.1001/jama.2012.362
9. Medicare for All Act, S 1506, full text. Accessed January 26, 2026. https://www.sanders.senate.gov/wp-content/uploads/TAM25280.pdf
10. Medicare for All Act, S 1506, full text. Accessed January 26, 2026. https://www.sanders.senate.gov/wp-content/uploads/TAM25280.pdf
11. Medicare for All Act, S 1506, full text. Accessed January 26, 2026. https://www.sanders.senate.gov/wp-content/uploads/TAM25280.pdf
12. Terry K. Physician-Led Healthcare Reform: A New Approach to Medicare For All. Washington, DC: American Association for Physician Leadership; 2020:7-10.
13. DeLauro, Schakowsky introduce Medicare for America. Rep. Rosa DeLauro. December 19, 2018. Accessed January 26, 2026. https://delauro.house.gov/media-center/press-releases/delauro-schakowsky-introduce-medicare-america
14. Terry K. Physician-Led Healthcare Reform: A New Approach to Medicare For All. Washington, DC: American Association for Physician Leadership; 2020:6-7.
15. Freed M, Biniek JF, Damico A, Neuman T. Medicare Advantage in 2024: enrollment data and key trends. Kaiser Family Foundation. August 8, 2024. Accessed January 26, 2026. https://www.kff.org/medicare/issue-brief/medicare-advantage-in-2024-enrollment-update-and-key-trends/
16. Ducas A, Lipschutz D. Trump could saddle seniors with a costly Medicare Advantage plan—whether they like it or not. MarketWatch. May 7, 2025. Accessed January 26, 2026. https://www.marketwatch.com/story/trumps-push-to-privatize-medicare-would-be-a-disaster-for-taxpayers-especially-seniors-b9cb8a69

17. Freed M, Ochieng N, Cubanski J, Neuman T. Key facts about Medigap enrollment and premiums for Medicare beneficiaries. Kaiser Family Foundation. October 18, 2024. Accessed January 26, 2026. https://www.kff.org/medicare/issue-brief/key-facts-about-medigap-enrollment-and-premiums-for-medicare-beneficiaries/
18. Butler SM. Medicare Advantage for all, perhaps? JAMA Health Forum. 2020;1(7):e200967. doi:10.1001/jamahealthforum.2020.0967
19. The Medicare Advantage program: status report. Medicare Payment Advisory Commission. March 2025:320. Accessed January 26, 2026. https://www.medpac.gov/wp-content/uploads/2025/03/Mar25_Ch11_MedPAC_Report_To_Congress_SEC.pdf
20. Terry K and Muhlestein D. Medicare Advantage For All? Not So Fast. Health Affairs Forefront, March 11, 2021. doi: 10.1377/forefront.20210304.136304
21. Einav L, Finkelstein A. We've Got You Covered: Rebooting American Health Care. New York, NY: Penguin Random House; 2023.
22. Clemens M. Technology and rising health care costs. Forbes. October 26, 2017. Accessed January 26, 2026. https://www.forbes.com/sites/forbestechcouncil/2017/10/26/technology-and-rising-health-care-costs/
23. Baicker K, Chandra A, Shepard M. Achieving universal health insurance coverage in the United States: addressing market failures or providing a social floor? J Econ Perspect. 2023;37(2):99-122. doi:10.1257/jep.37.2.99
24. Johnson DW, Kusserow P. The Coming Healthcare Revolution: 10 Forces That Will Cure America's Health Crisis. Hoboken, NJ: Wiley; 2024.
25. Terry K. Has the time come for hospital at home? Next Avenue. October 23, 2020. Accessed January 26, 2026. https://www.nextavenue.org/hospital-at-home/
26. Zikr HE, Schriger DL, Kilaru AS. Hospital participation in the acute hospital care at home waiver program. JAMA. 2025;333(8):718-720. doi:10.1001/jama.2024.26368
27. Zikr HE, Schriger DL, Kilaru AS. Hospital participation in the acute hospital care at home waiver program. JAMA. 2025;333(8):718-720. doi:10.1001/jama.2024.26368
28. Calendar year (CY) 2026 home health prospective payment system final rule. Centers for Medicare & Medicaid Services. November 28, 2025. Accessed January 26, 2026. https://www.cms.gov/newsroom/fact-sheets/calendar-year-cy-2026-home-health-prospective-payment-system-final-rule-cms-1828-f
29. Zikr HE, Schriger DL, Kilaru AS. Hospital participation in the acute hospital care at home waiver program. JAMA. 2025;333(8):718-720. doi:10.1001/jama.2024.26368
30. Schneider EC, Shah A, Doty MM, Tikkanen R, Fields K, Williams RD II. Mirror, mirror 2021: reflecting poorly. Commonwealth Fund. August 4, 2021. Accessed

January 26, 2026. https://www.commonwealthfund.org/publications/fund-reports/2021/aug/mirror-mirror-2021-reflecting-poorly

31. Federal judge upholds hospital rate transparency rule. National Academy for State Health Policy. July 6, 2020. Accessed January 26, 2026. https://nashp.org/federal-judge-upholds-hospital-rate-transparency-rule/
32. Vogel S. Hospital price transparency compliance dips: report. Healthcare Dive. March 4, 2024. Accessed January 26, 2026. https://www.healthcaredive.com/news/hospital-price-transparency-requirements-patient-rights-advocate/709168/
33. Departments of Labor, Health and Human Services, Treasury announce move to strengthen healthcare price transparency. Centers for Medicare & Medicaid Services. May 22, 2025. Accessed January 26, 2026. https://www.cms.gov/newsroom/press-releases/departments-labor-health-and-human-services-treasury-announce-move-strengthen-healthcare-price
34. Adams K. Hospitals are facing new price transparency requirements, but will they truly help patients shop for care? Medcity News. September 18, 2024. Accessed January 26, 2026. https://medcitynews.com/2024/12/healthcare-price-transparency-hospital-consumer/
35. Transcarent completes merger with Accolade. Transcarent. April 8, 2025. Accessed January 26, 2026. https://transcarent.com/press-releases/transcarent-completes-merger-with-accolade
36. Amazon One Medical overview. Accessed January 26, 2026. https://www.onemedical.com/business/
37. Anastasijevic D. Mayo Clinic launches advanced care at home model of care. Mayo Clinic. June 25, 2020. Accessed January 26, 2026. https://newsnetwork.mayoclinic.org/discussion/mayo-clinic-launches-advanced-care-at-home-model-of-care/
38. Home services. Intermountain Healthcare. Accessed January 26, 2026. https://intermountainhealthcare.org/services/home-services
39. Klasko SK. Feelin' Alright: How The Message In the Music Can Make Healthcare Healthier. Chicago, IL: Health Administration Press; 2023.
40. Robert Wachter, A Giant Leap: How AI Is Transforming Healthcare and What That Means For Our Future. (New York: Penguin Books, 2026).
41. Ibid. 261
42. Teddy Rosenbluth, "Health Advice from A.I. chatbots Is Frequently Wrong, Study Shows," New York Times, Feb. 12, 2026. https://www.nytimes.com/2026/02/09/well/chatgpt-health-advice.html?campaign_id=9&emc=edit_nn_20260211&instance_id=170910&nl=the-morning&regi_id=69318529&segment_id=215096&user_id=de63455830b2f67ef5f1e6e7b9de441d

Chapter 5

1. For more information on health system investments, see Allen A. Financialization in health care: history, current trends, and impacts on patients. Healthcare Value Hub. December 3, 2024. Accessed January 26, 2026. https://healthcarevaluehub.org/resource/2024/financialization-in-health-care-history-current-trends-and-impacts-on-patients/]
2. Chase D, Arensmeyer J. The Affordable Care Act's impact on small business. Kaiser Family Foundation. October 1, 2018. Accessed January 26, 2026. https://www.commonwealthfund.org/publications/issue-briefs/2018/oct/affordable-care-act-impact-small-business
3. Who pays for long-term care? LongTermCare.gov. Accessed January 26, 2026. https://acl.gov/ltc/costs-and-who-pays/who-pays-long-term-care
4. Dually eligible individuals—categories. Centers for Medicare & Medicaid Services. Accessed January 26, 2026. https://www.cms.gov/medicare-medicaid-coordination/medicare-and-medicaid-coordination/medicare-medicaid-coordination-office/downloads/medicaremedicaidenrolleecategories.pdf
5. State Medicaid programs. Centers for Medicare & Medicaid Services. Accessed January 26, 2026. https://acl.gov/ltc/medicare-medicaid-and-more/medicaid
6. Eastabrook D. How private investment is becoming a driving force behind PACE. Modern Healthcare. December 23, 2024. Accessed January 26, 2026. https://www.modernhealthcare.com/providers/seen-health-habitat-health-pace-programs-kaiser-permanente-2025/
7. Claxton G, Rae M, Winger A. Employer-sponsored health insurance 101. Kaiser Family Foundation. May 28, 2024. Accessed January 26, 2026. https://www.kff.org/health-policy-101-employer-sponsored-health-insurance/?entry=table-of-contents-introduction
8. Ortaliza J, Cox C. 2024 medical loss ratio rebates. Kaiser Family Foundation. June 5, 2024. Accessed January 26, 2026. https://www.kff.org/private-insurance/medical-loss-ratio-rebates/
9. Newitt P. Optum physicians are paid 17% more than peers: study. Becker's ASC Review. November 7, 2025. Accessed January 26, 2026. https://www.beckersasc.com/asc-transactions-and-valuation-issues/optum-physicians-are-paid-17-more-than-peers-study/
10. Guardado JR, Kane CK. Competition in health insurance: a comprehensive study of U.S. markets, 2025 update. American Medical Association. Accessed January 26, 2026. https://www.ama-assn.org/system/files/competition-health-insurance-us-markets.pdf
11. Most of this section has been reproduced, with the author's permission, from Steve Klasko's book, Feelin' Alright: How The Message in the Music Can Make Healthcare Healthier.

12. Jain A, Levy J, Polsky D, Anderson KE. Medicare Advantage and the Maryland all-payer model. Health Affairs Forefront. March 18, 2022. doi:10.1377/forefront.20220316.50044
13. Emanuel EJ, Johnson DW, Guido M, Goozner M. Meaningful value-based payment reform, part 1: Maryland leads the way. Health Affairs Forefront. February 9, 2022. doi:10.1377/forefront.20220205.211264
14. Murray R. Setting hospital rates to control costs and boost quality: the Maryland experience. Health Aff. 2009;28(5):1395-1405. doi:10.1377/hlthaff.28.5.1395
15. Kilaru AS, Crider CR, Chiang J. Health care leaders' perspectives on the Maryland all-payer model. JAMA Health Forum. 2022;3(2):e214920. doi:10.1001/jamahealthforum.2021.4920
16. Haber S, Beil H, Morrison M, *et al.* Evaluation of the Maryland all-payer model, volume 1: final report. November 2019. Accessed January 26, 2026. https://downloads.cms.gov/files/md-allpayer-finalevalrpt.pdf
17. Haber S, Bell H, Zheng X, *et al.* Evaluation of the Maryland all-payer model, volume 1: final report. November 2019. Accessed January 26, 2026. https://downloads.cms.gov/files/md-allpayer-finalevalrpt.pdf
18. Galarraga J, Pines JM. The challenging transformation of health care under Maryland's global budgets. Health Affairs Forefront. December 19, 2017. doi:10.1377/forefront.20171214.96251
19. Maryland Total Cost of Care Model. Centers for Medicare & Medicaid Services. Accessed January 26, 2026. https://innovation.cms.gov/innovation-models/md-tccm
20. Brennan TA. Maryland hospital all-payer model: can it be emulated? Health Affairs Forefront. May 31, 2022. doi:10.1377/forefront.20220526.939479
21. Emanuel EJ, Johnson DW, Guido M, Goozner M. Meaningful value-based payment reform, part 2: expanding the Maryland model to other states. Health Affairs Forefront. February 10, 2022. doi:10.1377/forefront.20220207.85767
22. Kacik A. States push hospital price caps to rein in spending. Modern Healthcare. June 12, 2025. Accessed January 26, 2026. https://www.modernhealthcare.com/politics-policy/hospital-price-caps-indiana-washington/
23. Brot-Goldberg Z, Cooper Z, Craig S, Klarnet L. Is there too little antitrust enforcement in the US hospital sector? Am Econ Rev Insights. 2024;6(4):595-611. doi:10.1257/aeri.20230481
24. Kocher R, Berwick DM. Policies for making health care in the United States better. Health Affairs Forefront. June 6, 2019. doi:10.1377/hblog20190530.216896
25. Chang D. How much will that surgery cost? Hospital prices remain largely unhelpful. Medpage Today. April 2, 2025. Accessed January 26, 2026. https://www.medpagetoday.com/hospitalbasedmedicine/generalhospitalpractice/114933

26. Findlay SD. Consumers' interest in provider ratings grows, and improved report cards and other steps could accelerate their use. Health Aff. 2016;35(4):688-696. doi:10.1377/hlthaff.2015.1654

Chapter 6

1. Koller CF, Betancourt JR, Miller ME. Out of balance: fixing our health system's neglect of primary care. Health Affairs Forefront. September 5, 2024. doi:10.1377/forefront.20240904.902880
2. Zu M, Saunders RS, Muhlestein D, Bleser WK, McClellan MB. The Medicare Shared Savings Program in 2020: positive movement (and uncertainty) during a pandemic. Health Affairs Forefront. October 14, 2021. doi:10.1377/forefront.20211008.785640
3. Greiner A, Muhlestein D, Kempski A, *et al.* Primary care: the MVP of MSSP. Primary Care Collaborative, Robert Graham Center, and Simple Healthcare. November 2024. Accessed January 26, 2026. https://www.graham-center.org/content/dam/rgc/documents/publications-reports/reports/primary-care-the-mvp-of-mssp-2024-evidence-report.pdf
4. Yetter EJ. Understanding corporate practice of medicine laws by state. Physicians First Healthcare Partners. August 25, 2017. Accessed January 26, 2026. https://www.physiciansfirst.com/blog/corporate-practice-of-medicine-laws-by-state/
5. Condon C. Physicians are doing more—but being paid less. Becker's Physician Leadership. Feb. 10, 2026. https://www.beckersphysicianleadership.com/compensation/the-physician-work-pay-gap-widens/?origin=PhysicianE&utm_source=PhysicianE&utm_medium=email&utm_content=newsletter&oly_enc_id=1405B9453478D7V
6. Insurer UnitedHealth to buy Everett Clinic operator for $4.9 billion as lines blur in health care. The Seattle Times. December 6, 2017. Accessed January 26, 2026. https://www.seattletimes.com/business/insurer-unitedhealth-to-buy-everett-clinic-operator-for-4-9-billion-as-lines-blur-in-health-care/
7. DePeau-Wilson M. Optum acquires Houston-based physician group for $2 billion. MedPage Today. September 2, 2022. Accessed January 26, 2026. https://www.medpagetoday.com/special-reports/exclusives/100531
8. Grumbach K, Cohen DJ, Jabbarpour Y. The failing experiment of primary care as a for-profit enterprise. Health Affairs Forefront. September 5, 2024. doi:10.1377/forefront.20240903.604079
9. Robeznieks A. Nearly 60% of doctors work in a practice that's part of an ACO. American Medical Association. October 30, 2023. Accessed January 26, 2026. https://www.ama-assn.org/practice-management/payment-delivery-models/nearly-60-doctors-work-practice-s-part-aco
10. Muhlestein D, Saunders RS, de Lisle K, *et al.* Growth of value-based care and accountable care organizations in 2022. Health Affairs Forefront. December 2, 2022. doi:10.1377/forefront.20221130.22253

11. Richards R, Leavitt Partners. Personal communication.
12. AMA examines decade of change in physician practice ownership and organization. American Medical Association. July 12, 2023. Accessed January 26, 2026. https://www.ama-assn.org/press-center/ama-press-releases/ama-examines-decade-change-physician-practice-ownership-and
13. Grace S, AMGA. Personal communication.
14. PAI-Avalere report on physician employment trends and acquisitions of medical practices: 2019-2023. Physicians Advocacy Institute. April 2024. Accessed January 26, 2026. https://www.physiciansadvocacyinstitute.org/PAI-Research/PAI-Avalere-Study-on-Physician-Employment-Practice-Ownership-Trends-2019-2023
15. Robeznieks A. Nearly 60% of doctors work in a practice that's part of an ACO. American Medical Association. October 30, 2023. Accessed January 26, 2026. https://www.ama-assn.org/practice-management/payment-delivery-models/nearly-60-doctors-work-practice-s-part-aco
16. Shared Savings Program participation options. Centers for Medicare & Medicaid Services. Accessed January 26, 2026. https://www.cms.gov/Medicare/Medicare-Fee-for-Service-Payment/sharedsavingsprogram/Downloads/ssp-aco-participation-options.pdf
17. Shared Savings Program fast facts—as of January 1, 2025. Centers for Medicare & Medicaid Services. Accessed January 26, 2026. https://www.cms.gov/files/document/2025-shared-savings-program-fast-facts.pdf
18. ACO REACH. Centers for Medicare & Medicaid Services. Accessed January 26, 2026. https://www.cms.gov/priorities/innovation/innovation-models/aco-reach
19. ACO REACH model: performance year 2023 financial and quality performance results' highlights. Centers for Medicare & Medicaid Services. November 8, 2024. Accessed January 26, 2026. https://www.cms.gov/priorities/innovation/aco-reach-py2023-financial-and-quality-performance-results-fact-sheet
20. Terry K. Rx for Health Care Reform. Nashville, TN: Vanderbilt University Press; 2007:172.
21. Farias V. No secret sauce: a proven, no-nonsense approach to MSSP. Group Practice Journal. April 2019. Accessed January 26, 2026. http://www.amga.org/wcm/SM/2019/04/68c0422.pdf
22. New York City's population estimates and trends. NYC Department of City Planning Population Division. May 2025. Accessed January 26, 2026. https://www.nyc.gov/assets/planning/downloads/pdf/our-work/reports/new-york-city-population-estimates-and-trends_may-2025.pdf
23. Quick facts. U.S. Census Bureau. Accessed January 26, 2026. https://www.census.gov/quickfacts/spokanecitywashington
24. New York physician supply and demand through 2030: executive summary. Center for Health Workforce Studies. March 2009. Accessed January 26, 2026. https://www.albany.edu/news/images/PhysicianShortagereport.pdf

25. Washington State's physician workforce in 2014. Center for Health Workforce Studies. Accessed January 26, 2026. http://depts.washington.edu/uwrhrc/uploads/CHWS_WA_Phys_Workforce_2014.pdf
26. Altschuler J, Margolius D, Bodenheimer T, Grumbach K. Estimating a reasonable patient panel size for primary care physicians with team-based task delegation. Ann Fam Med. 2012, 10;5:396-400. doi: 10.1370/afm.1400. http://www.annfammed.org/content/10/5/396.full).
27. Raffoul M, Moore M, Kamerow D, Bazemore A. A primary care panel size of 2500 is neither accurate nor reasonable. J Am Board Fam Med 2016;29:496–499. DOI: https://doi.org/10.3122/jabfm.2016.04.150317
28. Terry K. Rx for Health Care Reform. Nashville, TN: Vanderbilt University Press; 2007:185-191.
29. Brook RH, McGlynn EA, Shekelle PG, *et al.* Report cards for health care: is anyone checking them? RAND Research Brief. 2002. https://www.rand.org/pubs/research_briefs/RB4544.html
30. Sinaiko AD, Eastman D, Rosenthal MB. How report cards on physicians, physician groups, and hospitals can have greater impact on consumer choices. Health Aff. 2012;31(3):602-611. doi:10.1377/hlthaff.2011.1197
31. Findlay SD. Consumers' interest in provider ratings grows, and improved report cards and other steps could accelerate their use. Health Aff. 2016;35(4):688-696. doi:10.1377/hlthaff.2015.1654
32. Findlay SD. Consumers' interest in provider ratings grows, and improved report cards and other steps could accelerate their use. Health Aff. 2016;35(4):688-696. doi:10.1377/hlthaff.2015.1654
33. Health care quality report cards, 2018-19 edition. California Office of the Patient Advocate. Accessed January 26, 2026. https://www.opa.ca.gov/reportcards/Pages/default.aspx
34. Measure summary. Wisconsin Collaborative for Healthcare Quality. Accessed January 26, 2026. https://reports.wchq.org/measure-summary
35. MN Community Measurement. Accessed January 26, 2026. https://mncm.org
36. Terry K. Online reviews most important factor in choosing a doctor: survey. Medscape. December 7, 2021. Accessed January 26, 2026. https://www.medscape.com/viewarticle/964264
37. Sinaiko AD, Eastman D, Rosenthal MB. How report cards on physicians, physician groups, and hospitals can have greater impact on consumer choices. Health Aff. 2012;31(3):602-611. doi:10.1377/hlthaff.2011.1197
38. Findlay SD. Consumers' interest in provider ratings grows, and improved report cards and other steps could accelerate their use. Health Aff. 2016;35(4):688-696. doi:10.1377/hlthaff.2015.1654
39. Sinaiko AD, Eastman D, Rosenthal MB. How report cards on physicians, physician groups, and hospitals can have greater impact on consumer choices. Health Aff. 2012;31(3):602-611. doi:10.1377/hlthaff.2011.1197

Chapter 7

1. Lemaire N, Singer SJ. Do independent physician-led ACOs have a future? NEJM Catalyst. February 22, 2018. Accessed January 26, 2026. https://catalyst.nejm.org/do-independent-physician-led-acos-have-a-future/
2. Phillips RS, Altman W, Friedman C, Song Z. A value-based primary care model that doubles primary care investment. Health Affairs Forefront. December 16, 2024. doi:10.1377/forefront.20241212.213721
3. Patel MS, Arron MJ, Sinsky TA, *et al*. Estimating the staffing infrastructure for a patient-centered medical home. Am J Manag Care. 2013;19(6):509-516. Accessed January 26, 2026. https://www.ajmc.com/view/estimating-the-staffing-infrastructure-for-a-patient-centered-medical-home
4. Primary care payment models. Health Care Payment Learning & Action Network. 2017. Accessed January 26, 2026. https://hcp-lan.org/workproducts/pcpm-whitepaper-final.pdf
5. Lightbeam Health. Accessed January 26, 2026. https://www.lightbeamhealth.com
6. Privia Health. Accessed January 26, 2026. http://www.priviahealth.com
7. Aledade. Accessed January 26, 2026. https://aledade.com
8. Arcadia. Accessed January 26, 2026. https://www.arcadia.io
9. Innovaccer. Accessed January 26, 2026. https://innovaccer.com
10. Elligint Health. Accessed January 26, 2026. https://elliginthealth.com
11. Health Catalyst. Accessed January 26, 2026. https://www.healthcatalyst.com
12. Partners in Care. Accessed January 26, 2026. https://www.piccorp.com/about
13. Keckley P. Is Phycor 2.0 ahead? The Keckley Report. July 11, 2016. Accessed January 26, 2026. https://www.paulkeckley.com/the-keckley-report/2016/7/11/is-phycor-20-ahead
14. Rooke-Ley H, Reddy M, Mehta N, *et al*. The corporate backdoor to medicine: how MSOs are reshaping physician practices. Millbank Memorial Fund Issue Brief. April 28, 2025. Accessed January 26, 2026. https://www.milbank.org/publications/the-corporate-backdoor-to-medicine-how-msos-are-reshaping-physician-practices/
15. Terry K. Tame the private equity beast by shifting its focus to value-based care. Health Affairs Forefront. May 8, 2024. doi:10.1377/forefront.20240506.636591
16. One Medical completes acquisition of Iora Health. Amazon One Medical. September 1, 2021. Accessed January 26, 2026. https://www.onemedical.com/mediacenter/one-medical-completes-acquisition-iora-health/
17. CVS Health to acquire Oak Street Health. CVS Health. February 8, 2023. Accessed January 26, 2026. https://www.sec.gov/Archives/edgar/data/64803/000094787123000133/ss1747225_ex9901.htm
18. Cutler DM, Song Z. The new role of private investment in health care delivery. JAMA Health Forum. 2024;5(2):e240164. doi:10.1001/jamahealthforum.2024.0164

19. Stewart E, Baker J. Private equity: the metastasizing disease threatening health care. Health Affairs Forefront. December 18, 2023. doi:10.1377/forefront.20231213.928665
20. Health Over Wealth Act discussion draft section by section summary. U.S. Senate. Accessed January 26, 2026. https://www.markey.senate.gov/imo/media/doc/health_over_wealth_act_section_x_section.pdf
21. Medicare Shared Savings Program & Medicare ACO Track 1+ model repayment mechanism arrangements. Centers for Medicare & Medicaid Services. April 2019. Accessed January 26, 2026. https://www.cms.gov/Medicare/Medicare-Fee-for-Service-Payment/sharedsavingsprogram/Downloads/Repayment-Mechanism-Guidance.pdf
22. Shared Savings Program participation options. Centers for Medicare & Medicaid Services. Accessed January 26, 2026. https://www.cms.gov/Medicare/Medicare-Fee-for-Service-Payment/sharedsavingsprogram/Downloads/ssp-aco-participation-options.pdf
23. Martin AB, Hartman M, Washington B, Catlin A. National health expenditures in 2023: faster growth as insurance coverage and utilization increased. Health Aff. 2025;44(1):12-22. doi:10.1377/hlthaff.2024.01375
24. NHE fact sheet. Centers for Medicare & Medicaid Services. Accessed January 26, 2026. https://www.cms.gov/research-statistics-data-and-systems/statistics-trends-and-reports/nationalhealthexpenddata/nhe-fact-sheet.html
25. Martin AB, Hartman M, Washington B, Catlin A. National health expenditures in 2023: faster growth as insurance coverage and utilization increased. Health Aff. 2025;44(1):12-22. doi:10.1377/hlthaff.2024.01375
26. Medicare Shared Savings Program: shared savings and losses and assignment methodology. Centers for Medicare & Medicaid Services. February 2019. Accessed January 26, 2026. https://www.cms.gov/Medicare/Medicare-Fee-for-Service-Payment/sharedsavingsprogram/Downloads/Shared-Savings-Losses-Assignment-Spec-V7.pdf

Chapter 8

1. Kallmes DF, Comstock BA, Heagerty PJ, *et al.* A randomized trial of vertebroplasty for osteoporotic spinal fractures. N Engl J Med. 2009;361(6):569-579. doi:10.1056/NEJMoa0900563
2. Buchbinder R, Osborne RH, Ebeling PR, *et al.* A randomized trial of vertebroplasty for painful osteoporotic vertebral fractures. N Engl J Med. 2009;361(6):557-568. doi:10.1056/NEJMoa0900429
3. Firanescu CE, de Vries J, Lodder P, *et al.* Vertebroplasty versus sham procedure for painful acute osteoporotic vertebral compression fractures (VERTOS IV): randomised sham controlled clinical trial. BMJ. 2018;361:k1551. doi:10.1136/bmj.k1551

4. Buchbinder R, Johnston RV, Rischin KJ, *et al*. Vertebroplasty for treating spinal fractures due to osteoporosis. Cochrane Database Syst Rev. 2018;11(11):CD006349. doi:10.1002/14651858.CD006349.pub4
5. Berwick DM, Hackbarth AD. Eliminating waste in US health care. JAMA. 2012;307(14):1513-1516. doi:10.1001/jama.2012.362
6. Shrank WH, Rogstad TL, Parekh N. Waste in the US health care system: estimated costs and potential savings. JAMA. 2019;322(15):1501-1509. doi:10.1001/jama.2019.13978
7. Institute of Medicine. *Crossing the Quality Chasm: A New Health System for the 21st Century*. Washington, DC: National Academy Press; 2001:3.
8. Fisher ES, Wennberg DE, Stukel TA, *et al*. The implications of regional variations in Medicare spending. Part 1: the content, quality, and accessibility of care. Ann Intern Med. 2003;138(4):273-287. doi:10.7326/0003-4819-138-4-200302180-00006
9. Fisher ES, Wennberg DE, Stukel TA, *et al*. The implications of regional variations in Medicare spending. Part 2: health outcomes and satisfaction with care. Ann Intern Med. 2003;138(4):288-298. doi:10.7326/0003-4819-138-4-200302180-00007
10. Fisher ES, Wennberg DE, Stukel TA, *et al*. The implications of regional variations in Medicare spending. Part 1: the content, quality, and accessibility of care. Ann Intern Med. 2003;138(4):273-287. doi:10.7326/0003-4819-138-4-200302180-00006
11. Chassin MR, Kosecoff J, Park RE, *et al*. Does inappropriate use explain geographic variations in the use of health care services? A study of three procedures. JAMA. 1987;258(18):2533-2537. doi:10.1001/jama.1987.03400180067028
12. Gawande A. The cost conundrum: what a Texas town can teach us about health care. The New Yorker. June 1, 2009. Accessed January 26, 2026. https://www.newyorker.com/magazine/2009/06/01/the-cost-conundrum
13. Molitor D. The evolution of physician practice styles: evidence from cardiologist migration. Am Econ J Econ Policy. 2018;10(1):326-356. doi:10.1257/pol.20160319
14. Gawande A. Overkill. The New Yorker. May 11, 2015. Accessed January 26, 2026. https://www.newyorker.com/magazine/2015/05/11/overkill-atul-gawande
15. Farias V. No secret sauce: a proven, no-nonsense approach to MSSP. Group Practice Journal. April 2019. Accessed January 26, 2026. http://www.amga.org/wcm/SM/2019/04/680422.pdf
16. Chassin MR. Quality of care: time to act. JAMA. 1991;266(24):3472-3473. doi:10.1001/jama.1991.03470240094040
17. McGlynn EA, Asch SM, Adams J, *et al*. Thc quality of health care delivered to adults in the United States. N Engl J Med. 2003;348(26):2635-2645. doi:10.1056/NEJMsa022615
18. Kohn LT, Corrigan JM, Donaldson MS, eds. To Err Is Human: Building a Safer Health System. Washington, DC: National Academies Press; 2000:1.

19. Rutherford PA, Provost LP, Kotagal UR, Luther K, Anderson A. Achieving hospital-wide patient flow. Institute for Healthcare Improvement White Paper. Cambridge, MA: Institute for Healthcare Improvement; 2017.
20. Newman-Toker DE, Nassery N, Schaffer AC, *et al.* Burden of serious harms from diagnostic error in the USA. BMJ Qual Saf. 2024;33(2):109-120. doi:10.1136/bmjqs-2021-014130
21. Terry K. Putting physicians at financial risk might reduce misdiagnosis. 4sight Health. January 14, 2025. Accessed January 26, 2026. https://www.4sighthealth.com/putting-physicians-at-financial-risk-might-reduce-misdiagnosis/
22. Committee on Quality of Health Care in America, Institute of Medicine. Crossing the Quality Chasm: A New Health System for the 21st Century. Washington, DC: National Academy Press; 2001:3.
23. Rutherford PA, Provost LP, Kotagal UR, Luther K, Anderson A. Achieving hospital-wide patient flow. Institute for Healthcare Improvement White Paper. Cambridge, MA: Institute for Healthcare Improvement; 2017.
24. Louden K. Creating a better discharge summary. ACP Hospitalist. March 2009. Accessed January 26, 2026. https://acphospitalist.org/archives/2009/03/discharge.htm
25. O'Malley AS, Reschovsky JD. Referral and consultation communication between primary care and specialist physicians: finding common ground. Arch Intern Med. 2011;171(1):56-65. doi:10.1001/archinternmed.2010.480
26. Berwick DM, Hackbarth AD. Eliminating waste in US health care. JAMA. 2012;307(14):1513-1516. doi:10.1001/jama.2012.362
27. Penm J, MacKinnon NJ, Strakowski SM, Ying J, Doty MM. Minding the gap: factors associated with primary care coordination of adults in 11 countries. Ann Fam Med. 2017;15(2):113-119. doi:10.1370/afm.2028
28. Shekelle P. Overview of clinical practice guidelines. UpToDate. Accessed January 26, 2026. https://www.uptodate.com/contents/overview-of-clinical-practice-guidelines
29. Steinberg EP, Luce BR. Evidence-based? Caveat emptor. Health Aff. 2005;24(1):80-92. doi:10.1377/hlthaff.24.1.80
30. Steinberg EP, Luce BR. Evidence-based? Caveat emptor. Health Aff. 2005;24(1):80-92. doi:10.1377/hlthaff.24.1.80
31. Weldring T, Smith SMS. Patient-reported outcomes (PROs) and patient-reported outcome measures (PROMs). Health Serv Insights. 2013;6:61-68. doi:10.4137/HSI.S11093
32. Wagle NW. Implementing patient-reported outcome measures. NEJM Catalyst. October 12, 2017. Accessed January 26, 2026. https://catalyst.nejm.org/implementing-proms-patient-reported-outcome-measures/
33. Wagle NW. Implementing patient-reported outcome measures. NEJM Catalyst. October 12, 2017. Accessed January 26, 2026. https://catalyst.nejm.org

/implementing-proms-patient-reported-outcome-measures/

34. Guggenheim R. Putting EBM to work (easier said than done). Manag Care. 2005;14(12):33-4, 41-3. PMID: 16405246.
35. Terry K. Rx for Health Care Reform. Nashville, TN: Vanderbilt University Press; 2007:103.
36. NQF's work in quality measurement. National Quality Forum. Accessed January 26, 2026. http://www.qualityforum.org/about_nqf/work_in_quality_measurement
37. Rosenthal MB, Frank RG, Li Z, *et al.* Early experience with pay-for-performance. JAMA. 2005;294(14):1788-1793. doi:10.1001/jama.294.14.1788
38. Pearson SD, Schneider EC, Kleinman KP, Coltin KL, Singer JA. The impact of pay-for-performance on health care quality in Massachusetts, 2001-2003. Health Aff. 2008;27(4):1167-1176. doi:10.1377/hlthaff.27.4.1167
39. Sorondo B, Allen A, Bayleran J, *et al.* Using a patient portal to transmit patient report health information into the electronic record: workflow implications and user experience. EGEMS (Wash DC). 2016;4(3):1237. doi:10.13063/2327-9214.1237
40. Regulatory nightmare threatens care for America's seniors. American Medical Association. October 14, 2014. Accessed January 26, 2026. www.ama-assn.org/ama/pub/news/2014/2014-10-21-regulatory-nightmare-threatens-seniors.page
41. Scirica B. Study shows remote patient monitoring improves blood pressure and cholesterol. Mass General Brigham News. April 4, 2023. Accessed January 26, 2026. https://www.massgeneralbrigham.org/en/about/newsroom/articles/remote-blood-pressure-monitoring
42. Smith T. Remote monitoring helps Type 2 diabetes patients manage a dangerous disease. UCHealth Today. March 5, 2022. Accessed January 26, 2026. https://www.uchealth.org/today/diabetes-remote-monitoring-program-helps-patients-manage-dangerous-disease/
43. Choosing Wisely: a report on the first five years. Choosing Wisely. Accessed January 26, 2026. http://www.choosingwisely.org/wp-content/uploads/2017/10/Choosing-Wisely-at-Five.pdf
44. Facts and figures. Choosing Wisely. Accessed January 26, 2026. http://www.choosingwisely.org/our-mission/facts-and-figures/
45. Patient resources. Choosing Wisely. Accessed January 26, 2026. http://www.choosingwisely.org/patient-resources/
46. Choosing Wisely: a report on the first five years. Choosing Wisely. Accessed January 26, 2026. http://www.choosingwisely.org/wp-content/uploads/2017/10/Choosing-Wisely-at-Five.pdf
47. Castellucci M. Low-value care persists five years into Choosing Wisely campaign. Modern Healthcare. October 24, 2017. Accessed January 26, 2026. https://www

.modernhealthcare.com/article/20171024/NEWS/171029944/low-value-care-persists-five-years-into-choosing-wisely-campaign

48. Kerr EA, Kullgren JT, Saini SD. Choosing Wisely: how to fulfill the promise in the next 5 years. Health Aff. 2017;36(11):2012-2018. doi:10.1377/hlthaff.2017.0953
49. Castellucci M. Spending on low-value services slowed from 2014 to 2016. Modern Healthcare. June 21, 2019. Accessed January 26, 2026. https://www.modernhealthcare.com/payment/spending-low-value-services-slowed-2014-2016
50. Choosing Wisely: a report on the first five years. Choosing Wisely. Accessed January 26, 2026. http://www.choosingwisely.org/wp-content/uploads/2017/10/Choosing-Wisely-at-Five.pdf
51. Kerr EA, Kullgren JT, Saini SD. Choosing Wisely: how to fulfill the promise in the next 5 years. Health Aff. 2017;36(11):2012-2018. doi:10.1377/hlthaff.2017.0953

Chapter 9

1. Farias V. No secret sauce: a proven, no-nonsense approach to MSSP. Group Practice Journal. April 2019. Accessed January 26, 2026. http://www.amga.org/wcm/SM/2019/04/680422.pdf
2. Hodach R, Grundy P, Jain A, Weiner M. Provider-Led Population Health Management: Key Strategies for Healthcare in the Cognitive Era. 2nd ed. Indianapolis, IN: John Wiley & Sons; 2016:14-15.
3. Bodenheimer T. Anatomy and physiology of primary care teams. JAMA Intern Med. 2019;179(1):61-62. doi:10.1001/jamainternmed.2018.5550
4. Altschuler J, Margolius D, Bodenheimer T, Grumbach K. Estimating a reasonable patient panel size for primary care physicians with team-based task delegation. Ann Fam Med. 2012;10(5):396-400. doi:10.1370/afm.1400
5. McGlynn EA, Asch SM, Adams J, *et al.* The quality of health care delivered to adults in the United States. N Engl J Med. 2003;348(26):2635-2645. doi:10.1056/NEJMsa022615
6. Terry K. Here comes more competition. Not-so-busy specialists are becoming generalists, too. Med Econ. 1996;73(13):200-210.
7. Betancourt J, Schneider E. The future of primary care, brought to you by AI. Modern Healthcare. August 11, 2025. Accessed January 26, 2026. https://www.modernhealthcare.com/opinion/mh-primary-care-future-ai-regulation/
8. The Starfield Signal: a shared vision and roadmap for AI in primary care. American Academy of Family Physicians and Rock Health. 2025. Accessed January 26, 2026. https://www.aafp.org/dam/AAFP/documents/practice_management/ai-road-map.pdf
9. The Starfield Signal: a shared vision and roadmap for AI in primary care. American Academy of Family Physicians and Rock Health. 2025. Accessed January

26, 2026. https://www.aafp.org/dam/AAFP/documents/practice_management/ai-road-map.pdf; Adams K. Which clinical documentation AI tools are health systems using? MedCity News. August 25, 2024. Accessed January 26, 2026. https://medcitynews.com/2024/08/clinical-documentation-healthcare-burnout/

10. DePeau M. ChatGPT writes good clinical notes, study finds. Medpage Today. July 17, 2023. Accessed January 26, 2026. https://www.medpagetoday.com/special-reports/exclusives/105510
11. Kulkarni PA, Singh H. Artificial intelligence in clinical diagnosis: opportunities, challenges and hype. JAMA. 2023;330(4):317-318. doi:10.1001/jama.2023.11440
12. Adams K. Popular AI chatbots are spreading false medical info, Mount Sinai researchers say. Medcity News. August 11, 2025. Accessed January 26, 2026. https://medcitynews.com/2025/08/ai-chatbots-healthcare/
13. Charlap S. Towards a future for semi-autonomous AI-powered primary care providers. KevinMD. October 14, 2024. Accessed January 26, 2026. https://kevinmd.com/2024/10/towards-a-future-for-semi-autonomous-ai-powered-primary-care-providers.html
14. Fox A. Stanford Health and Qualtrics to build artificial patient experience agents. Healthcare IT News. August 15, 2025. Accessed January 26, 2026. https://www.healthcareitnews.com/news/stanford-health-and-qualtrics-build-artificial-patient-experience-agents
15. AI and the future primary care workforce. California Healthcare Foundation Issue Brief. June 2025. Accessed January 26, 2026. https://www.chcf.org/wp-content/uploads/2025/07/AIFuturePrimaryCareWorkforce_IssueBrief.pdf
16. Carmouche D. Why flashy AI tools won't fix health care without real infrastructure. KevinMD. June 10, 2025. Accessed January 26, 2026. https://kevinmd.com/2025/06/why-flashy-ai-tools-wont-fix-health-care-without-real-infrastructure.html
17. Hodach R, Grundy P, Jain A, Weiner M. Provider-Led Population Health Management: Key Strategies for Healthcare in the Cognitive Era. 2nd ed. Indianapolis, IN: John Wiley & Sons; 2016:7.
18. Health care costs: a primer. Kaiser Family Foundation. May 1, 2012. Accessed January 26, 2026. https://www.kff.org/report-section/health-care-costs-a-primer-2012-report
19. Hodach R, Grundy P, Jain A, Weiner M. Provider-Led Population Health Management: Key Strategies for Healthcare in the Cognitivc Era. 2nd ed. Indianapolis, IN: John Wiley & Sons; 2016:105.
20. Hodach R, Grundy P, Jain A, Weiner M. Provider-Led Population Health Management: Key Strategies for Healthcare in the Cognitive Era. 2nd ed. Indianapolis, IN: John Wiley & Sons; 2016:104.

21. Terry K. Physician-Led Healthcare Reform: A New Approach to Medicare for All. Washington, DC: American Association for Physician Leadership; 2020:104-106.
22. Davy C, Bleasel J, Liu H, *et al*. Effectiveness of chronic care models: opportunities for improving healthcare practice and health outcomes: a systematic review. BMC Health Serv Res. 2015;15:194. doi:10.1186/s12913-015-0854-8
23. Davy C, Bleasel J, Liu H, *et al*. Effectiveness of chronic care models: opportunities for improving healthcare practice and health outcomes: a systematic review. BMC Health Serv Res. 2015;15:194. doi:10.1186/s12913-015-0854-8
24. Stellefson M, Dipnarine K, Stopka C. The chronic care model and diabetes management in US primary care settings: a systematic review. Prev Chronic Dis. 2013;10:120180. doi:10.5888/pcd10.120180
25. Reducing care fragmentation. Group Health Cooperative Institute. Accessed January 26, 2026. http://www.improvingchroniccare.org/downloads/reducing_care_fragmentation.pdf
26. Terry K. Rx for Health Care Reform. Nashville, TN: Vanderbilt University Press; 2007:100.
27. 2024 Employer health benefits survey. Kaiser Family Foundation. October 9, 2024. Accessed January 26, 2026. https://www.kff.org/health-costs/2024-employer-health-benefits-survey/
28. Barnett ML, Song Z, Bitton A, Rose S, Landon BE. Gatekeeping and patterns of outpatient care post healthcare reform. Am J Manag Care. 2018;24(10):e312-e316. https://www.ajmc.com/view/gatekeeping-and-patterns-of-outpatient-care-post-healthcare-reform
29. Cohen K. New West Physicians' journey to becoming a high-performing health system. Group Practice Journal. March 2016. Accessed January 26, 2026. http://www.amga.org/wcm/PI/Acclaim/2015/newWest.pdf
30. Parekh AK. Winning their trust. N Engl J Med. 2011;364(24):e51. doi:10.1056/NEJMp1105645
31. Pearson T. The prevention of cardiovascular disease: have we really made progress? Health Aff. 2007;26(1):49-60. doi:10.1377/hlthaff.26.1.49
32. Pearson T. The prevention of cardiovascular disease: have we really made progress? Health Aff. 2007;26(1):49-60. doi:10.1377/hlthaff.26.1.49
33. Hibbard JH. Moving toward a more patient-centered health care delivery system. Health Aff. 2004. doi:10.1377/hlthaff.var.133
34. A new definition of patient engagement: what is patient engagement and why is it important? Center for Advancing Health. 2010. https://catalog.nyam.org/bib/253487.
35. Prochaska JO, Norcross JC, DiClemente CC. Changing for Good. New York, NY: HarperCollins; 1995, 2002.

36. Glanz K, Rimer BK, Viswanath KJ. Health Behavior and Health Education. 3rd ed. San Francisco, CA: Jossey-Bass Inc; 2002.
37. Glanz K, Rimer BK, Viswanath KJ. Health Behavior and Health Education. 3rd ed. San Francisco, CA: Jossey-Bass Inc; 2002.
38. Nielsen-Bohlman L, Panzer AM, Kindig DA, eds. Health Literacy: A Prescription to End Confusion. Washington, DC: National Academies Press; 2004.
39. The world health report 2002—reducing risks, promoting healthy life. World Health Organization. Accessed January 26, 2026. https://www.who.int/whr/2002/en/

Chapter 10

1. Cottrill A, Cubanski J, Neuman T. What to know about Medicare coverage of telehealth. Kaiser Family Foundation. October 2, 2024. Accessed January 26, 2026. https://www.kff.org/medicare/what-to-know-about-medicare-coverage-of-telehealth/
2. In April, telehealth utilization increased nationally and in South, but decreased in other regions. FAIR Health. July 15, 2024. Accessed January 26, 2026. https://www.fairhealth.org/press-release/in-april-telehealth-utilization-increased-nationally-and-in-south-but-decreased-in-other-regions-telehealth-utilization-in-south-increased-by-7-2-percent-from-march-to-april
3. Gage AD, Knight MA, Bintz C, *et al.* Disparities in telemedicine uses and payment policies in the United States between 2019 and 2023. Commun Med (Lond). 2025;5:52. doi:10.1038/s43856-025-00757-2
4. Jercich K. AMA survey: majority of physicians say telehealth enables more comprehensive quality data. Healthcare IT News. April 25, 2022. Accessed January 26, 2026. https://www.healthcareitnews.com/news/ama-survey-majority-physicians-say-telehealth-enables-more-comprehensive-quality-care
5. Littrell A. 30% of all U.S. medical care could be virtual by 2026. Medical Economics. May 23, 2025. Accessed January 26, 2026. https://www.medicaleconomics.com/view/30-of-all-u-s-medical-care-could-be-virtual-by-2026
6. Cottrill A, Cubanski J, Neuman T. What to know about Medicare coverage of telehealth. Kaiser Family Foundation. October 2, 2024. Accessed January 26, 2026. https://www.kff.org/medicare/what-to-know-about-medicare-coverage-of-telehealth/
7. Telehealth policy updates. Department of Health and Human Services. Accessed January 26, 2026. https://telehealth.hhs.gov/providers/telehealth-policy/telehealth-policy-updates
8. Uscher-Pines L, Mehrotra A. The effect of telehealth on spending—reframing the debate. JAMA. 2024;332(18):1513-1514. doi:10.1001/jama.2024.16157
9. Reed M, Huang J, Somers M, *et al.* Telemedicine versus in-person primary care: treatment and followup visits. Ann Intern Med. 2023;176(10):1349-1357. doi:10.7326/M23-1335

10. Funding Package Signed by President Trump Extends Key Telehealth Provisions for Multiple Years, Ends Partial Government Shutdown. American Telemedicine Association. Feb. 5, 2026. https://www.americantelemed.org/press-releases/funding-package-signed-by-president-trumpextendskey-telehealth-provisions-for-multiple-years-ends-partial-government-shutdow/
11. Private insurance coverage for telehealth. Department of Health and Human Services. Accessed January 26, 2026. https://telehealth.hhs.gov/providers/billing-and-reimbursement/private-insurance-coverage-for-telehealth
12. Fox A. Report shows overwhelming doctor support for virtual care. Healthcare IT News. December 17, 2024. Accessed January 26, 2026. https://www.healthcareitnews.com/news/report-shows-overwhelming-doctor-support-virtual-care
13. Mehrotra A, Perkins J. Congress can unlock the full potential of telehealth through a permanent fix. Health Affairs Forefront. March 4, 2025. doi:10.1377/forefront.20250303.724320
14. Littrell A. 30% of all U.S. medical care could be virtual by 2026. Medical Economics. May 23, 2025. Accessed January 26, 2026. https://www.medicaleconomics.com/view/30-of-all-u-s-medical-care-could-be-virtual-by-2026
15. Fox A. Report shows overwhelming doctor support for virtual care. Healthcare IT News. December 17, 2024. Accessed January 26, 2026. https://www.healthcareitnews.com/news/report-shows-overwhelming-doctor-support-virtual-care
16. "Alliance for Connected Care Leads Health Care Stakeholders Urging Congress to Extend Medicare Telehealth Access Before September 2025 Deadline." Alliance for Connected Care. August 11, 2025. https://connectwithcare.org/alliance-for-connected-care-leads-350-health-care-stakeholders-urging-congress-to-extend-medicare-telehealth-access-before-september-2025-deadline/
17. Terry K. Has the time come for hospital at home? Next Avenue. October 23, 2020. Accessed January 26, 2026. https://www.nextavenue.org/hospital-at-home/
18. Michael McAuliff. PBM, telehealth, hospital-at-home measures clear Congress. Modern Healthcare. February 3, 2026. https://www.modernhealthcare.com/politics-regulation/mh-congress-government-funding-bill-pbm-telehealth/?utm_content=article1-readmore&utm_source=modern-healthcare-daily-dose&utm_medium=email&utm_campaign=20260203
19. Eastabrook D. In-home emergency care cuts costs, but needs more payer buy-in. Modern Healthcare. June 27, 2024. Accessed January 26, 2026. https://www.modernhealthcare.com/providers/emergency-room-care-at-home-growth-challenges/
20. Siwicki B. Texas Health Resources' virtual-first focus is paying dividends. Healthcare IT News. August 21, 2025. Accessed January 26, 2026. https://www

.healthcareitnews.com/news/texas-health-resources-virtual-first-focus-paying-dividends

21. Adler-Milstein J, Mehrotra A. Paying for digital health care—problems with the fee-for-service system. N Engl J Med. 2021;385(10):871-873. doi:10.1056/NEJMp2107879
22. Henderson J. Modest decline in patient portal messages after billing initiative launched. MedPage Today. December 30, 2024. Accessed January 26, 2026. https://www.medpagetoday.com/practicemanagement/informationtechnology/113589
23. Adler-Milstein J, Mehrotra A. Paying for digital health care—problems with the fee-for-service system. N Engl J Med. 2021;385(10):871-873. doi:10.1056/NEJMp2107879
24. Henderson J. Modest decline in patient portal messages after billing initiative launched. MedPage Today. December 30, 2024. Accessed January 26, 2026. https://www.medpagetoday.com/practicemanagement/informationtechnology/113589
25. Rotenstein L, Landman A, Bates DW. The electronic inbox—benefits, questions, and solutions for the road ahead. JAMA. 2023;330(18):1735-1736. doi:10.1001/jama.2023.19195
26. Day S, Seninger C, Kothari M, *et al.* Digital health consumer adoption report 2019. Rock Health. Accessed January 26, 2026. https://rockhealth.docsend.com/view/i6j4ieu
27. Wells C, Spry C. An overview of smartphone apps. Canadian Journal of Health Technologies. 2022;2(2). doi:10.51731/cjht.2022.269
28. Klasko SK, Terry K. Feelin' Alright: How the Message in the Music Can Make Healthcare Healthier. Chicago, IL: Health Administration Press; 2023:25.
29. Klasko SK, Terry K. Feelin' Alright: How the Message in the Music Can Make Healthcare Healthier. Chicago, IL: Health Administration Press; 2023:24-25.
30. Perna G. Remote patient monitoring poised to grow if reimbursement remains. Modern Healthcare. April 26, 2023. Accessed January 26, 2026. https://www.modernhealthcare.com/policy/remote-patient-monitoring-reimbursement-patient-outcome-rural-healthcare/
31. Perna G. Remote patient monitoring poised to grow if reimbursement remains. Modern Healthcare. April 26, 2023. Accessed January 26, 2026. https://www.modernhealthcare.com/policy/remote-patient-monitoring-reimbursement-patient-outcome-rural-healthcare/
32. Perna G. Hospitals navigate the high cost of remote patient monitoring. Modern Healthcare. August 30, 2024. Accessed January 26, 2026. https://www.modernhealthcare.com/digital-health/remote-patient-monitoring-costs-mayo-clinic-ochsner-providence/

33. Smith T. Remote monitoring helps type 2 diabetes patients manage a dangerous disease. UC Health Today. March 5, 2022. Accessed January 26, 2026. https://www.uchealth.org/today/diabetes-remote-monitoring-program-helps-patients-manage-dangerous-disease/

34. Johnson EL, Miller E. Remote patient monitoring in diabetes: how to acquire, manage, and use all of the data. Diabetes Spectr. 2022;35(1):43-56. doi:10.2337/dsi21-0015

35. Ginsburg GS, Picard RW, Friend SH. Key issues as wearable digital health technologies enter clinical care. N Engl J Med. 2024;390(12):1118-1127. doi:10.1056/NEJMra2307160

36. Siwicki B. Can AI power progress with remote patient monitoring technology? Healthcare IT News. October 7, 2024. Accessed January 26, 2026. https://www.healthcareitnews.com/news/can-ai-power-progress-remote-patient-monitoring-technology

37. Hall SD. Geisinger finds telemedicine cuts readmissions, costs for heart failure patients. Fierce Healthcare. October 3, 2014. Accessed January 26, 2026. https://www.fiercehealthcare.com/it/geisinger-finds-telemedicine-cuts-readmissions-costs-for-heart-failure-patients

38. The best use cases for remote patient monitoring. Thorough Care. Accessed January 26, 2026. https://www.thoroughcare.net/blog/remote-patient-monitoring-use-cases

39. Telehealth and remote patient monitoring. Department of Health and Human Services. Accessed January 26, 2026. https://telehealth.hhs.gov/providers/best-practice-guides/telehealth-and-remote-patient-monitoring/using-remote-patient

40. Topol EJ. The Patient Will See You Now: The Future of Medicine Is In Your Hands. New York, NY: Basic Books; 2015:8.

Chapter 11

1. Rural health: addressing barriers to care. NICHM Foundation. October 25, 2023. Accessed January 26, 2026. https://nihcm.org/publications/rural-health-addressing-barriers-to-care

2. Kacik A. Rural hospitals bid to save maternity care. Modern Healthcare. April 16, 2025. Accessed January 26, 2026. https://www.modernhealthcare.com/providers/rural-obstetric-units-rmoms-grants-funding

3. Amboree TL, Damgacioglu H, Chiao EY, *et al.* Rural-urban disparities in cervical cancer incidence and mortality among US women. JAMA Netw Open. 2025;8(3):e2462634. doi:10.1001/jamanetworkopen.2024.62634

4. Campanella T. Working-age people living in rural areas are 43% more likely to die from natural causes than in urban areas. LinkedIn. August 6, 2025. Accessed

January 26, 2026. https://www.linkedin.com/pulse/working-age-people-living-rural-areas-43-more-likely-die-campanella-b8quc/

5. Rural health: addressing barriers to care. NICHM Foundation. October 25, 2023. Accessed January 26, 2026. https://nihcm.org/publications/rural-health-addressing-barriers-to-care
6. Haught R, Coleman A, Dobson A, *et al.* The impact of proposed federal Medicaid work requirements on hospital revenues and financial margins. Commonwealth Fund. September 18, 2025. Accessed January 26, 2026. https://www.commonwealthfund.org/publications/issue-briefs/2025/sep/impact-medicaid-work-requirements-hospital-revenues-margins
7. Howren MB, Hansen JR. The One Big Beautiful Bill Act—implications for rural health care. JAMA. 2025;334(13):1143-1144. doi:10.1001/jama.2025.13518
8. Howren MB, Hansen JR. The One Big Beautiful Bill Act—implications for rural health care. JAMA. 2025;334(13):1143-1144. doi:10.1001/jama.2025.13518
9. Adams K. Why more than 30% of rural hospitals are at risk of closure. MedCity News. August 8, 2024. Accessed January 26, 2026. https://medcitynews.com/2024/08/rural-hospital-healthcare-finance/
10. Kacik A. Medicare Advantage plans are crippling rural hospitals, CEO says. Modern Healthcare. December 28, 2023. Accessed January 26, 2026. https://www.modernhealthcare.com/providers/medicare-advantage-rural-hospital-emergency-program
11. Lee JD, Mullens CL, Markovitz AA, Probst JC. The rapid growth of Medicare Advantage poses challenges to rural hospitals. Health Affairs Forefront. July 21, 2025. doi:10.1377/forefront.20250718.900838
12. Burda D. The simple reason why rural hospitals close. 4sight Health. June 23, 2021. Accessed January 26, 2026. https://www.4sighthealth.com/the-simple-reason-why-rural-hospitals-close/
13. Parker K, Horowitz JM, Brown A, *et al.* Demographic and economic trends in urban, suburban, and rural communities. Pew Research Center. May 22, 2018. Accessed January 26, 2026. https://www.pewresearch.org/social-trends/2018/05/22/demographic-and-economic-trends-in-urban-suburban-and-rural-communities/
14. Lagasse J. Almost half of rural hospitals in the red, data shows. Healthcare Finance. February 18, 2025. Accessed January 26, 2026. https://www.healthcarefinancenews.com/news/almost-half-rural-hospitals-red-data-shows
15. Carroll C, Euhus R, Beaulieu N, Chernew ME. Hospital survival in rural markets: closures, mergers, and profitability. Health Aff. 2023;42(4):498-507. doi:10.1377/hlthaff.2022.01191
16. Howren MB, Hansen JR. The One Big Beautiful Bill Act—implications for rural health care. JAMA. 2025;334(13):1143-1144. doi:10.1001/jama.2025.13518

17. Mann C, Striar A. How differences in Medicaid, Medicare, and commercial health insurance payment rates impact access, health equity, and cost. Commonwealth Fund Blog. August 17, 2022. Accessed January 26, 2026. https://www.commonwealthfund.org/blog/2022/how-differences-medicaid-medicare-and-commercial-health-insurance-payment-rates-impact
18. Conley K. Rural healthcare needs more than just telehealth. Medcity News. October 6, 2024. Accessed January 26, 2026. https://medcitynews.com/2024/10/rural-healthcare-needs-more-than-just-telehealth/
19. Lee JD, Mullens CL, Markovitz AA, Probst JC. The rapid growth of Medicare Advantage poses challenges to rural hospitals. Health Affairs Forefront. July 21, 2025. doi:10.1377/forefront.20250718.900838
20. Lee JD, Mullens CL, Markovitz AA, Probst JC. The rapid growth of Medicare Advantage poses challenges to rural hospitals. Health Affairs Forefront. July 21, 2025. doi:10.1377/forefront.20250718.900838
21. Kacik A. Rural hospitals bid to save maternity care. Modern Healthcare. April 16, 2025. Accessed January 26, 2026. https://www.modernhealthcare.com/providers/rural-obstetric-units-rmoms-grants-funding
22. Rural emergency hospitals. Centers for Medicare & Medicaid Services. Accessed January 26, 2026. https://www.cms.gov/files/document/rural-emergency-hospitals-factsheet-september-2024.pdf
23. Rural emergency hospitals (REHs). Rural Health Information Hub. Accessed January 26, 2026. https://www.ruralhealthinfo.org/topics/rural-emergency-hospitals
24. Rural hospitals risk of closing. Center for Healthcare Quality & Payment Reform. August 2025. Accessed January 26, 2026. https://ruralhospitals.chqpr.org/downloads/Rural_Hospitals_at_Risk_of_Closing.pdf
25. Howren MB, Hansen JR. The One Big Beautiful Bill Act—implications for rural health care. JAMA. 2025;334(13):1143-1144. doi:10.1001/jama.2025.13518
26. Campanella T. Working-age people living in rural areas are 43% more likely to die from natural causes than in urban areas. LinkedIn. August 6, 2025. Accessed January 26, 2026. https://www.linkedin.com/pulse/working-age-people-living-rural-areas-43-more-likely-die-campanella-b8quc/
27. Carroll C, Euhus R, Beaulieu N, Chernew ME. Hospital survival in rural markets: closures, mergers, and profitability. Health Aff. 2023;42(4):498-507. doi:10.1377/hlthaff.2022.01191
28. Bose N, Gerhart J, Kandru G, *et al.* Rural healthcare in crisis: innovations for a brighter future. Modern Healthcare. January 6, 2025. Accessed January 26, 2026. https://www.modernhealthcare.com/opinion/rural-healthcare-telehealth-payment-technology
29. Bose N, Gerhart J, Kandru G, *et al.* Rural healthcare in crisis: innovations for a brighter future. Modern Healthcare. January 6, 2025. Accessed January 26,

2026. https://www.modernhealthcare.com/opinion/rural-healthcare-telehealth-payment-technology

30. Lichtenwald I. Make broadband the first salvo in a rural renaissance. Medsphere Blog. November 11, 2021. Accessed January 26, 2026. https://www.medsphere.com/blog/make-broadband-the-first-salvo-in-a-rural-renaissance/
31. Kacik A. Rural Wisconsin hospitals join clinically integrated network boom. Modern Healthcare. September 18, 2025. Accessed January 26, 2026. https://www.modernhealthcare.com/providers/mh-rural-hospital-wisconsin-clinically-integrated/
32. Kacik A. More rural hospitals mulling clinically integrated networks. Modern Healthcare. December 14, 2023. Accessed January 26, 2026. https://www.modernhealthcare.com/providers/clinically-integrated-networks-rural-hospitals-rough-rider-high-value-nathan-white
33. Kacik A. 26 hospitals band together on a clinically integrated network. Modern Healthcare. April 17, 2025. Accessed January 26, 2026. https://www.modernhealthcare.com/providers/ohio-west-virginia-clinically-integrated-network
34. Rural health: addressing barriers to care. NIHCM Foundation. October 25, 2023. Accessed January 26, 2026. https://nihcm.org/publications/rural-health-addressing-barriers-to-care
35. Zients A. Rural ERs are increasingly run without doctors, experts say. Modern Healthcare. August 15, 2022. Accessed January 26, 2026. https://www.modernhealthcare.com/providers/mh-rural-emergency-rooms-sanford-health/
36. Federally Qualified Health Centers (FQHCs) and the health center program. Rural Health Information Hub. Accessed January 26, 2026. https://www.ruralhealthinfo.org/topics/federally-qualified-health-centers
37. Community health centers: a lifeline for rural America. National Association of Community Health Centers. May 2025. Accessed January 26, 2026. https://www.nachc.org/wp-content/uploads/2025/01/chcs_lifeline-for-rural-america_may-2025.pdf
38. Johnson C. Recent events have made primary care more fragile—further challenges lie ahead. Health Affairs Forefront. March 4, 2025. doi:10.1377/forefront.20250302.257604
39. Tribble SJ, Larweh H. Deep staff cuts at a little known federal agency pose trouble for droves of local health programs. KFF Health News. August 1, 2025. Accessed January 26, 2026. https://kffhealthnews.org/news/article/hrsa-federal-staff-cuts-affect-health-programs-grants/
40. The state of rural provider compensation in 2024. NRHA, Stroudwater Associates. Accessed January 26, 2026. https://www.stroudwater.com/white-paper/the-state-of-rural-provider-compensation-in-2024/

41. Family medicine salary report 2025. AMN Healthcare. Accessed January 26, 2026. https://www.amnhealthcare.com/blog/physician/locums/family-medicine-salary-report-2025/
42. Stephenson J. $1.5 billion issued by Biden administration to boost health care workforce size, diversity. JAMA Health Forum. 2021;2(11):e214785. doi:10.1001/jamahealthforum.2021.4785
43. The National Health Service Corps. Congressional Research Service. January 4, 2022. Accessed January 26, 2026. https://crsreports.congress.gov/product/pdf/R/R44970/15
44. Rural J-1 visa waiver. Rural Health Information Hub. Accessed January 26, 2026. https://www.ruralhealthinfo.org/topics/j-1-visa-waiver
45. Twenter P. Nurse practitioner, RN shortage to hit 362,000 by 2032. Becker's Clinical Leadership. September 17, 2025. Accessed January 26, 2026. https://www.beckershospitalreview.com/quality/nursing/nurse-practitioner-rn-shortage-to-hit-362000-by-2032/
46. Aledade announces expansion of Humana value-based care agreement to serve federally qualified health centers and rural health clinics. Aledade. March 20, 2025. Accessed January 26, 2026. https://aledade.com/newsroom/aledade-news/aledade-announces-expansion-of-humana-value-based-care-agreement/
47. Health center program: impact and growth. Health Resources and Services Administration. Accessed January 26, 2026. https://bphc.hrsa.gov/about-health-centers/health-center-program-impact-growth
48. Hinton E, Stolyar L. 10 things to know about Medicaid managed care. Kaiser Family Foundation. February 23, 2022. Accessed January 26, 2026. https://www.kff.org/medicaid/issue-brief/10-things-to-know-about-medicaid-managed-care/
49. Rosenbaum S, Shin P, Sharac J, Bedenbaugh C. Community health centers and Medicaid: a deeper dive into FQHC alternative payment. Health Affairs Forefront. January 27, 2023. doi:10.1377/forefront.20230126.640615
50. Houston R, Smithey A, Brykman K. Medicaid population-based payment: the current landscape, early insights, and considerations for policymakers. Center for Health Care Strategies. November 2022. Accessed January 26, 2026. https://www.chcs.org/media/Medicaid-Population-Based-Payment-Current-Landscape-Early-Insights-and-Considerations-for-Policymakers_111622.pdf
51. Houston R, Smithey A, Brykman K. Medicaid population-based payment: the current landscape, early insights, and considerations for policymakers. Center for Health Care Strategies. November 2022. Accessed January 26, 2026. https://www.chcs.org/media/Medicaid-Population-Based-Payment-Current-Landscape-Early-Insights-and-Considerations-for-Policymakers_111622.pdf
52. Hostetter M, Klein S. The perils and payoffs of alternative payment models for community health centers. The Commonwealth Fund. January 19, 2022.

Accessed January 26, 2026. https://www.commonwealthfund.org/publications/2022/jan/perils-and-payoffs-alternate-payment-models-community-health-centers

53. Howe G, McGinnis T. How health centers can improve patient care through value-based payment models. California Healthcare Foundation Issue Brief. June 2020. Accessed January 26, 2026. https://www.chcf.org/wp-content/uploads/2020/05/HealthCentersImproveCareValueBasedPayment.pdf
54. Burke LG, Stack CD, Pope JV. Declining interhospital transfers—a symptom of strained hospital capacity. JAMA Netw Open. 2025;8(5):e2512306. doi:10.1001/jamanetworkopen.2025.12306
55. Roberts ET, Hatfield LA, McWilliams JM, *et al.* Changes in hospital utilization three years into Maryland's global budget program for rural hospitals. Health Aff. 2018;37(4):644-653. doi:10.1377/hlthaff.2018.0112
56. Chatterjee P, Wang M, Chen X, *et al.* Mixed evidence that rural hospitals' finances improved with participation in the Pennsylvania rural health model. Health Aff. 2025;44(7):788-795. doi:10.1377/hlthaff.2024.01559
57. Campanella T. Working-age people living in rural areas are 43% more likely to die from natural causes than in urban areas. LinkedIn. August 6, 2025. Accessed January 26, 2026. https://www.linkedin.com/pulse/working-age-people-living-rural-areas-43-more-likely-die-campanella-b8quc/

Chapter 12

1. Foden-Vencil K. How Oregon is getting 'frequent flyers' out of hospital ERs. Kaiser Health News. July 10, 2013. Accessed January 26, 2026. https://khn.org/news/emergency-room-frequent-flyers/
2. The world health report 2002—reducing risks, promoting healthy life. World Health Organization. Accessed January 26, 2026. https://www.who.int/whr/2002/en/
3. Insights from McKinsey's consumer social determinants of health survey. McKinsey & Company. April 2019. Accessed January 26, 2026. https://www.mckinsey.com/industries/healthcare-systems-and-services/our-insights/insights-from-the-mckinsey-2019-consumer-social-determinants-of-health-survey
4. Khullar D, Chokshi DA. Health, income & poverty: where we are & what could help. Health Affairs Health Policy Brief. October 4, 2018. doi:10.1377/hpb20180817.901935
5. McGinnis JM, Williams-Russo P, Knickman JR. The case for more active policy attention to health promotion. Health Aff. 2002;21(2):78-93. doi:10.1377/hlthaff.21.2.78
6. Integrating social care into the delivery of health care: moving upstream to improve the nation's health. National Academies of Sciences, Engineering and

Medicine. September 2019. Accessed January 26, 2026. https://www.nap.edu/catalog/25467/integrating-social-care-into-the-delivery-of-health-care-moving

7. Hodach R, Grundy P, Jain A, Weiner M. Provider-Led Population Health Management: Key Strategies for Healthcare in the Cognitive Era. 2nd ed. Indianapolis, IN: John Wiley & Sons; 2016:203.
8. Castellucci M. Fee-for-service limits long-term work on social determinants, execs warn. Modern Healthcare. June 15, 2019. Accessed January 26, 2026. https://www.modernhealthcare.com/providers/fee-service-limits-long-term-work-social-determinants-execs-warn
9. Williford J, Rosenthal S, Kim D. Global budgeting in New York State: lessons from Montefiore Health System. Health Affairs Forefront. November 18, 2024. doi:10.1377/forefront.20241115.569586
10. Terry K. Why physicians must step up, address social determinants of health. Medical Economics. February 25, 2017. Accessed January 26, 2026. https://www.medicaleconomics.com/view/why-physicians-must-step-address-social-determinants-health
11. Kacik A. Looming uninsured surge may overwhelm ERs. Here's who can help. Modern Healthcare. August 18, 2025. Accessed January 26, 2026. https://www.modernhealthcare.com/providers/mh-medicaid-cuts-er-overcrowdfng-kaiser-permanente/
12. Drabo EF, Eckel G, Ross SL, *et al.* A social-return-on-investment analysis of Bon Secours Hospital's 'Housing for Health' affordable housing program. Health Aff. 2021;40(3):513-520. doi:10.1377/hlthaff.2020.00998
13. Ryan JL, Franklin SM, Canterberry M, *et al.* Association of health-related social needs with quality and utilization outcomes in a Medicare Advantage population with diabetes. JAMA Netw Open. 2023;6(4):e239316. doi:10.1001/jamanetworkopen.2023.9316
14. Berkowitz SA, Archibald J, Yu Z, *et al.* Medicaid spending and health-related social needs in the North Carolina Healthy Opportunities Pilots Program. JAMA. 2025;333(12):1041-1050. doi:10.1001/jama.2025.1042
15. Whitman A, De Lew N, Chappel A, *et al.* Addressing social determinants of health: examples of successful evidence-based strategies and current federal efforts. HHS Office of Health Policy. April 1, 2022. Accessed January 26, 2026. https://aspe.hhs.gov/sites/default/files/documents/e2b650cd64cf84aae8ff0fae7474af82/SDOH-Evidence-Review.pdf
16. Whitman A, De Lew N, Chappel A, *et al.* Addressing social determinants of health: examples of successful evidence-based strategies and current federal efforts. HHS Office of Health Policy. April 1, 2022. Accessed January 26, 2026. https://aspe.hhs.gov/sites/default/files/documents/e2b650cd64cf84aae8ff0fae7474af82/SDOH-Evidence-Review.pdf

17. Palar K, Cox C. Modeling the value of 'food is medicine': challenges and opportunities for scaling up medically tailored meals. Health Aff. 2025;44(4):443-448. doi:10.1377/hlthaff.2025.00161
18. DeSilva H. Where food-is-medicine programs are heading. Modern Healthcare. August 20, 2025. Accessed January 26, 2026. https://www.modernhealthcare.com/providers/mh-food-is-medicine-programs-nachc/
19. DSRIP overview. New York State Department of Health. Accessed January 26, 2026. https://www.health.ny.gov/health_care/medicaid/redesign/dsrip/overview.htm
20. Bachrach D, Bernstein W, Augenstein J, Lipson M, Ellis R. Implementing New York's DSRIP program: implications for Medicaid payment and delivery system reform. Commonwealth Fund. April 2016. Accessed January 26, 2026. https://www.commonwealthfund.org/sites/default/files/documents/___media_files_publications_fund_report_2016_apr_1871_bachrach_implementing_new_york_dsrip_v4.pdf
21. Lindenfeld Z, Chen K, Kapur S, Chang JE. Assessing differences in social determinants of health screening rates in a large, urban safety-net health system. J Prim Care Community Health. 2023;14:21501319231207713. doi:10.1177/21501319231207713
22. Health care's blind side: the overlooked connection between social needs and good health. Robert Wood Johnson Foundation. Accessed January 26, 2026. http://www.rwjf.org/content/dam/farm/reports/surveys_and_polls/2011/rwjf71795
23. Mechanic R, Fitch A. Working with ACOs to address social determinants of health. Health Affairs Forefront. January 23, 2023. doi:10.1377/forefront.20230119.448380
24. Murray GF, Rodriguez HP, Lewis VA. Upstream with a small paddle: how ACOs are working against the current to meet patients' social needs. Health Aff. 2020;39(2):199-206. doi:10.1377/hlthaff.2019.01266
25. Community health centers leveraging the social determinants of health. Institute for Alternative Futures. March 2012. Accessed January 26, 2026. https://kresge.org/sites/default/files/IAF-CHCsLeveragingSDH.pdf
26. Hodach R, Grundy P, Jain A, Weiner M. Provider-Led Population Health Management: Key Strategies for Healthcare in the Cognitive Era. 2nd ed. Indianapolis, IN: John Wiley & Sons; 2016:203.
27. Johnson KO, Barolin N, Ogbue C, Verlander K. Lessons from five years of the CMS Accountable Health Communities Model. Health Affairs Forefront. August 8, 2022. doi:10.1377/forefront.20220805.764159
28. Accountable Health Communities (AHC) model evaluation. RTI International. December 2020. Accessed January 26, 2026. https://innovation.cms.gov/data-and-reports/2020/ahc-first-eval-rpt

29. Johnson SR. Kaiser to launch social care network. Modern Healthcare. May 6, 2019. Accessed January 26, 2026. https://www.modernhealthcare.com/care-delivery/kaiser-launch-social-care-network
30. Johnson SR. CVS and Aetna to launch social care network. Modern Healthcare. July 24, 2019. Accessed January 26, 2026. https://www.modernhealthcare.com/providers/cvs-and-aetna-launch-social-care-network
31. Minemyer P. Why UnitedHealthcare wants to expand diagnostic codes to the social determinants of health. FierceHealthcare. February 11, 2019. Accessed January 26, 2026. https://www.fiercehealthcare.com/payer/why-unitedhealthcare-wants-to-expand-diagnostic-codes-to-social-determinants-health
32. Miliard M. New BCBS Institute working with Lyft, CVS, Walgreens to tackle social determinants. Healthcare IT News. March 16, 2018. Accessed January 26, 2026. https://www.healthcareitnews.com/news/new-bcbs-institute-working-lyft-cvs-walgreens-tackle-social-determinants
33. Minemyer P. Why New Jersey's top insurer wants to expand its work on the social determinants of health in 2019. Fierce Healthcare. February 25, 2019. Accessed January 26, 2026. https://www.fiercehealthcare.com/payer/why-horizon-bcbsnj-wants-to-expand-its-work-social-determinants-health-2019
34. Whitman A, De Lew N, Chappel A, *et al.* Addressing social determinants of health: examples of successful evidence-based strategies and current federal efforts. HHS Office of Health Policy. April 1, 2022. Accessed January 26, 2026. https://aspe.hhs.gov/sites/default/files/documents/e2b650cd64cf84aae8ff0fae7474af82/SDOH-Evidence-Review.pdf
35. Duddy-Tenbrunsel R, Donthi S, Fruman B, Fix A. More Medicare Advantage plans will offer non-medical benefits in 2022. Avalere. October 19, 2021. Accessed January 26, 2026. https://avalere.com/insights/more-medicare-advantage-plans-will-offer-non-medical-benefits-in-2022
36. Tepper N. Medicare Advantage plans edge away from supplemental benefits. Modern Healthcare. September 25, 2025. Accessed January 26, 2026. https://www.modernhealthcare.com/insurance/mh-medicare-advantage-supplemental-benefits-2026/
37. Hinton E, Diana A. Medicaid authorities and options to address social determinants of health. Kaiser Family Foundation. January 29, 2024. Accessed January 26, 2026. https://www.kff.org/medicaid/medicaid-authorities-and-options-to-address-social-determinants-of-health-sdoh/
38. Whitman A, De Lew N, Chappel A, *et al.* Addressing social determinants of health: examples of successful evidence-based strategies and current federal efforts. HHS Office of Health Policy. April 1, 2022. Accessed January 26, 2026. https://aspe.hhs.gov/sites/default/files/documents/e2b650cd64cf84aae8ff0fae7474af82/SDOH-Evidence-Review.pdf

39. Foden-Vencil K. Oregon's $2 billion Medicaid bet. Kaiser Health News. May 30, 2012. Accessed January 26, 2026. https://khn.org/news/oregon-cco/
40. Aney K. Former Oregon governor believes new approach needed on health care. Blue Mountain Eagle. September 23, 2019. Accessed January 26, 2026. https://www.bluemountaineagle.com/news/former-oregon-governor-believes-new-approach-needed-on-health-care/article_b026a73a-f7ea-5cd1-a769-17734367cae2.html
41. Terry K. Why physicians must step up, address social determinants of health. Medical Economics. February 25, 2017. Accessed January 26, 2026. https://www.medicaleconomics.com/health-law-and-policy/why-physicians-must-step-address-social-determinants-health
42. Statewide "boots on the ground" and demonstrated ROI. Community Care of North Carolina. Accessed January 26, 2026. https://www.communitycarenc.org/what-we-do/care-management
43. Livingston S. Social determinants are core of North Carolina's Medicaid overhaul. Modern Healthcare. August 3, 2018. Accessed January 26, 2026. https://www.modernhealthcare.com/article/20180803/TRANSFORMATION01/180809944/social-determinants-are-core-of-north-carolina-s-medicaid-overhaul
44. Ndugga N, Hill L, Pillai D, Artiga S. Race, inequality, and health. Kaiser Family Foundation. October 8, 2025. Accessed January 26, 2026. https://www.kff.org/racial-equity-and-health-policy/health-policy-101-race-inequality-and-health/
45. Zambrana RE, Williams DR. The intellectual roots of current knowledge on racism and health: relevance to policy and the national equity discourse. Health Aff. 2022;41(12):163-170. doi:10.1377/hlthaff.2021.01439
46. Beach MC, Harrigian K, Chee B, *et al.* Racial bias in clinician assessment of patient credibility: evidence from electronic health records. PLoS One. 2025;20(8):e0328134. doi:10.1371/journal.pone.0328134
47. Gangopadhyaya A. Do Black and white patients experience similar rates of adverse safety events at the same hospital? Robert Wood Johnson Foundation. July 2021. Accessed January 26, 2026. https://www.rwjf.org/en/insights/our-research/2021/07/do-black-and-white-patients-experience-similar-rates-of-adverse-safety-events-at-the-same-hospital.html
48. Klasko SK. Feelin' Alright: How The Message In The Music Can Make Healthcare Healthier. Chicago, IL: Health Administration Press; 2023:213.
49. Radley DC, Shah A, Collins SR, *et al.* Advancing racial equity in U.S. health care. Commonwealth Fund. April 18, 2024. Accessed January 26, 2026. https://www.commonwealthfund.org/publications/fund-reports/2024/apr/advancing-racial-equity-us-health-care
50. Caratala S, Maxwell C. Health disparities by race and ethnicity. Center for American Progress. May 7, 2020. Accessed January 26, 2026. https://www.americanprogress.org/article/health-disparities-race-ethnicity/

51. Klasko SK. Feelin' Alright: How The Message In The Music Can Make Healthcare Healthier. Chicago, IL: Health Administration Press; 2023:213-214.
52. Caratala S, Maxwell C. Health disparities by race and ethnicity. Center for American Progress. May 7, 2020. Accessed January 26, 2026. https://www.americanprogress.org/article/health-disparities-race-ethnicity/
53. Frieden J. U.S. has made little progress with health equity, expert says. Medpage Today. December 17, 2024. Accessed January 26, 2026. https://www.medpagetoday.com/publichealthpolicy/equity-in-medicine/113442
54. Euhus R, Williams E, Burns A, Rudowitz R. Allocating CBO's estimates of federal Medicaid spending reductions across the states: enacted reconciliation package. Kaiser Family Foundation. July 23, 2025. Accessed January 26, 2026. https://www.kff.org/medicaid/allocating-cbos-estimates-of-federal-medicaid-spending-reductions-across-the-states-enacted-reconciliation-package/
55. Setting the Record Straight on Premium Tax Credit Enhancements. Center on Budget and Policy Priorities. January 12, 2026. Accessed January 26, 2026. https://www.cbpp.org/blog/setting-the-record-straight-on-premium-tax-credit-enhancements
56. Fraze TK, Brewster AL, Lewis VA, Beidler LB, Murray GF, Colla CH. Prevalence of screening for food insecurity, housing instability, utility needs, transportation needs, and interpersonal violence by US physician practices and hospitals. JAMA Netw Open. 2019;2(9):e1911514. doi:10.1001/jamanetworkopen.2019.11514
57. Terry K. Physician-Led Healthcare Reform: A New Approach to Medicare For All. Washington, DC: American Association for Physician Leadership; 2020:125.
58. Terry K. Physician-Led Healthcare Reform: A New Approach to Medicare For All. Washington, DC: American Association for Physician Leadership; 2020:125.
59. Klein S, Hostetter M. In focus: integrating behavioral health and primary care. Commonwealth Fund Quality Matters Archive. August/September 2014. Accessed January 26, 2026. http://www.commonwealthfund.org/publications/newsletters/quality-matters/2014/august-september/in-focus
60. Mental health by the numbers. National Alliance on Mental Illness. Accessed January 26, 2026. https://www.nami.org/learn-more/mental-health-by-the-numbers
61. Integrating behavioral health into primary care. SAMHSA-HRSA Center for Integrated Health Systems. Accessed January 26, 2026. http://www.integration.samhsa.gov/integrated-care-models/behavioral-health-in-primary-care
62. Freda B, Kozick D, Spencer A. For health: lessons for bridging community-based organizations and health care organizations. Center for Health Care Strategies. January 2018. Accessed January 26, 2026. https://www.chcs.org/media/CBO-HCO_Partnership_update_032018.pdf
63. Terry K. Physician-Led Healthcare Reform: A New Approach to Medicare For All. Washington, DC: American Association for Physician Leadership; 2020:129.

64. Hodach R, Grundy P, Jain A, Weiner M. Provider-Led Population Health Management: Key Strategies for Healthcare in the Cognitive Era. 2nd ed. Indianapolis, IN: John Wiley & Sons; 2016:197-198.
65. Abrams MK, Schneider EC. Fostering a high-performance health system that serves our nation's sickest and frailest. Commonwealth Fund Blog. October 29, 2015. Accessed January 26, 2026. https://www.commonwealthfund.org/blog/2015/fostering-high-performance-health-system-serves-our-nations-sickest-and-frailest

Chapter 13

1. Rakshit S, Winger A, Cotter L, *et al.* How has U.S. spending on healthcare changed over time? Peterson-KFF Health System Tracker. December 20, 2024. Accessed January 26, 2026. https://www.healthsystemtracker.org/chart-collection/u-s-spending-healthcare-changed-time/
2. NHE fact sheet, historical NHE: 2023. Centers for Medicare & Medicaid Services. Accessed January 26, 2026. https://www.cms.gov/data-research/statistics-trends-and-reports/national-health-expenditure-data/nhe-fact-sheet
3. Terry K. Technology: the biggest healthcare cost driver of all: can we curb its rise? Medical Economics. March 21, 1994.
4. Eddy DM. Health system reform: will controlling costs require rationing services? JAMA. 1994;272(4):324-328. doi:10.1001/jama.1994.03520040088055
5. Terry K. Technology: the biggest healthcare cost driver of all: can we curb its rise? Medical Economics. March 21, 1994.
6. Minimally invasive surgery. Mayo Clinic. Accessed January 26, 2026. https://www.mayoclinic.org/tests-procedures/minimally-invasive-surgery/about/pac-20384771
7. Bukowski B. Advanced technologies, techniques redefine hip and knee replacements. Mayo Clinic Blog. April 11, 2024. Accessed January 26, 2026. https://www.mayoclinichealthsystem.org/hometown-health/speaking-of-health/advances-in-hip-and-knee-replacement
8. Bukowski B. Advanced technologies, techniques redefine hip and knee replacements. Mayo Clinic Blog. April 11, 2024. Accessed January 26, 2026. https://www.mayoclinichealthsystem.org/hometown-health/speaking-of-health/advances-in-hip-and-knee-replacement
9. Ailaney N, Schloemann DT, Wegman SJ, *et al.* Trends in outpatient primary total hip and knee replacement from the hospital outpatient department and ambulatory surgery center settings in New York State. Arthroplasty Today. 2025;33:101695. doi:10.1016/j.artd.2025.101695
10. Shichman I, Roof M, Askew N, *et al.* Projections and epidemiology of primary hip and knee arthroplasty in Medicare patients to 2040-2060. JB JS Open Access. 2023;8(1):e22.00112. doi:10.2106/JBJS.OA.22.00112

11. Fischer K. How much does a hip replacement cost? GoodRx. August 29, 2022. Accessed January 26, 2026. https://www.goodrx.com/health-topic/joints/how-much-does-a-hip-replacement-cost
12. Does Medicare cover hip replacement? Humana. July 9, 2024. Accessed January 26, 2026. https://www.humana.com/medicare/medicare-resources/does-medicare-cover-hip-replacement
13. Pauly MV. Should we be worried about high real medical spending growth in the United States? Health Aff. 2003;22(Suppl1 Web Exclusives). doi:10.1377/hlthaff.W3.15
14. Terry K. Rx For Healthcare Reform. Nashville, TN: Vanderbilt University Press; 2007:287.
15. Shryock T. Medical device industry projected to grow 9.8% from 2024 through 2029. Medical Economics. April 2, 2025. Accessed January 26, 2026. https://www.medicaleconomics.com/view/medical-device-industry-projected-to-grow-9-8-from-2024-through-2029
16. Pulse of the MedTech industry report 2025. EY. Accessed January 26, 2026. https://www.ey.com/content/dam/ey-unified-site/ey-com/en-us/noindex/documents/ey-pulse-of-the-medtech-industry-2025-report.pdf
17. Terry K. FDA-cleared medical devices lack proper vetting, doctors say. WebMD. October 16, 2024. Accessed January 26, 2026. https://www.webmd.com/heart-disease/news/20241016/cm/fda-cleared-medical-devices-lack-proper-vetting
18. See C, Mooghali M, Dhruva SS, *et al.* Class I recalls of cardiovascular devices between 2013 and 2022: a cross-sectional analysis. Ann Intern Med. 2024;177(11):1499-1508. doi:10.7326/ANNALS-24-00724
19. Ardaugh BM, Graves SE, Redberg RF. The 510(k) ancestry of a metal-on-metal hip implant. N Engl J Med. 2013;368(2):97-100. doi:10.1056/NEJMp1211581
20. Dhruva SS, Tingley SR, Incze M, *et al.* Evaluation of payer policies to reduce low-value medical device–based procedure use. JAMA Health Forum. 2025;6(10):e253898. doi:10.1001/jamahealthforum.2025.3898
21. Iglesias CP. Does assessing the value for money of therapeutic medical devices require a flexible approach? Expert Rev Pharmacoecon Outcomes Res. 2015;15(1):21-32. doi:10.1586/14737167.2015.982098
22. Terry K. Rx for Health Care Reform. Nashville, TN: Vanderbilt University Press; 2007:228.
23. Schaffer EM, Su RGS, Chay J, *et al.* Cost-effectiveness of left ventricular assist device for transplant-ineligible patients. JAMA Netw Open. 2025;8(4):e254483. doi:10.1001/jamanetworkopen.2025.4483
24. Heart donation. Donate Life America. Accessed January 26, 2026. https://donatelife.net/donation/organs/heart-donation/
25. McDermott M, Robinson W, Smith K. Skin substitutes: a case for how ACOs can help prevent fraud, waste, and abuse. Health Affairs Forefront. October 7, 2025. doi:10.1377/forefront.20251006.704299

26. McDermott M, Robinson W, Smith K. Skin substitutes: a case for how ACOs can help prevent fraud, waste, and abuse. Health Affairs Forefront. October 7, 2025. doi:10.1377/forefront.20251006.704299
27. Medicare Part B payment trends for skin substitutes raises major concerns about fraud, waste and abuse. Department of Health and Human Services Office of Inspector General. September 2025. Accessed January 26, 2026. https://oig.hhs.gov/documents/evaluation/10939/OEI-BL-24-00420.pdf
28. Calendar year (CY) 2026 Medicare physician fee schedule final rule. Centers for Medicare & Medicaid Services. October 31, 2025. Accessed January 26, 2026. https://www.cms.gov/newsroom/fact-sheets/calendar-year-cy-2026-medicare-physician-fee-schedule-final-rule-cms-1832-f
29. Palmer K. Medicare will pay more than $1,000 for AI to analyze a heart scan. Is that too much? STAT. November 11, 2025. Accessed January 26, 2026. https://www.statnews.com/2025/11/11/medicare-coverage-ai-heart-scans-heartflow-cleerly-elucid/
30. Jeffries E. Mayo Clinic uses AI to detect heart condition early. Becker's Health IT. November 10, 2025. Accessed January 26, 2026. https://www.beckershospitalreview.com/healthcare-information-technology/ai/mayo-clinic-uses-ai-to-detect-heart-condition-early/
31. Nguyen D, Murayama A, Li T, *et al*. Payments to health care professionals and teaching hospitals by AI- and machine learning–enabled medical device manufacturers. JAMA. 2025;334(18):1669-1672. doi:10.1001/jama.2025.14813
32. Nguyen D, Murayama A, Li T, *et al*. Payments to health care professionals and teaching hospitals by AI- and machine learning–enabled medical device manufacturers. JAMA. 2025;334(18):1669-1672. doi:10.1001/jama.2025.14813
33. Palmer K. Medicare will pay more than $1,000 for AI to analyze a heart scan. Is that too much? STAT. November 11, 2025. Accessed January 26, 2026. https://www.statnews.com/2025/11/11/medicare-coverage-ai-heart-scans-heartflow-cleerly-elucid/
34. Palmer K. Medicare will pay more than $1,000 for AI to analyze a heart scan. Is that too much? STAT. November 11, 2025. Accessed January 26, 2026. https://www.statnews.com/2025/11/11/medicare-coverage-ai-heart-scans-heartflow-cleerly-elucid/
35. Health at a glance 2023: diagnostic technologies. Organisation for Economic Co-operation and Development. Accessed January 26, 2026. https://www.oecd.org/en/publications/2023/11/health-at-a-glance-2023_e04f8239/full-report/diagnostic-technologies_23088ad0.html
36. Emery DJ, Shojania KG, Forster AJ, *et al*. Overuse of magnetic resonance imaging. JAMA Intern Med. 2013;173(9):823-825. doi:10.1001/jamainternmed.2013.3804
37. Mukkamala L, Schaffer SL, Weber MG, *et al*. Is magnetic resonance imaging overused among patients undergoing total knee arthroplasty? J Am Acad Orthop Surg Glob Res Rev. 2024;8(10):e24.00258. doi:10.5435/JAAOSGlobal-D-24-00258

38. Müskens JLJM, Kool RB, van Dulmen SA, Westert GP. Overuse of diagnostic testing in healthcare: a systematic review. BMJ Qual Saf. 2022;31(1):54-63. doi:10.1136/bmjqs-2020-012576
39. Growth in U.S. health spending remains slow in 2010. Centers for Medicare & Medicaid Services. January 9, 2012. Accessed January 26, 2026. https://www.cms.gov/newsroom/press-releases/growth-us-health-spending-remains-slow-2010
40. NHE fact sheet: historical NHE, 2023. Centers for Medicare & Medicaid Services. Accessed January 26, 2026. https://www.cms.gov/data-research/statistics-trends-and-reports/national-health-expenditure-data/nhe-fact-sheet
41. Merritt D. How big pharma blocks access to low-cost generic drugs. Blue Cross Blue Shield Association Blog. September 24, 2025. Accessed January 26, 2026. https://www.bcbs.com/news-and-insights/article/big-pharma-blocks-access-to-low-cost-generic-drugs
42. Legasse J. Medicare Part D drug prices up nearly 100%. Healthcare Finance. January 14, 2025. Accessed January 26, 2026. https://www.healthcarefinancenews.com/news/medicare-part-d-drug-prices-nearly-100
43. Rakshit S, Winger A, Cotter L, *et al.* How has U.S. spending on healthcare changed over time? Peterson-KFF Health System Tracker. December 20, 2024. Accessed January 26, 2026. https://www.healthsystemtracker.org/chart-collection/u-s-spending-healthcare-changed-time/
44. Legasse J. Medicare Part D drug prices up nearly 100%. Healthcare Finance. January 14, 2025. Accessed January 26, 2026. https://www.healthcarefinancenews.com/news/medicare-part-d-drug-prices-nearly-100
45. Drug pricing overview 119th Congress. The Campaign for Sustainable Rx Pricing. Accessed January 26, 2026. https://www.csrxp.org/wp-content/uploads/2025/03/CSRxP-New-Congress-Toolkit-March-2025-Final.pdf
46. Comparing U.S. and international market size and average pricing for prescription drugs, 2017-2022. Department of Health and Human Services, Assistant Secretary for Planning and Evaluation, Office of Science & Data Policy. December 2024. Accessed January 26, 2026. https://aspe.hhs.gov/sites/default/files/documents/4326cc7fe43bc11770598cf2a13f478c/international-market-size-prices.pdf
47. Comparing U.S. and international market size and average pricing for prescription drugs, 2017-2022. Department of Health and Human Services, Assistant Secretary for Planning and Evaluation, Office of Science & Data Policy. December 2024. Accessed January 26, 2026. https://aspe.hhs.gov/sites/default/files/documents/4326cc7fe43bc11770598cf2a13f478c/international-market-size-prices.pdf
48. Comparing U.S. and international market size and average pricing for prescription drugs, 2017-2022. Department of Health and Human Services, Assistant Secretary for Planning and Evaluation, Office of Science & Data Policy.

December 2024. Accessed January 26, 2026. https://aspe.hhs.gov/sites/default/files/documents/4326cc7fe43bc11770598cf2a13f478c/international-market-size-prices.pdf

49. Merritt D. How big pharma blocks access to low-cost generic drugs. Blue Cross Blue Shield Association Blog. September 24, 2025. Accessed January 26, 2026. https://www.bcbs.com/news-and-insights/article/big-pharma-blocks-access-to-low-cost-generic-drugs
50. Merritt D. How big pharma blocks access to low-cost generic drugs. Blue Cross Blue Shield Association Blog. September 24, 2025. Accessed January 26, 2026. https://www.bcbs.com/news-and-insights/article/big-pharma-blocks-access-to-low-cost-generic-drugs
51. Effect of market entry on generic drug prices: Medicare data 2007-2022. Department of Health and Human Services, Assistant Secretary for Planning and Evaluation. January 16, 2025. Accessed January 26, 2026. https://aspe.hhs.gov/sites/default/files/documents/510e964dc7b7f00763a7f8a1dbc5ae7b/aspe-ib-generic-drugs-competition.pdf
52. Gupta R, Shah ND, Ross JS. Generic drugs in the United States: policies to address pricing and competition. Clin Pharmacol Ther. 2019;105(2):329-337. doi:10.1002/cpt.1314
53. Hassan C, Christensen J. Biogen discontinues Alzheimer's medication Aduhelm. CNN Health. January 31, 2024. Accessed January 26, 2026. https://www.cnn.com/2024/01/31/health/aduhelm-alzheimers-biogen
54. Salloway S, Chalkias S, Barkhof F, *et al*. Amyloid-related imaging abnormalities in 2 phase 3 studies evaluating aducanumab in patients with early Alzheimer disease. JAMA Neurol. 2022;79(1):13-21. doi:10.1001/jamaneurol.2021.4161
55. Buntz B. 2024's blockbusters: top 50 drugs by sales. Drug Discovery & Development. April 4, 2025. Accessed January 26, 2026. https://www.drugdiscoverytrends.com/2024s-blockbusters-top-50-pharmaceuticals-by-sales/
56. Keytruda: cost, insurance & financial help. Merck. Accessed January 26, 2026. https://www.keytruda.com/financial-support/
57. Ventola CL. Direct-to-consumer pharmaceutical advertising: therapeutic or toxic? P T. 2011;36(10):669-684. https://www.ncbi.nlm.nih.gov/pmc/articles/PMC3278148/
58. Rosenthal E. With TV drug ads, what you see is not necessarily what you get. Journal of Health Economics and Outcomes Research. September 24, 2024. Accessed January 26, 2026. https://jheor.org/post/2674-with-tv-drug-ads-what-you-see-is-not-necessarily-what-you-get
59. Rosenthal E. With TV drug ads, what you see is not necessarily what you get. Journal of Health Economics and Outcomes Research. September 24, 2024. Accessed January 26, 2026. https://jheor.org/post/2674-with-tv-drug-ads-what-you-see-is-not-necessarily-what-you-get

60. Kantor ED, Rehm CD, Haas JS, *et al.* Trends in prescription drug use among adults in the United States from 1999-2012. JAMA. 2015;314(17):1818-1830. doi:10.1001/jama.2015.13766

61. QuickStats: percentage of adults aged ≥18 who took prescription medication during the past 12 months, by sex and age group—National Health Interview Survey, United States, 2021. MMWR Morb Mortal Wkly Rep. 2023;72(16):450. doi:10.15585/mmwr.mm7216a7

62. Rosenbluth H. Banning DTC ads won't work, but reforming them could. STAT News. March 18, 2025. Accessed January 26, 2026. https://www.statnews.com/2025/03/18/direct-to-consumer-drug-ads-ban-rfk-jr-reform/

63. Alpert A, Sood N. Assessing the case against direct-to-consumer drug advertisements. JAMA Health Forum. 2025;6(11):e255325. doi:10.1001/jamahealthforum.2025.5325

64. Woloshin S, Fischhoff B. 'Dancing patients' aren't the biggest problem with drug ads. Washington Post. October 16, 2025. Accessed January 26, 2026. https://www.washingtonpost.com/opinions/2025/10/16/fda-prescription-drug-ads-benefits-harms/

65. Graham M. Advertising to consumers. Wall Street Journal. Accessed January 26, 2026. https://www.msn.com/en-us/money/companies/senators-to-propose-ban-on-drug-advertising-to-consumers/ar-AA1GB7zg

66. Wouters OJ, McKee M, Luyten J. Estimated research and development investment needed to bring a new medicine to market, 2009-2018. JAMA. 2020;323(9):844-853. doi:10.1001/jama.2020.1166

67. Sertkaya A, Beleche T, Jessup A, Sommers BD. Costs of drug development and research and development intensity in the US, 2000-2018. JAMA Netw Open. 2024;7(6):e2415445. doi:10.1001/jamanetworkopen.2024.15445

68. Sertkaya A, Beleche T, Jessup A, Sommers BD. Costs of drug development and research and development intensity in the US, 2000-2018. JAMA Netw Open. 2024;7(6):e2415445. doi:10.1001/jamanetworkopen.2024.15445

69. Biggs S, Long D. Insights into the 2023 U.S. pharmaceutical market. IQVIA Blog. July 25, 2023. Accessed January 26, 2026. https://www.iqvia.com/locations/united-states/blogs/2023/07/insights-into-the-2023-us-pharmaceutical-market

70. Understanding the use of medicines in the U.S., 2025: evolving standards of care, patient access, and spending. IQVIA Institute. Accessed January 26, 2026. https://www.iqvia.com/insights/the-iqvia-institute/reports-and-publications/reports/understanding-the-use-of-medicines-in-the-us-2025

71. Martin K. What pharmacy benefit managers do, and how they contribute to drug spending. KFF Explainer. March 17, 2025. Accessed January 26, 2026. https://www.commonwealthfund.org/publications/explainer/2025/mar/what-pharmacy-benefit-managers-do-how-they-contribute-drug-spending

72. Martin K. What pharmacy benefit managers do, and how they contribute to drug spending. KFF Explainer. March 17, 2025. Accessed January 26, 2026. https://www.commonwealthfund.org/publications/explainer/2025/mar/what-pharmacy-benefit-managers-do-how-they-contribute-drug-spending

73. Berryman L. Big 3 PBMs reaped $7.3B from generic specialty drug markups: FTC. Modern Healthcare. January 14, 2025. Accessed January 26, 2026. https://www.modernhealthcare.com/politics-policy/cvs-caremark-express-scripts-optumrx-drug-markups-ftc-report

74. Biggs S, Long D. Insights into the 2023 U.S. pharmaceutical market. IQVIA Blog. July 25, 2023. Accessed January 26, 2026. https://www.iqvia.com/locations/united-states/blogs/2023/07/insights-into-the-2023-us-pharmaceutical-market

75. Grothaus M. Why are pharmacies closing? Hundreds have disappeared since PBM reform was abandoned. Fast Company. March 12, 2025. Accessed January 26, 2026. https://www.fastcompany.com/91296236/walgreens-pharmacy-store-closings-hundreds-vanish-blame-pbm

76. Firth S. Trump Signs Bill With Major Reforms for Pharmacy Middlemen. Medpage Today. February 5, 2026. https://www.medpagetoday.com/washington-watch/reform/119762?xid=nl_mpt_DHE_2026-02-07&mh=b4e385c060e6d1df87e6be98fa56639c&zdee=gAAAABm4u-E9x25WDwGKRsOhxiUzVI_4ZrDZluVHy2ojnGrlqpBVFYURjqGjS0wGZf_i5v00SsiNXpcuO1dgZ1EVj_q78v9WquSKopJuxidCU4_dvNMjXU%3D&utm_source=Sailthru&utm_medium=email&utm_campaign=Weekly%20Review%202026-02-07&utm_term=NL_DHE_Weekly_Active

77. Allen A. Medicare drug pricing reform cuts costs as pharma lawyers up. Modern Healthcare. February 16, 2024. Accessed January 26, 2026. https://www.modernhealthcare.com/policy/biden-medicare-drug-price-negotiations-pharmaceutical-astrazeneca-farxiga-ira-cms-pbm

78. Frieden J. Medicare unveils first 10 negotiated drug prices. Medpage Today. August 15, 2024 (updated December 10). Accessed January 26, 2026. https://www.medpagetoday.com/publichealthpolicy/medicare/111523

79. Martin K. Medicare drug price negotiations: all you need to know. Commonwealth Fund. May 15, 2025. Accessed January 26, 2026. https://www.commonwealthfund.org/publications/explainer/2025/may/medicare-drug-price-negotiations-all-you-need-know

80. Frieden J. Medicare unveils first 10 negotiated drug prices. Medpage Today. August 15, 2024 (updated December 10). Accessed January 26, 2026. https://www.medpagetoday.com/publichealthpolicy/medicare/111523

81. Tollen L. The Medicare drug price negotiation program, year two: effects on access and innovation. Health Affairs Forefront. June 3, 2025. doi:10.1377/forefront.20250602.732579

82. Robbins R. U.S. announces negotiated prices for 15 drugs under Medicare. New York Times. November 25, 2025. Accessed January 26, 2026. https://www.nytimes.com/2025/11/25/health/drugs-prices-medicare.html
83. Frieden J. Medicare prices to drop up to 85% on drugs for weight-loss, cancer, asthma, and more. Medpage Today. November 26, 2025. Accessed January 26, 2026. https://www.medpagetoday.com/publichealthpolicy/medicare/118727
84. Kelkar AH, Cliff ERS. Reducing drug prices—the most favored nation policy vs price negotiation. JAMA. 2025;334(9):761-762. doi:10.1001/jama.2025.11614
85. Robbins R, Sanger-Katz M. Trump announces deal with Pfizer to sell drugs to Medicaid at European prices. New York Times. September 30, 2025. Accessed January 26, 2026. https://www.nytimes.com/2025/09/30/health/trump-pfizer-trumprx-medications.html
86. Whoriskey P, Gilbert D. Trump claimed a win on drug prices, but Big Pharma also scored. The Washington Post. October 2, 2025. Accessed January 26, 2026. https://www.washingtonpost.com/health/2025/10/02/drug-prices-trump-pharma-europe/
87. Robbins R, Sanger-Katz M. Trump announces pricing deals with nine drugmakers. New York Times. December 19, 2025. Accessed January 26, 2026. https://www.nytimes.com/2025/12/19/health/trump-drug-pricing-deals.html
88. Goldman M. More than half of TrumpRx drugs have a cheaper alternative. Axios. Feb. 6, 2026. https://www.axios.com/2026/02/06/trumprx-list-drugs-website-cheaper-prices?utm_source=4sight+Health+Readers&utm_campaign=8b1182c755-EMAIL_CAMPAIGN_2018_08_29_09_53_COPY_01&utm_medium=email&utm_term=0_96b6d85309-8b1182c755-147472109
89. Gondi S, Papanicolas I, Rome BN. Lowering drug prices in the US—look within, not abroad. JAMA. 2025;334(9):765-766. doi:10.1001/jama.2025.12324
90. Ukeomah K, Japinga M, Arad N, *et al.* How value-based payment can improve drug spending, utilization, and equity. Commonwealth Fund Blog. July 12, 2023. Accessed January 26, 2026. https://www.commonwealthfund.org/blog/2023/how-value-based-payment-can-improve-drug-spending-utilization-and-equity
91. Robinson JC. On US and foreign drug prices, 'most favored nation' policy is an unreasonable answer to a reasonable question. Health Affairs Forefront. May 23, 2025. doi:10.1377/forefront.20250520.477038

Chapter 14

1. Budgetary effects of policies that would increase hepatitis C treatment. Congressional Budget Office. June 2024. Accessed January 26, 2026. https://www.cbo.gov/publication/60407
2. Treatment of hepatitis C. Centers for Disease Control and Prevention. December 20, 2023. Accessed January 26, 2026. https://www.cdc.gov/hepatitis-c/treatment/index.html

3. Ruder K. As semaglutide's popularity soars, rare but serious adverse effects are emerging. JAMA. 2023;330(22):2140-2142. doi:10.1001/jama.2023.16620
4. Lincoff AM, Brown-Frandsen K, Colhoun HM, *et al.* Semaglutide and cardiovascular outcomes in obesity without diabetes. N Engl J Med. 2023;389(24):2221-2232. doi:10.1056/NEJMoa2307563
5. Monaco K. Wegovy approved for major heart disease prevention. MedPage Today. March 8, 2024. Accessed January 26, 2026. https://www.medpagetoday.com/cardiology/prevention/109090
6. Vinluan F. New FDA approval adds chronic kidney disease to Ozempic's label. MedCity News. January 29, 2025. Accessed January 26, 2026. https://medcitynews.com/2025/01/ozempic-fda-approval-chronic-kidney-disease-ckd-novo-nordisk-nvo/
7. Monaco K. GLP-1 agents' risks and benefits broader than previously thought. Medpage Today. January 20, 2025. Accessed January 26, 2026. https://www.medpagetoday.com/endocrinology/diabetes/113847
8. Ruder K. As semaglutide's popularity soars, rare but serious adverse effects are emerging. JAMA. 2023;330(22):2140-2142. doi:10.1001/jama.2023.16620
9. Moiz A, Filion KB, Toutounchi H, *et al.* Efficacy and safety of glucagon-like peptide-1 receptor agonists for weight loss among adults without diabetes. Ann Intern Med. 2025;178(2):199-217. doi:10.7326/ANNALS-24-01590
10. Lincoff AM, Brown-Frandsen K, Colhoun HM, *et al.* Semaglutide and cardiovascular outcomes in obesity without diabetes. N Engl J Med. 2023;389(24):2221-2232. doi:10.1056/NEJMoa2307563
11. Adult obesity facts. Centers for Disease Control and Prevention. May 14, 2024. Accessed January 26, 2026. https://www.cdc.gov/obesity/adult-obesity-facts/index.html
12. Emerson J. Sanders: weight loss drugs could bankrupt healthcare system. Becker's Hospital Review. May 16, 2024. Accessed January 26, 2026. https://www.beckershospitalreview.com/glp-1s/sanders-weight-loss-drug-could-bankrupt-healthcare-system/
13. Thorpe KE, Joski PJ. Estimated reduction in health care spending associated with weight loss in adults. JAMA Netw Open. 2024;7(12):e2449200. doi:10.1001/jamanetworkopen.2024.49200
14. Lin GA, Lee W, Fahim SM, *et al.* Semaglutide and tirzepatide for obesity: effectiveness and value; evidence report. Institute for Clinical and Economic Review. October 29, 2025. Accessed January 26, 2026. https://icer.org/wp-content/uploads/2025/10/ICER_Obesity_Evidence-Report_For-Publication_102925.pdf
15. Tsipas S, Khan T, Loustalot F, *et al.* Spending on glucagon-like peptide-1 receptor agonists among US adults. JAMA Netw Open. 2025;8(4):e252964. doi:10.1001/jamanetworkopen.2025.2964

16. Robbins R, Sanger-Katz M, Blum D. Obesity drugs may drop to as little as $149 a month. New York Times. November 6, 2025. Accessed January 26, 2026. https://www.nytimes.com/2025/11/06/health/obesity-drug-prices-trump.html
17. Robbins R, Sanger-Katz M, Blum D. Obesity drugs may drop to as little as $149 a month. New York Times. November 6, 2025. Accessed January 26, 2026. https://www.nytimes.com/2025/11/06/health/obesity-drug-prices-trump.html
18. BALANCE (Better Approaches to Lifestyle and Nutrition for Comprehensive Health) Model. Centers for Medicare & Medicaid Services. Accessed January 26, 2026. https://www.cms.gov/priorities/innovation/innovation-models/balance
19. Ippolito B, Levy JF. Expanding Medicare coverage of anti-obesity medicines could increase annual spending by $3.1 billion to $6.1 billion. Health Aff. 2024;43(9). doi:10.1377/hlthaff.2024.00356
20. Adult obesity facts. Centers for Disease Control and Prevention. May 14, 2024. Accessed January 26, 2026. https://www.cdc.gov/obesity/adult-obesity-facts/index.html
21. Freedhoff Y. If new obesity medications work, why do so many stop them? Medscape. January 31, 2025. Accessed January 26, 2026. https://www.medscape.com/viewarticle/if-new-obesity-medications-work-why-do-so-many-stop-them-2025a10002ak
22. Muth N. States are walking back Medicaid coverage for GLP-1s. Medpage Today. July 15, 2025. Accessed January 26, 2026. https://www.medpagetoday.com/opinion/second-opinions/116512
23. Berryman L. GLP-1 costs drive employers to specialty benefits vendors. Modern Healthcare. September 25, 2024. Accessed January 26, 2026. https://www.modernhealthcare.com/insurance/wegovy-glp-1-costs-vendors-personify-health-business-group/
24. Cutler DM. The pathology of US health care—the example of weight loss medications. JAMA Health Forum. 2024;5(8):e243052. doi:10.1001/jamahealthforum.2024.3052
25. Berryman L. Blue Cross Blue Shield plans reverse course on GLP-1 coverage. Modern Healthcare. May 28, 2025. Accessed January 26, 2026. https://www.modernhealthcare.com/insurance/bcbs-plans-michigan-massachusetts-glp1-coverage/
26. Berryman L. Blue Cross Blue Shield plans reverse course on GLP-1 coverage. Modern Healthcare. May 28, 2025. Accessed January 26, 2026. https://www.modernhealthcare.com/insurance/bcbs-plans-michigan-massachusetts-glp1-coverage/
27. Nelson R. 'Low-value' prostate cancer screening prevalent in primary care. MDEdge. January 9, 2023. Accessed January 26, 2026. https://www.mdedge.com/oncologypractice/article/260528/preventive-care/low-value-prostate-cancer-screening-prevalent

28. Hall AM, Aubrey-Bassler K, Thorne B, Maher CG. Do not routinely offer imaging for uncomplicated low back pain. BMJ. 2021;372:n291. doi:10.1136/bmj.n291
29. Vena cava filters. Cleveland Clinic. Accessed January 26, 2026. https://my.clevelandclinic.org/health/treatments/17609-vena-cava-filters
30. DeMarco C. Should you get a full-body scan to look for cancer? MD Anderson Cancer Center. November 10, 2023. Accessed January 26, 2026. https://www.mdanderson.org/cancerwise/should-you-get-a-full-body-scan-to-look-for-cancer.h00-159623379.html
31. Garber AM, Sox HC. The role of costs in comparative effectiveness research. Health Aff. 2010;29(10):1805-1811. doi:10.1377/hlthaff.2010.0647
32. Garber AM, Sox HC. The role of costs in comparative effectiveness research. Health Aff. 2010;29(10):1805-1811. doi:10.1377/hlthaff.2010.0647
33. Paulden M. Recent amendments to NICE's value-based assessment of health technologies: implicitly inequitable? Expert Rev Pharmacoecon Outcomes Res. 2017;17(3):239-242. doi:10.1080/14737167.2017.1330152
34. Dranove D. What's Your Life Worth? Upper Saddle River, NJ: Financial Times Prentice Hall; 2003:98-104.
35. Paulden M. Recent amendments to NICE's value-based assessment of health technologies: implicitly inequitable? Expert Rev Pharmacoecon Outcomes Res. 2017;17(3):239-242. doi:10.1080/14737167.2017.1330152
36. Robbins R, Nelson E. To avoid tariffs, U.K. agrees to Trump's demand to pay more for drugs. New York Times. December 1, 2025. Accessed January 26, 2026. https://www.nytimes.com/2025/12/01/business/us-uk-pharma-tariffs-prices.html
37. Claxton K, Martin S, Soares M, *et al*. Methods for the estimation of the National Institute for Health and Care Excellence cost-effectiveness threshold. Health Technol Assess. 2015;19(14):1-503. doi:10.3310/hta19140
38. Claxton K, Martin S, Soares M, *et al*. Methods for the estimation of the National Institute for Health and Care Excellence cost-effectiveness threshold. Health Technol Assess. 2015;19(14):1-503. doi:10.3310/hta19140
39. Cameron D, Ubels J, Norstrom F. On what basis are medical cost-effectiveness thresholds set? Clashing opinions and an absence of data: a systematic review. Glob Health Action. 2018;11(1):1447828. doi:10.1080/16549716.2018.1447828
40. Cameron D, Ubels J, Norstrom F. On what basis are medical cost-effectiveness thresholds set? Clashing opinions and an absence of data: a systematic review. Glob Health Action. 2018;11(1):1447828. doi:10.1080/16549716.2018.1447828
41. Raferty J. Ever higher cancer drug prices—driven by US policies and genetic sequencing. BMJ Opinion. July 1, 2015. Accessed January 26, 2026. https://blogs.bmj.com/bmj/2015/07/01/james-raftery-ever-higher-cancer-drug-prices-driven-by-us-policies-and-genetic-sequencing/

42. Canada announces regulations to cut price of prescription drugs. The Guardian. August 9, 2019. Accessed January 26, 2026. https://www.theguardian.com/world/2019/aug/09/canada-prescription-drugs-cut-cost
43. About CADTH. Canadian Agency for Drugs and Technology. Accessed January 26, 2026. https://www.cadth.ca/about-cadth/what-we-do/products-services
44. Cameron D, Ubels J, Norstrom F. On what basis are medical cost-effectiveness thresholds set? Clashing opinions and an absence of data: a systematic review. Glob Health Action. 2018;11(1):1447828. doi:10.1080/16549716.2018.1447828
45. CADTH Canadian Drug Expert Committee recommendation for lanadelumab. Accessed January 26, 2026. https://www.cadth.ca/sites/default/files/cdr/complete/SR0618%20Takhzyro%20-%20CDEC%DecemerDecember20Final%20Recommendation%20November%2022%2C%202019_for%20posting.pdf
46. CADTH Canadian Drug Expert Committee recommendation for lanadelumab. Accessed January 26, 2026. https://www.cadth.ca/sites/default/files/cdr/complete/SR0618%20Takhzyro%20-%20CDEC%DecemerDecember20Final%20Recommendation%20November%2022%2C%202019_for%20posting.pdf
47. Robinson JC, Ex P, Panteli D. Single-payer drug pricing in a multipayer health system: does Germany offer a model for the US? Health Affairs Forefront. March 22, 2019. doi:10.1377/forefront.20190318.475434
48. Neumann PJ, Chambers JD. Medicare's reset on "coverage with evidence development." Health Affairs Forefront. April 1, 2013. doi:10.1377/hblog20130401.029345
49. Coverage with evidence development. Centers for Medicare & Medicaid Services. Accessed January 26, 2026. https://www.cms.gov/Medicare/Coverage/Coverage-with-Evidence-Development/index
50. CMS proposes coverage with evidence development for chimeric antigen receptor (CAR) T-cell therapy. Centers for Medicare & Medicaid Services. February 15, 2019. Accessed January 26, 2026. https://www.cms.gov/newsroom/press-releases/cms-proposes-coverage-evidence-development-chimeric-antigen-receptor-car-t-cell-therapy
51. Pear R. Medicare aims to expand coverage of cancer care. But is it enough? New York Times. April 13, 2019. Accessed January 26, 2026. https://www.nytimes.com/2019/04/13/us/politics/medicare-car-t-cancer.html
52. CMS expands coverage of CAR T-cell therapy for Medicare beneficiaries. ASCO Post. September 25, 2019. Accessed January 26, 2026. https://ascopost.com/issues/september-25-2019/cms-expands-coverage-of-car-t-cell-therapy-for-medicare-beneficiaries/
53. Medicare Evidence Development & Coverage Advisory Committee. Centers for Medicare & Medicaid Services. Accessed January 26, 2026. https://www.cms.gov/medicare/regulations-guidance/advisory-committees/evidence-development-coverage

54. Gray BH, Gusmano MK, Collins SR. AHCPR and the changing politics of health services. Health Aff. 2003;22(Suppl1):W3-283-W3-307. doi:10.1377/hlthaff.W3.283

55. Vogel L. Trump administration shutters clinical guidelines database. CMAJ. 2018;190(27):E841. doi:10.1503/cmaj.109-5624

56. Allen A. What's lost: Trump whacks tiny agency that works to make the nation's health care safer. KFF Health News. April 4, 2025. Accessed January 26, 2026. https://www.cnn.com/2025/04/04/health/health-care-cuts-agency-kff-health-news

57. Terry K. Rx For Healthcare Reform. Nashville, TN: Vanderbilt University Press; 2007:290-291.

58. Pizzi LT. The Institute for Clinical and Economic Review and its growing influence on US healthcare. Am Health Drug Benefits. 2016;9(1):9-10. https://pmc.ncbi.nlm.nih.gov/articles/PMC4822973/

59. Payers report that ICER analyses increasingly guide US price negotiations. ICON. November 15, 2019. Accessed January 26, 2026. https://www.iconplc.com/insights/blog/2019/11/15/payers-report-that-icer-analyses-increasingly-guide-us-price-negotiations/

60. NICE Citizens Council Reports. National Institute for Health and Care Excellence. Accessed January 26, 2026. https://www.ncbi.nlm.nih.gov/books/NBK402014/

61. Gulland A. NICE proposals for citizens council condemned by patients. BMJ. 2002;325(7361):406. doi:10.1136/bmj.325.7361.406/a

62. Get involved: we want you to be involved in our work. National Institute for Health and Care Excellence. Accessed January 26, 2026. https://www.nice.org.uk/get-involved

63. Heart valve disease presenting in adults: investigation and management: lay member. NICE Recruitment Notice. Accessed January 26, 2026. https://www.nice.org.uk/get-involved/our-committees/join-a-committee/nice-committee-vacancies-for-patients--service-users--carers-and-lay-people#!/job/UK/London/Virtual/NICE_National_Institute_Health_Care_Excellence/Lay_Member/Lay_Member-v7626561

64. Eddy DM. What care is 'essential'? What services are 'basic'? JAMA. 1991;265(6):782, 786-788. doi:10.1001/jama.265.6.782

65. Lecanemab approved for treatment of early Alzheimer's disease. Alzheimer's Association. Accessed January 26, 2026. https://www.alz.org/alzheimers-dementia/treatments/lecanemab-leqembi

66. Donanemab approved for treatment of early Alzheimer's disease. Alzheimer's Association. Accessed January 26, 2026. https://www.alz.org/alzheimers-dementia/treatments/donanemab

67. Report: more than 7 million Americans living with Alzheimer's. American Hospital Association. May 7, 2025. Accessed January 26, 2026. https://www.aha.org/news/headline/2025-05-07-report-more-7-million-americans-living-alzheimers
68. Brensocatib for non-cystic fibrosis bronchiectasis: effectiveness and value. Institute for Clinical and Economic Review. October 30, 2025. Accessed January 26, 2026. https://icer.org/wp-content/uploads/2025/10/ICER_NCFB-Final-Report_For-Publication_103025.pdf